2012

cpt® Reference Guide
for Cardiovascular Coding

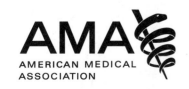

AMA
AMERICAN MEDICAL
ASSOCIATION

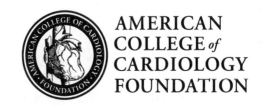

AMERICAN
COLLEGE *of*
CARDIOLOGY
FOUNDATION

American Medical Association

Executive Vice President, Chief Executive Officer: James L. Madara, MD
Chief Operating Officer: Bernard L. Hengesbaugh
Senior Vice President, Publishing and Business Services: Robert A. Musacchio, PhD
Vice President, Business Operations: Vanessa Hayden
Vice President, CPT and Physician Practice Solutions: Jay T. Ahlman
Manager, Book and Product Development and Production: Nancy C. Baker
Senior Developmental Editor: Lisa Chin-Johnson
Production Specialist: Mary Ann Albanese
Director, Coding Editorial and Regulatory Services: Marie Mindeman
Director, CPT Education and Information Services: Danielle Pavlovski
Senior Clinical Coding Specialist: Grace M. Kotowicz
Director, Sales, Marketing and Strategic Relationships: Joann Skiba
Director, Sales and Business Products: Mark Daniels
Manager, Marketing and Strategic Planning: Erin Kalitowski
Marketing Manager: Leigh Adams

Internet address: www.ama-assn.org

The American Medical Association ("AMA") has consulted sources believed to be knowledgeable in their fields. However, the AMA does not warrant that the information is in every respect accurate and/or complete. The AMA assumes no responsibility for use of the information contained in this publication. The AMA shall not be responsible for, and expressly disclaims liability for, damages of any kind arising out of the use of, reference to, or reliance on, the content of this publication. This publication is for informational purposes only. The AMA does not provide medical, legal, financial, or other professional advice and readers are encouraged to consult a professional advisor for such advice.

The Center for Medicare and Medicaid Services is responsible for the Medicare content contained in this publication and no endorsement by the AMA is intended or should be implied. Readers are encouraged to refer to the current official Medicare program provisions contained in relevant laws, regulations, and rulings.

For information regarding the reprinting or licensing of **CPT® Reference Guide for Cardiovascular Coding 2012**, please contact:
  CPT Intellectual Property Services
  American Medical Association
  515 N. State St.
  Chicago, IL 60654
  312 464-5022

Additional copies of this book may be ordered by calling: 800 621-8335 or from the secure AMA Web site at www.amabookstore.com. Refer to product number OP076011.

ISBN: 978-1-60359-634-3
AC51: 12-P-095:12/11

American College of Cardiology

Chief Executive Officer: Jack Lewin, MD
Senior Vice-President Advocacy Division: James Fasules, MD, FACC
Senior Director, Regulatory Affairs: Rebecca Kelly
Associate Director, Regulatory Affairs: Brian Whitman
Senior Specialist, Coding and Reimbursement: Debra Mariani
Associate Director, Regulatory Affairs: Lisa Goldstein
Associate Director, Payer Advocacy: Richard Punsalan

The American Medical Association and the American College of Cardiology would like to extend our appreciation to the volunteer physicians, who provided their assistance in preparing this book. Thanks are due to the **ACC Coding Task Force:**

Chair: Robert N. Piana, MD, FACC
CoChair: Patrick Frias, MD, FACC
Kenneth P. Brin, MD, FACC
Michael Mansour, MD, FACC
Jerold Saef, MD, FACC
Douglas S. Segar, MD, FACC
Amit C. Shanker, MD, FACC
Randall C. Thompson, MD, FACC
Diane E. Wallis, MD, FACC
Donna McSpadden, FACMPE

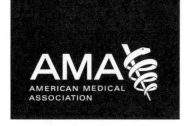
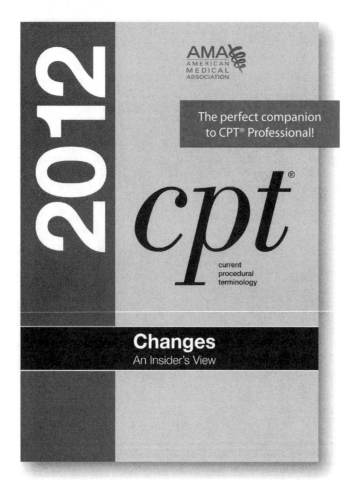

Table of Contents

Introduction

The American College of Cardiology (ACC) and the American Medical Association (AMA) have joined forces to publish the *CPT® Reference Guide for Cardiovascular Coding*, an easy-to-use reference guide to Current Procedural Terminology (CPT®) coding for cardiovascular procedures and services. *CPT® Reference Guide for Cardiovascular Coding* is intended to be a supplement to, not a substitute for, *CPT® 2012*. The book is intended to help cardiovascular professionals and their practice staff code correctly. It provides an authoritative interpretation of CPT for cardiovascular services.

The appendixes provide current adjunctive information. Topics affecting reporting include the use of the National Correct Coding Initiative (NCCI), CPT Category II codes for the Physician Quality Reporting System (PQRS) in the Medicare program, the transition from ICD-9-CM to ICD-10-CM diagnosis reporting, and excerpted instruction for reporting to the Centers for Medicare & Medicaid Services (CMS). Also referenced are regulatory issues such as the American Recovery and Reinvestment Act of 2009 (ARRA), which made significant changes to the Health Insurance Portability and Accountability Act (HIPAA). Other appendixes include an updated listing of the addresses of the CMS CMD Directory and a summary of CPT codes with technical and professional components.

The ACC and AMA hope you will find the *CPT® Reference Guide for Cardiovascular Coding* to be a useful resource. We welcome your feedback and suggestions for making future editions even better.

Instructions for Use of the Reference Guide

The book begins with an introduction to CPT that will be useful reading for physicians and novice and experienced cardiology coders alike.

Subsequent chapters parallel the organization of the *CPT 2012* codebook. The services in the *CPT® Reference Guide for Cardiovascular Coding* are listed in numerical order for easy location.

The Table of Contents on page v provides listing of the hierarchy in families of services to assist in location of services and codes by page number. Once a code has been located, code descriptors are highlighted in light blue and listed either alone (eg, 34803 *endovascular repair of abdominal aortic aneurysm*; page 96) or by code family (eg, 78451-78454 *myocardial perfusion imaging*; page 114).

Guidelines

Chapters 2 to 5 include specific CPT code language, along with relevant excerpts from CPT introductory language, guidelines, and instructions. Specific guidelines are presented at the beginning of the major subsections of Cardiology (eg, Intracardiac Electrophysiologic Procedures/Studies; page 193; Noninvasive Vascular Diagnostic Studies; page 208). These guidelines define items that are necessary to appropriately interpret and report the procedures and services contained in that section. For example, in the **Intracardiac Electrophysiologic Procedures/Services** section, specific instructions are provided to indicate that modifier 51 is not applicable to append to codes

93600-93603, 93610, 93612, 93615-93618, and 93631 for designation of performance of multiple procedures at the same session. Guidelines also provide explanations regarding terms that apply only to a particular section. These major sections are followed by subsection titles, codes and code descriptors highlighted in light blue.

The **Myocardial Perfusion Imaging** subsection (page 114) is a good illustration of the subsection organization model for this Reference Guide. In this subsection, the title, **"Myocardial Perfusion Imaging"** is followed by an overview of the intent of the entire family of codes. This is followed by subheads that discuss the intent of each code individually (78451, 78452, 78453, 78454), followed by the **Description of Service** for the code.

When other information is available, these subheads may be followed by either a **Coding Tip** (additional information for reporting a code) or a **Payment Policy Alert** to illustrate significant payer policy related to the code (eg, see page 128 for codes 92980, 92981). In some subsections, the **Description of Service, Coding Tip,** or **Payment Policy Alert** may not be provided if that category of information is not available for the code. The clinical examples and descriptions of service that are included for many codes were developed as part of the CPT Editorial Panel code development process and the AMA/Specialty Society RVS Update Committee (RUC) valuation process. Information on cardiology basics for coders and numerous medical illustrations also appear throughout the book.

CHAPTER 1

CPT® in Perspective

Physicians' Current Procedural Terminology (CPT®) is a set of codes, descriptions, and guidelines intended to describe procedures and services performed by physicians and other health care providers. The goal is to provide a uniform language for the accurate description of physicians' medical, surgical, diagnostic, and therapeutic services. Used consistently, the CPT format facilitates understanding by physicians and third-party payers.

The Coding Cycle

CPT codes were first published in 1966 and underwent three major revisions between 1966 and 1982. In 1983, the fourth edition (CPT-4) was published, and it has since been updated annually. The Centers for Medicare & Medicaid Services (CMS) adopted CPT codes for use in the Medicare and Medicaid programs in 1983. Because Medicare is the largest third-party payer, it was logical that the CPT code set would eventually be adopted by the health insurance industry. CPT codes have thus become the national standard for describing and reporting physicians' services by the health insurance industry as well.

All physicians and their agents for billing and reimbursement are required to become familiar with the codes and coding conventions used in the CPT codebook. Without this understanding, accurate and appropriate coding for physicians' services cannot be translated into equitable and appropriate reimbursement.

There are three levels of CPT codes. Category I, Category II, and Category III. Category I codes, identified with a numeric five-digit CPT code and a descriptor, are used for commonly identified services and procedures performed by large numbers of physicians in clinical practice over a broad geographic distribution. In 1992, the American Medical Association (AMA), with input from the specialty societies, added cognitive or evaluation and management (E/M) services to the CPT codebook (Chapter 2). Category II codes facilitate reporting of services related to performance measures, and Category III codes are for tracking new services and procedures that use emerging technologies.

Category II codes were added in 2004 as supplemental tracking codes. This category was created, in part, to facilitate documentation by providers of their compliance with nationally recognized performance guidelines on an individual patient basis. It is anticipated that proper use of these codes will one day facilitate documentation of performance measures that may be mandated by outside entities, such as monitoring agencies and health plans. Category II codes, published online as the Alphabetical Clinical Topics Listing and in the Category II section of the CPT codebook, are assigned an alphanumeric identifier with the letter "F" in the last field (eg, **0001F**). These codes may be used in quality reporting programs such as Medicare's Physician Quality Reporting Initiative. The Performance Measures Advisory Group is a standing workgroup of the AMA CPT Editorial Panel that assists the panel in review and maintenance of the Category II codes. This workgroup, includes representatives of the CPT Editorial Panel, is involved in the development of performance measures, in addition to AMA CPT staff, clinical quality improvement staff, and other knowledgeable experts. Tracking codes for performance measurement are released three times yearly following approval of the panel minutes after each Editorial Panel meeting (March 15, June 15, and November 15) on the AMA CPT Web site, www. ama-assn.org/go/cpt, and are published annually in the CPT codebook as part of the general CPT code set. Physician Quality Reporting System (PQRS) measures that are relevant to cardiology include Acute

Myocardial Infarction, Chest Pain (Non-traumatic), Coronary Artery Bypass Graft (CABG), and other diagnoses/clinical conditions (see www.ama-assn.org/apps/listserv/x-check/qmeasure.cgi?submit=PQRS).

Category III (emerging technology) codes facilitate data collection and reporting of new services and procedures that do not yet meet the criteria for Category I codes. Procedures using emerging technology or procedures that are performed in only a few regions of the country typically are assigned Category III CPT codes. Category III codes are assigned an alphanumeric identifier with the letter 'T' in the last field (eg, **0001T**), similar to Category II codes. They are also located in the section following the CPT Category II codes near the end of the CPT codebook; introductory language in this section explains the purpose and use of these codes. The approval process for coding proposals for a Category III code follows the existing procedures for new or revised CPT codes. Category III codes are not referred to the Relative Value Update Committee (RUC), an advisory committee made up of AMA specialty society representatives who make recommendations to CMS on the relative values for work and practice expenses to be assigned to new or revised codes. Category III codes may be reimbursed on a case-by-case basis, depending on policy decisions by local carriers or individual payers. Approved Category III codes are biannually published on the AMA CPT Web site. If a Category III code is not converted to a Category I code within 5 years, the panel determines whether the usefulness of the code requires that it is still needed or whether the code should be archived.

The users of CPT codes should be aware that changes in the editorial process have resulted in more frequent updates to the AMA CPT Web site than the annual print revision of the CPT codebook. Therefore, a search of the CPT Web site (www.ama-assn.org/go/cpt) should always be considered if the answer to a coding question is not immediately found in the printed version of the CPT codebook.

When selecting a code to describe the procedure(s) or service(s) performed, the name that accurately identifies the service should be selected. It is not appropriate to select a CPT code that merely approximates the service(s) provided. Occasionally, procedures or services may not be accurately described by any of the CPT codes. In such cases, an appropriate "unlisted services" code such as **93799** (Unlisted cardiovascular service or procedure) can be used. A complete description of the service rendered must accompany that bill, and payment will be dependent on the policies of the specific payer.

The inclusion of a code (descriptor language and code number) in the CPT code set or codebook is the result of careful review by the AMA CPT Editorial Panel to ascertain whether the service or procedure is generally accepted as a contemporary medical practice by physicians in all parts of the country. It must be emphasized that inclusion of a code in the CPT code set does not imply nor guarantee automatic coverage and reimbursement by insurers. Payers may elect to exclude codes from coverage, require specific documentation of medical necessity, and/or limit the billing frequency of certain codes.

The AMA CPT Editorial Panel meets three times a year in February, May, and October. Codes approved at the final meeting of the publication year (in February) go into effect the following year. Codes approved in May and October must wait another full calendar year. Deadlines for submission are 12 weeks before the meeting. The schedule and deadlines to submit an application for establishment of a new CPT code or revision of an existing CPT code are available at www.ama-assn.org/resources/doc/cpt/cpt-code-change-request.doc.

The AMA CPT Editorial Panel considers and decides on updates and revisions of the code set each time it meets. This panel has the authority to make additions, deletions, and modifications to any of the existing CPT codes or descriptors. With the exception of the Web publication of Category I vaccine codes, Category II codes, and Category III codes, these changes are published annually. Several criteria must be met before submitting a request for a new Category I code to the AMA CPT Editorial Panel. First, the suggested service or procedure should represent a distinct physician service. Second, the procedure or service should be performed by many physicians throughout the country, not by just a few physicians regionally or locally. When a code request includes a new drug or device, approval by the Food and Drug Administration is necessary. Finally, the applicant is required to submit five article references to support the clinical efficacy of the described service or procedure and meet the application literature requirements (US peer-reviewed, discrete patient populations, US studies).

FIGURE 1-1. The AMA CPT Code Process

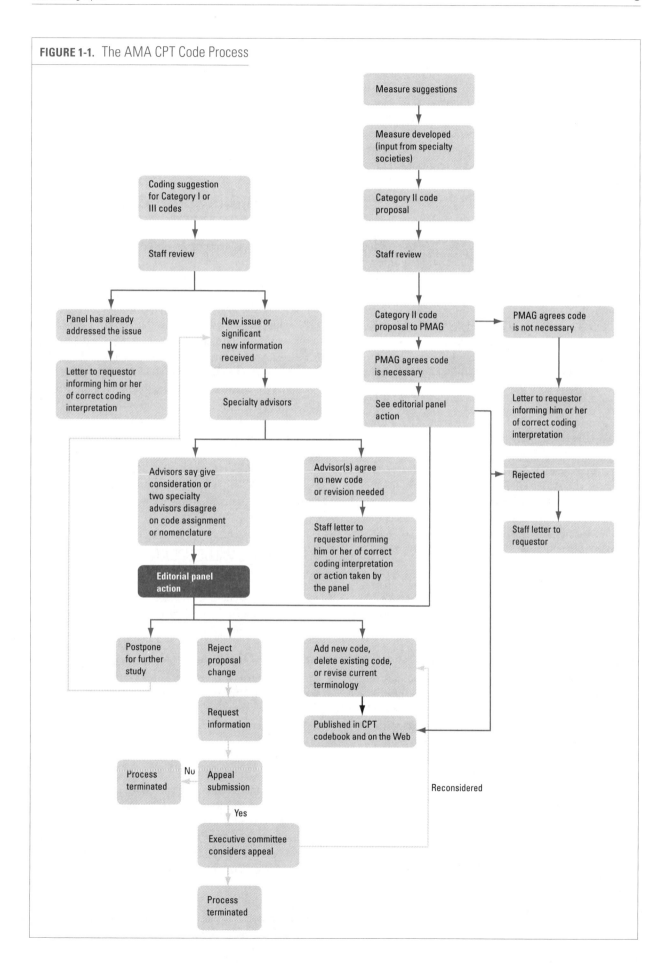

Procedure(s) or service(s) still in the emerging-technology stage are eligible for consideration as Category III codes until the aforementioned criteria can be met. In consideration of requests for these emerging services, the Panel takes into consideration whether a protocol of the study or procedure being performed is available; the level of support from the specialties that would use this procedure; the availability of published US peer-reviewed literature; and the availability of descriptions of current US trials outlining the efficacy of the procedure or service.

The online CPT Process booklet, *CPT® Process—How a Code Becomes a Code* (www.ama-assn.org/ama/pub/physician-resources/solutions-managing-your-practice/coding-billing-insurance/cpt/cpt-process-faq/code-becomes-cpt.page), and the CPT Application Process FAQs (www.ama-assn.org/ama/pub/physician-resources/solutions-managing-your-practice/coding-billing-insurance/cpt/cpt-process-faq.page?) should be consulted for more detailed information on the process for applying for CPT codes.

The American College of Cardiology (ACC) Coding Task Force actively participates in the development of new and revised coding proposals. First, the task force routinely proposes and reviews new codes for consideration by the AMA CPT Editorial Panel. Second, the chair of the ACC Coding Task Force serves as a member of the AMA CPT Advisory Committee and, in such capacity, has the opportunity to comment on any new code being proposed.

Any medical society, manufacturer, individual physician, or provider may request CPT code changes through the AMA or the CPT Advisory Committee members listed in the CPT codebook. For requests for codes to describe new cardiology services, the ACC encourages submission of applications for new cardiovascular codes or changes to existing codes to the ACC Coding Task Force for discussion and consideration. All changes, including minor wording or punctuation changes, must go through the editorial process because even the placement of an indentation or a semicolon can change the entire meaning of a code or code-change proposal.

Such requests should be mailed to:

> Chair
> Coding Task Force
> American College of Cardiology
> 2400 N St., NW
> Washington, DC 20037

The ACC Coding Task Force comprises a broad selection of members of the College. In addition, the task force works closely with cardiology and other subspecialty organizations to facilitate the development of specific cardiovascular coding proposals and to ensure consistency in coding recommendations.

The Reimbursement Cycle

CPT CODES AND THE MEDICARE FEE SCHEDULE

The advent of the Medicare physician fee schedule created a greater need for accurate codes and descriptors to describe physician work. Although individual CPT codes do not establish reimbursement for a service or procedure, an accurate CPT code descriptor is necessary in assigning relative value units (RVUs) to codes in the Medicare fee schedule. The AMA Specialty Society Relative Value Update Committee (RUC) develops RVUs for new or revised services and procedures. The ACC continues to work closely with the CPT Editorial Panel to advocate changes in, and additions to, CPT codes. Furthermore, the ACC has instituted a process for provision of accurate data to assist the RUC and CMS in their activities for development of recommendations for work and practice expense values.

THE RELATIVE VALUE UPDATE PROCESS

The RUC is composed of 29 member representatives of the medical specialties, one of whom is appointed by the ACC. The RUC receives input from an advisory committee made up of representatives from more than 80 specialty societies, all of whom hold seats in the AMA House of Delegates. The members of the advisory committee work as advocates for their respective specialties and present the results of their organizations' surveys for the development of accurate RVU recommendations to the RUC.

The RUC meets three times a year, at least 3 months after each of the three CPT Editorial Panel meetings. The RUC staff summarizes the coding panel's actions and asks each specialty society representative to indicate their organization's level of interest in developing a physician and practice expense RVU proposal for each new or revised code. The organization can then survey its membership to obtain primary data, comment on the recommendations of other organizations, decide that the coding revision requires no RVU change, or take no action. Often, two or more specialty societies are involved in developing a recommendation.

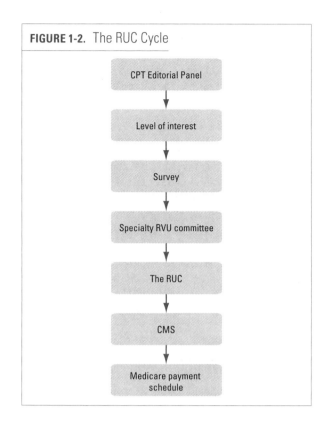

FIGURE 1-2. The RUC Cycle

ACC develops its recommendations through its Cardiovascular Relative Value Update Committee, which oversees the process of surveying physicians concerning new and revised codes to which RVUs need to be assigned.

The ACC urges anyone who receives an RUC survey to complete it. The RUC considers 30 responses to be an important threshold for validity.

The RUC can decide to accept or modify a specialty society's recommendation or refer it back to the organization. The RUC then forwards its recommendations to the CMS by May of each year for inclusion in the next year's fee schedule. The CMS accepts more than 90% of the RUC's recommendations.

The ACC provides RVUs and coding advice for all commonly billed CPT codes on its Web site (*see Advocacy, Issues, Physician Payment, Medicare Physician Payment*).

The AMA and the ACC encourage all members to participate actively in the advocacy process, particularly as it addresses the issues relating to physician reimbursement. Details can be found at the ACC Web site (www.cardiosource.org) under the Advocacy tab, through the ACC Advocacy Department at (800) 435-9203, or at the AMA Web site (www.ama-assn.org/ama/pub/advocacy.shtml).

NATIONAL CORRECT CODING INITIATIVE

In an effort to promote correct coding and reduce inappropriate payment, the CMS established the National Correct Coding Initiative (NCCI) in 1995. The Initiative is intended to save Medicare hundreds of millions of dollars by identifying and rejecting mutually incompatible sets of codes and the use of multiple CPT codes for billing in place of one comprehensive code (a practice known as "unbundling"). The NCCI edits apply only to code pairs billed for the same date of service and the same provider.

The NCCI recognizes, however, that for some code pairs there may be occasions when the codes may be appropriately submitted together. For these situations, a modifier may be appropriate to indicate that the services are independent or distinct and the reporting of both codes on the same claim form reflects appropriate coding.

Physicians should understand that documentation in the medical record must accurately describe the services provided, the necessity and appropriateness of the services, and the circumstances that warrant the use of both codes together, along with a modifier (see Chapter 6). Payer policies related to the use of modifiers are subject to frequent change. Physicians and their billing agents should frequently consult announcements from Medicare Part B carriers and Medicare administrative contractors to ensure the appropriate use of modifiers as related to the NCCI edits.

The NCCI provides the opportunity for input on proposed NCCI edits from the national medical specialty societies and the AMA with continual refinement to ensure correct coding. The ACC responds to proposed edits it believes to be inappropriate, which has resulted in deletion of many code pairs from the list of "forbidden" code pairs. This has prevented many inappropriate rejections of provider claims for Medicare cardiovascular services. The NCCI edits are released on a quarterly basis and available at www.cms.gov/NationalCorrectCodInitEd.

MEDICALLY UNLIKELY EDITS

Medically unlikely edits (MUEs) were implemented by the CMS on January 1, 2007, in an effort to reduce the paid claims error rate. The MUEs are maximum units of service that a provider could report for a single beneficiary on a single date of service. The MUEs do not exist for all CPT/Healthcare Common Procedure Coding System (HCPCS) codes. As with the NCCI edits, the CMS provides the opportunity for input on proposed MUEs from the national medical specialty societies and the AMA.

The MUEs are released on a quarterly basis; however, some edits remain confidential and are not published on the CMS Web site. The MUEs that are public are available at the CMS Web site at www.cms.gov/NationalCorrectCodInitEd/08_MUE.asp.

Non-CPT Coding and Payment Systems

In addition to CPT codes, several other procedural coding systems exist. They are discussed only briefly here, but it is important to remember that private carriers may elect to use such alternative systems. Physicians and their billing agents must be continually alert to the specific requirements for reimbursement by the carriers that function as fiscal intermediaries.

HEALTHCARE COMMON PROCEDURE CODING SYSTEM

The CPT coding system is only one part of the broader Healthcare Common Procedure Coding System (HCPCS). This system has three levels of codes. Level I codes consist of CPT codes and descriptions. Level II codes are published nationally by the CMS to provide more precise codes for areas such as durable medical equipment, ambulance, and injectable drugs. Level III codes are established by local carriers and are often characterized by variations, duplicate codes, and other nuances. Among its many provisions, the Health Insurance Portability and Accountability Act (HIPAA) requires that local codes be eliminated and replaced by standard codes (eg, CPT Category III and HCPCS Level II codes). The CMS staff is revising the HCPCS to comply with the provisions of HIPAA. There may be circumstances in which a physician is instructed to use a Level II HCPCS code instead of a CPT code to report a service due to legislation, payment policy, or coverage decisions by the CMS.

For example, the CMS may choose to create a Level II HCPCS G-code (eg, **G0275** Renal angiography, non-selective, one or both kidneys, performed at the same time as cardiac catheterization) to track a specific procedure outside the CPT editorial process. Circumstances in which a G-code may be created include the following: (1) expediting a new or revised Medicare benefit assignment; (2) departure from CPT-described use that conflicts with a Medicare policy or benefit; (3) new technology, not currently reportable with CPT codes; and (4) more specific delineation of a service or procedure that is not fully delineated in the existing CPT descriptor nomenclature. Through the CPT process, existing G-codes are reviewed and recommendations made for each code to be retained, revised, or converted to an approved CPT code.

INTERNAL CODING SYSTEMS

Regional and local carriers such as Blue Cross and Blue Shield (BCBS) may use other coding conventions that were developed internally. However, in most instances, major carriers use the CPT code set. The AMA is particularly concerned when local coding systems are inconsistent with the rules established for use of CPT coding. Physicians who encounter problems with local coding systems should contact the AMA CPT Network (www.cptnetwork.com) for clarification on the actual intent of the CPT code or the ACC Advocacy Division at (800) 435-9203.

INTERNATIONAL CLASSIFICATION OF DISEASES, NINTH EDITION, CLINICAL MODIFICATION

Medicare and Medicaid as well as many private carriers require that claims include diagnosis codes based on the International Classification of Diseases, Ninth Edition, Clinical Modification (ICD-9-CM), in addition to CPT procedure codes. Together, these codes inform the insurance payer of the service or procedure provided and the associated diagnosis. For many services, insurance payers base payment on medical necessity criteria. In this manner, reimbursement for a given service (CPT code) is provided only if the ICD-9 diagnosis submitted with the claim is included in the payer's list of diagnoses that meet criteria for medical necessity according to that payer's policy. If the submitted diagnosis is not on the medical necessity list, the claim is generally rejected. However, in most cases, the claim may be resubmitted with an appeal letter and medical justification, a process that is costly and time-consuming. A systematic review of payers' explanation-of-benefits forms should help to determine local payer policies. Most Medicare intermediaries have published these medical necessity criteria in the form of local coverage determinations (LCDs). For further information on these LCDs, refer to www.cms.gov/medicare-coverage-database/#LCDsAndChallenges and to the relevant Medicare carrier Web sites listed at www.cms.gov/medicareprovidersupenroll/downloads/contact_list.pdf.

More than one diagnosis may be submitted for a single CPT code, particularly if more than one body system or medical condition has been addressed during a single patient visit (eg, detailed history and examination, and medical decision making of low complexity [**99203**]). Documentation supporting the use of multiple ICD-9-CM codes must be consistent with current documentation guidelines (www.cms.gov/MLNEdWebGuide/25_EMDOC.asp).

The ICD-9-CM system, which will continue to be in use through 2012, uses a three-, four- or five-digit coding mechanism, and Medicare requires diagnoses to be coded to the greatest degree of specificity. If a more specific four-digit code is available to describe a patient's diagnosis or problem, it must be used in place of a three-digit code. Likewise, if appropriate, a more specific five-digit code must be used in place of a four-digit code. (See Appendix C for more information on ICD-9-CM coding.)

CODING TIP The Department of Health and Human Services has adopted the new version of diagnosis codes, ICD-10-CM. This change will take effect on October 1, 2013.

CPT: The Basics

The CPT code set is intended to provide a uniform language that accurately describes medical, surgical, and diagnostic services and thereby serves as an effective means for reliable nationwide communication among physicians and other health care providers, patients, and third parties. As such, it is a compendium of more than 9,000 services provided by physicians in all specialties and other qualified health care providers.

The main body of the CPT code set is organized into six sections that are further divided into various subsections with anatomic, procedural, condition, or descriptor subheadings. This categorization is for organizational purposes only, and the use of codes within a section is not restricted to specific specialties or physicians. For example, complete reporting of nuclear stress tests requires that codes be reported from both the Radiology and Medicine sections of the CPT codebook.

The six CPT Category I subsections and the range of their numeric codes are shown in Table 1-1.

TABLE 1-1. CPT Category I Subsections

CPT Category I Subsections	Code Range
Evaluation and Management	99201-99499
Anesthesia	00100-01999
Surgery	10021-69990
Radiology	70010-79999
Pathology and Laboratory	80047-89398
Medicine	90281-99607

GUIDELINES

At the beginning of each of the six sections in the CPT codebook, a set of broad introductory guidelines for interpretation and reporting of the codes listed in that section is given. For instance, guidelines in the Anesthesiology section define terms unique to that section of the CPT codebook, such as "time reporting." Introductory paragraphs to subsections of the CPT codebook also provide important information for CPT code users. Cardiovascular-related services may be found in many subsections of the CPT codebook.

CPT TERMINOLOGY AND FORMAT

The CPT codes are numerically coded descriptions of individual medical services and procedures. The descriptor for each code is a unique definition of the relevant procedure or service. However, in the print format, complete descriptors may not be repeated for some codes when they refer back to a common portion of the preceding code, which is punctuated with a semicolon. Such codes can be identified when an entry is followed by one or more codes that are indented. For example:

93015 Cardiovascular stress test using maximal or submaximal treadmill or bicycle exercise, continuous electrocardiographic monitoring, and/or pharmacological stress; with physician supervision, with interpretation and report

93016 physician supervision only, without interpretation and report

Note that the common part of code **93015** (ie, all of the descriptor preceding the semicolon) should be considered part of code **93016**, which reads in full, "Cardiovascular stress test using maximal or sub-maximal treadmill or bicycle exercise, continuous electrocardiographic monitoring, and/or pharma-cological stress; physician supervision only, without interpretation and report."

Parenthetical statements are often instructional or exclusionary statements to aid in correct coding, par-ticularly when there has been an interim change or a new code has been added.

CODE CHANGES

The CPT coding system is revised annually by the AMA. Among the several hundred annual changes are new codes, deleted codes, and changes in code num-bers and descriptions. Physicians and their coding staff should always obtain and use the current edition of the CPT codebook to ensure accuracy in coding and to avoid unnecessary denials of claims. The ▶◀ symbol is used to indicate new and revised text other than the procedure descriptors. These symbols indicate CPT Editorial Panel actions. When a new procedure code is added, the ● symbol is placed before the code number in the year in which it first appears. If a revision has resulted in substantially altered terminology that year, the ▲ symbol is placed before the code number. The CPT add-on codes are annotated by a ✚ symbol and are listed in Appendix D of the CPT codebook. The ⊘ symbol is used to identify codes that are exempt from the use of modifier 51 but have not been designated as CPT add-on procedures or services. A list of codes exempt from modifier 51 use is included in Appendix E of the CPT codebook. The ⚡ symbol is used to identify codes for vaccines that are pending Food and Drug Administration approval. A listing of all changes in each new edition can be found in Appendix B of the CPT codebook. The ⊙ symbol identifies codes for which moderate sedation may not be submitted in addition to the code when moderate sedation is per-formed by the same physician. (See Appendix G of the CPT codebook for further details.)

A list of codes that include moderate sedation is provided in Appendix G of the CPT codebook. The ○ symbol is used to identify codes that are reinstated. Resequenced codes that are not placed numerically are identified with the # symbol, and a cross-reference note is placed where the code should have been numeri-cally (eg, "Code is out of numerical sequence. See . . .") as a navigational alert to direct the user to the location of the out-of-sequence code. Resequencing is used to allow placement of related concepts in appropriate locations within the families of codes regardless of the availability of numbers for sequential numeric placement.

Add-On Codes

Some of the listed procedures are commonly carried out in addition to the primary procedure performed. These additional or supplemental procedures are desig-nated as add-on codes with the ✚ symbol, and they are listed in Appendix D of the CPT codebook. Add-on codes in the CPT codebook can be readily identi-fied by specific descriptor nomenclature that includes phrases such as "each additional" or "(List separately in addition to primary procedure)."

The add-on code concept in the CPT codebook applies only to add-on procedures or services performed by the same physician. Add-on codes describe additional intraservice work associated with the primary proce-dure (eg, additional digit[s], lesion[s], neurorrhaphy[s], vertebral segment[s], tendon[s], joint[s]).

Add-on codes are always performed in addition to the primary service or procedure and must never be reported as a stand-alone code. All add-on codes in the CPT codebook are exempt from the multiple procedure concept (see the modifier 51 definition in Appendix A of the CPT codebook).

Unlisted Procedures

The CPT Editorial Panel acknowledges that there may be certain services or procedures that are not included in the CPT codebook. For this reason, there are a number of specific codes designated for report-ing unlisted procedures. Refer to the specific section of the CPT codebook under "Guidelines." When an unlisted–procedure code is submitted on a claim form, the service or procedure should be described in a writ-ten report sent with the claim form to the third-party payer. Code **93799** is reported for an unlisted cardio-vascular service or procedure.

CHAPTER 2

Evaluation and Management Services

Evaluation and management (E/M) services apply to outpatient and inpatient encounters for visits and consultations. According to the CPT guidelines, E/M codes describe purely cognitive services; neither testing nor procedures are included. Because these codes describe cognitive clinical services provided by physicians (eg, the history and physical examination), a physician rather than a staff member will most accurately code these services. Thus, to secure appropriate reimbursement, a thorough understanding of E/M codes is crucial to physicians, regardless of specialty. This is particularly important for the cardiologist who frequently performs complex cognitive services for patients with multiple confounding multisystem diseases. Documentation of E/M services establishes the medical necessity not only of the visit or consultation itself, but also of the diagnostic and/or therapeutic services that are ordered or performed. This chapter details the clinical documentation required for E/M services.

Documentation of E/M Services

The E/M coding system has evolved since its introduction in 1992, when it used largely qualitative descriptions of coding and documentation. In 1995 and 1997, the documentation guidelines introduced qualitative measures to assist physicians and to add necessary reliability to audits. According to the CMS *Evaluation and Management Services Guide* (MLN Educational Web Guide), "The most substantial differences between the two versions occur in the examination documentation section. Either version of the documentation guidelines, not a combination of the two, may be used by the provider for a patient encounter." The following excerpt is taken from the Centers for Medicare and Medicaid Services' (CMS) *1997 Documentation Guidelines for Evaluation and Management Services.* For the more complete document, go to the US Department of Health and Human Services, CMS Web site at www.cms.gov/MLNProducts/Downloads/MASTER1.pdf.

WHAT IS DOCUMENTATION, AND WHY IS IT IMPORTANT?

Medical record documentation is required to record pertinent facts, findings, and observations about an individual's health history including past and present illnesses, examinations, tests, treatments, and outcomes. The medical record chronologically documents the care of the patient and is an important element contributing to high-quality care. The medical record facilitates:

- the ability of the physician and other health care professionals to evaluate and plan the patient's immediate treatment, and to monitor his/her health care over time;

- communication and continuity of care among physicians and other health care professionals involved in the patient's care;

- accurate and timely claims review and payment;

- appropriate utilization review and quality of care evaluations; and

- collection of data that may be useful for research and education.

An appropriately documented medical record can reduce many of the "hassles" associated with claims processing and may serve as a legal document to verify the care provided, if necessary.

WHAT DO PAYERS WANT AND WHY?

Because payers have a contractual obligation to enrollees, they may require reasonable documentation that services are consistent with the insurance coverage provided. They may request information to validate:

- the site of service;

- the medical necessity and appropriateness of diagnostic and/or therapeutic services; and/or

- that services provided have been accurately reported.

GENERAL PRINCIPLES OF MEDICAL RECORD DOCUMENTATION

The principles of documentation listed below are applicable to all types of medical and surgical services in all settings. For Evaluation and Management (E/M) services, the nature and amount of physician work and documentation varies by type of service, place of service, and the patient's status. The general principles listed below may be modified to account for these variable circumstances in providing E/M services.

1. The medical record should be complete and legible.

2. The documentation of each patient encounter should include:

   - reason for the encounter and relevant history, physical examination findings, and prior diagnostic test results;

   - assessment, clinical impression, or diagnosis;

   - plan for care; and

   - date and legible identity of the observer.

3. If not documented, the rationale for ordering diagnostic and other ancillary services should be easily inferred.

4. Past and present diagnoses should be accessible to the treating and/or consulting physician.

5. Appropriate health risk factors should be identified.

6. The patient's progress, response to and changes in treatment, and revision of diagnosis should be documented.

7. The CPT and ICD-9-CM codes reported on the health insurance claim form or billing statement should be supported by the documentation in the medical record.

SOAP DOCUMENTATION

Table 2-1 details the SOAP method of documentation of a patient encounter.

TABLE 2-1. SOAP Method of Documentation

S = Subjective	What the patient tells the physician: history
O = Objective	What the physician observes: examination
A = Assessment	What the physician decides: medical decision making and nature of patient's problem
P = Plan	What action the physician takes: treatment

Remember, from a documentation perspective: If it is not documented, it was not done! If it is not legible, it does not exist!

DOCUMENTATION OF E/M SERVICES

This publication provides definitions and documentation guidelines for the three key components of E/M services and for visits that consist predominantly of counseling or coordination of care. The three *key* components—history, examination, and medical decision making—appear in the descriptors for office and other outpatient services, hospital observation services, hospital inpatient services, consultations, emergency department services, nursing facility services, domiciliary care services, and home services. While some of the text of the CPT codebook has been repeated in this publication, the reader should refer to the CPT codebook for the complete descriptors for E/M services and instructions for selecting a level of service. Documentation guidelines are identified by the symbol •DG.

The descriptors for the levels of E/M services recognize seven components that are used in defining the levels of E/M services. These components are:

- history;

- examination;

- medical decision making;

- counseling;

- coordination of care;

- nature of presenting problem; and

- time.

The first three of these components (ie, history, examination, and medical decision making) are the key components in selecting the level of E/M services. In the case of visits that consist predominantly of counseling or coordination of care, time is the key or controlling factor to qualify for a particular level of E/M service. Because the level of E/M service is dependent on two or three key components, performance and documentation of one component (eg, examination) at the highest level does not necessarily mean that the encounter in its entirety qualifies for the highest level of E/M service.

These Documentation Guidelines for E/M services reflect the needs of the typical adult population. For certain groups of patients, the recorded information may vary slightly from that described here. Specifically, the medical records of infants, children, adolescents, and pregnant women may have additional or modified information recorded in each history and examination area. As an example, newborn records may include under history of present illness (HPI) the details of the mother's pregnancy

and the infant's status at birth; social history will focus on family structure; family history will focus on congenital anomalies and hereditary disorders in the family. In addition, the content of a pediatric examination will vary with the age and development of the child. Although not specifically defined in these documentation guidelines, these patient group variations on history and examination are appropriate.

DOCUMENTATION OF HISTORY

The levels of E/M services are based on four types of history (Problem Focused, Expanded Problem Focused, Detailed, and Comprehensive). Each type of history includes some or all of the following elements:

- Chief complaint (CC);

- History of present illness (HPI);

- Review of systems (ROS); and

- Past, family and/or social history (PFSH).

The extent of history of present illness, review of systems, and past, family and/or social history that is obtained and documented is dependent upon clinical judgment and the nature of the presenting problem(s).

Table 2-2 shows the progression of the elements required for each type of history. To qualify for a given type of history, all three elements in the table must be met. (A chief complaint is indicated at all levels.)

TABLE 2-2. Element Required for History

History of Present Illness	Review of Systems	Past, Family, and/or Social History	Type of History
Brief	N/A	N/A	*Problem focused*
Brief	Problem pertinent	N/A	*Expanded problem focused*
Extended	Extended	Pertinent	*Detailed*
Extended	Complete	Complete	*Comprehensive*
Brief	N/A	N/A	*Problem focused*
Brief	Problem pertinent	N/A	*Expanded problem focused*

N/A indicates not applicable.

Modified from *1997 Documentation Guidelines for Evaluation and Management Services.*
Available at: www.cms.gov/MLNProducts/Downloads/MASTER1.pdf. Accessed December 2010.

- *DG: The CC, ROS, and PFSH may be listed as separate elements of history, or they may be included in the description of the history of present illness.*

- *DG: A[n] ROS and/or a PFSH obtained during an earlier encounter does not need to be re-recorded if there is evidence that the physician reviewed and updated the previous information. This may occur when a physician updates his or her own record or in an institutional setting or group practice where many physicians use a common record. The review and update may be documented by:*

  - *describing any new ROS and/or PFSH information or noting there has been no change in the information; and*

  - *noting the date and location of the earlier ROS and/or PFSH.*

- *DG: The ROS and/or PFSH may be recorded by ancillary staff or on a form completed by the patient. To document that the physician reviewed the information, there must be a notation supplementing or confirming the information recorded by others.*

- *DG: If the physician is unable to obtain a history from the patient or other source, the record should describe the patient's condition or other circumstance that precludes obtaining a history.*

Definitions and specific documentation guidelines for each of the elements of history are listed below.

Chief Complaint (CC)

The CC is a concise statement describing the symptom, problem, condition, diagnosis, physician recommended return, or other factor that is the reason for the encounter, usually stated in the patient's words.

- *DG: The medical record should clearly reflect the chief complaint.*

History of Present Illness (HPI)

The HPI is a chronological description of the development of the patient's present illness from the first sign and/or symptom or from the previous encounter to the present. It includes the following elements:

- location,

- quality,

- severity,

- duration,

- timing,

- context,

- modifying factors, and

- associated signs and symptoms.

Brief and *extended* HPIs are distinguished by the amount of detail needed to accurately characterize the clinical problem(s).

A *brief* HPI consists of one to three elements of the HPI.

- *DG: The medical record should describe one to three elements of the present illness (HPI).*

An *extended* HPI consists of at least four elements of the HPI or the status of at least three chronic or inactive conditions.

- *DG: The medical record should describe at least four elements of the present illness (HPI), or the status of at least three chronic or inactive conditions.*

Review of Systems (ROS)

A[n] ROS is an inventory of body systems obtained through a series of questions seeking to identify signs and/or symptoms that the patient may be experiencing or has experienced. For purposes of the ROS, the following systems are recognized:

- Constitutional symptoms (eg, fever, weight loss)

- Eyes

- Ears, nose, mouth, throat

- Cardiovascular

- Respiratory

- Gastrointestinal

- Genitourinary

- Musculoskeletal

- Integumentary (skin and/or breast)

- Neurological

- Psychiatric

- Endocrine

- Hematologic/lymphatic

- Allergic/immunologic

A *problem-pertinent* ROS inquires about the system directly related to the problem(s) identified in the HPI.

•DG: *The patient's positive responses and pertinent negatives for the system related to the problem should be documented.*

An *extended* ROS inquires about the system directly related to the problem(s) identified in the HPI and a limited number of additional systems.

•DG: *The patient's positive responses and pertinent negatives for two to nine systems should be documented.*

A *complete* ROS inquires about the system(s) directly related to the problem(s) identified in the HPI *plus* all additional body systems.

•DG: *At least ten organ systems must be reviewed. Those systems with positive or pertinent negative responses must be individually documented. For the remaining systems, a notation indicating all other systems are negative is permissible. In the absence of such a notation, at least ten systems must be individually documented.*

Past, Family and/or Social History (PFSH)

The PFSH consists of a review of three areas:

* past history (the patient's past experiences with illnesses, operations, injuries, and treatments);

* family history (a review of medical events in the patient's family, including diseases that may be hereditary or place the patient at risk); and

* social history (an age-appropriate review of past and current activities).

For certain categories of E/M services that include only an interval history, it is not necessary to record information about the PFSH. Those categories are subsequent hospital care, follow-up inpatient consultations, and subsequent nursing facility care.

A *pertinent* PFSH is a review of the history area(s) directly related to the problem(s) identified in the HPI.

* DG: *At least one specific item from any of the three history areas must be documented for a pertinent PFSH.*

A *complete* PFSH is a review of two or all three of the PFSH history areas, depending on the category of the E/M service. A review of all three history areas is required for services that by their nature include a comprehensive assessment or reassessment of the patient. A review of two of the three history areas is sufficient for other services.

•DG: *At least one specific item from two of the three history areas must be documented for a complete PFSH for the following categories of E/M services: office or other outpatient services, established patient; emergency department; domiciliary care, established patient; and home care, established patient.*

•DG: *At least one specific item from each of the three history areas must be documented for a complete PFSH for the following categories of E/M services: office or other outpatient services, new patient; hospital observation services; hospital inpatient services, initial care; consultations; comprehensive nursing facility assessments; domiciliary care, new patient; and home care, new patient.*

DOCUMENTATION OF EXAMINATION

The levels of E/M services are based on four types of examination:

* *Problem Focused*—a limited examination of the affected body area or organ system.

* *Expanded Problem Focused*—a limited examination of the affected body area or organ system and any other symptomatic or related body area(s) or organ system(s).

* *Detailed*—an extended examination of the affected body area(s) or organ system(s) and any other symptomatic or related body area(s) or organ system(s).

* *Comprehensive*—a general multi-system examination, or complete examination of a single organ system and other symptomatic or related body area(s) or organ system(s).

These types of examinations have been defined for general multi-system and the following single organ systems:

* Cardiovascular

* Ears, nose, mouth, and throat

* Eyes

* Genitourinary (female)

* Genitourinary (male)

* Hematologic/lymphatic/immunologic

* Musculoskeletal

* Neurological

- Psychiatric

- Respiratory

- Skin

A general multi-system examination or a single organ system examination may be performed by any physician regardless of specialty. The type (general multi-system or single organ system) and content of examination are selected by the examining physician and are based upon clinical judgment, the patient's history, and the nature of the presenting problem(s).

The content and documentation requirements for each type and level of examination are summarized below and described in detail in [Tables 2-3 and 2-4]. In these tables, organ systems and body areas recognized in the CPT codebook for purposes of describing examinations are shown in the left column. The content, or individual elements, of the examination pertaining to that body area or organ system are identified by bullets (•) in the right column.

Parenthetical examples, "(eg, . . .)", are used for clarification and to provide guidance regarding documentation. Documentation for each element must satisfy any numeric requirements (such as "Measurement of *any three of the following seven . . .*") included in the description of the element. Elements with multiple components but with no specific numeric requirement (such as "Examination of *liver* and *spleen*") require documentation of at least one component. It is possible for a given examination to be expanded beyond what is defined here. When that occurs, findings related to the additional systems and/or areas should be documented.

- •DG: *Specific abnormal and relevant negative findings of the examination of the affected or symptomatic body area(s) or organ system(s) should be documented. A notation of "abnormal" without elaboration is insufficient.*

- •DG: *Abnormal or unexpected findings of the examination of any asymptomatic body area(s) or organ system(s) should be described.*

- •DG: *A brief statement or notation indicating "negative" or "normal" is sufficient to document normal findings related to unaffected area(s) or asymptomatic organ system(s).*

GENERAL MULTI-SYSTEM EXAMINATIONS

General multi-system examinations are described in detail [in Table 2-3]. To qualify for a given level of multi-system examination, the following content and documentation requirements should be met:

- *Problem Focused Examination*—should include performance and documentation of one to five elements identified by a bullet (•) [in Table 2-3] in one or more organ system(s) or body area(s).

- *Expanded Problem Focused Examination*—should include performance and documentation of at least six elements identified by a bullet (•) [in Table 2-3] in one or more organ system(s) or body area(s).

- *Detailed Examination*—should include at least six organ systems or body areas. For each system/area selected, performance and documentation of at least two elements [in Table 2-3] identified by a bullet (•) is expected. Alternatively, a detailed examination may include performance and documentation of at least twelve elements identified by a bullet (•) in two or more organ systems or body areas.

- *Comprehensive Examination*—should include at least nine organ systems or body areas. For each system/area selected, all elements of the examination identified [in Table 2-3] by a bullet (•) should be performed, unless specific directions limit the content of the examination. For each area/system, documentation of at least two elements identified by a bullet is expected.

TABLE 2-3. General Multi-System Examinations

System/Body Area	Elements of Examination
Constitutional	• Measurement of any **three of the following seven** vital signs: 1) sitting or standing blood pressure, 2) supine blood pressure, 3) pulse rate and regularity, 4) respiration, 5) temperature, 6) height, 7) weight (may be measured and recorded by ancillary staff) • General appearance of patient (eg, development, nutrition, body habitus deformities, attention to grooming)
Eyes	• Inspection of conjunctivae and lids (eg, xanthelasma) • Examination of pupils and irises (eg, reaction to light and accommodation, size, and symmetry) • Ophthalmoscopic examination of optic discs (eg, size, C/D ratio, appearance) and posterior segments (eg, vessel changes, exudates, hemorrhages)
Ears, Nose, Mouth and Throat	• External inspection of ears and nose (eg, overall appearance, scars, lesions, masses) • Otoscopic examination of auditory canals and tympanic membranes • Assessment of hearing (eg, whispered voice, finger rub, tuning fork) • Inspection of nasal mucosa, septum, and turbinates • Inspection of lips, teeth, and gums
Neck	• Examination of neck (eg, masses, overall appearance, symmetry, tracheal position, crepitus) • Examination of thyroid (eg, enlargement, tenderness, mass)
Respiratory	• Assessment of respiratory effort (eg, intercostal retractions, use of accessory muscles, diaphragmatic movement) • Percussion of chest (eg, dullness, flatness, hyperresonance) • Palpation of chest (eg, tactile fremitus) • Auscultation of lungs (eg, breath sounds, adventitious sounds, rubs)
Cardiovascular	• Palpation of heart (eg, location, size, thrills) • Auscultation of heart with notation of abnormal sounds and murmurs Examination of: • carotid arteries (eg, pulse amplitude, bruits) • abdominal aorta (eg, size, bruits) • femoral arteries (eg, pulse amplitude, bruits) • pedal pulses (eg, pulse amplitude) • extremities for peripheral edema and/or varicosities
Chest (Breasts)	• Inspection of breasts (eg, symmetry, nipple discharge) • Palpation of breasts and axillae (eg, masses or lumps, tenderness)
Gastrointestinal (Abdomen)	• Examination of abdomen with notation of presence or masses or tenderness • Examination of liver and spleen • Examination for presence or absence of hernia • Examination (when indicated) of anus, perineum and rectum, including sphincter tone, presence of hemorrhoids, rectal masses • Obtain stool sample for occult blood test when indicated

continued

CHAPTER 2

TABLE 2-3. General Multi-System Examinations *(continued)*

System/Body Area	Elements of Examination
Genitourinary	**Male:** • Examination of the scrotal contents (eg, hydrocele, spermatocele, tenderness of cord, testicular mass) • Examination of the penis • Digital rectal examination of prostate gland (eg, size, symmetry, nodularity, tenderness) **Female:** • Pelvic examination (with or without specimen collection for smears and cultures), including: • Examination of external genitalia (eg, general appearance, hair distribution, lesions) and vagina (eg, general appearance, estrogen effect, discharge, lesions, pelvic support, cystocele, rectocele) • Examination of urethra (eg, masses, tenderness, scarring) • Examination of bladder (eg, fullness, masses, tenderness) • Cervix (eg, general appearance, lesions, discharge) • Uterus (eg, size, contour, position, mobility, tenderness, consistency, descent or support) • Adnexa/parametria (eg, masses, tenderness, organomegaly, nodularity)
Lymphatic	Palpation of lymph nodes in **two or more** areas: • Neck • Axillae • Groin • Other
Musculoskeletal	• Examination of gait and station • Inspection and/or palpation of digits and nails (eg, clubbing, cyanosis, inflammatory conditions, petechiae, ischemia, infections, nodes) • Examination of joints, bones and muscles of **one or more of the following six** areas: 1) head and neck; 2) spine, ribs, and pelvis; 3) right upper extremity; 4) left upper extremity; 5) right lower extremity; and 6) left lower extremity. The examination of a given area includes: • inspection and/or palpation with notation of presence of any misalignment, asymmetry, crepitation, defects, tenderness, masses, effusions • assessment of range of motion with notation of any pain, crepitation or contracture • assessment of stability with notation of any dislocation (luxation), subluxation or laxity • assessment of muscle strength and tone (eg, flaccid, cog wheel, spastic) with notation of any atrophy or abnormal movements
Skin	• Inspection of skin and subcutaneous tissue (eg, rashes, lesions, ulcers) • Palpation of skin and subcutaneous tissue (eg, induration, subcutaneous nodules, tightening)
Neurologic	• Test cranial nerves with notation of any deficits • Examination of deep tendon reflexes with notation of pathological reflexes (eg, Babinski) • Examination of sensation (eg, by touch, pin, vibration, proprioception)

continued

TABLE 2-3. General Multi-System Examinations *(continued)*

System/Body Area	Elements of Examination
Psychiatric	• Description of patient's judgment and insight Brief assessment of mental status including: • orientation to time, place, and person • recent and remote memory • mood and affect (eg, depression, anxiety, agitation)

For the original *1997 Documentation Guidelines for Evaluation and Management Services*, go to: www.cms.gov/MLNProducts/Downloads/MASTER1.pdf. Accessed December 2010.

TABLE 2-4. Content* and Documentation Requirements: General Multi-System

Level of Exam	Perform and Document
Problem Focused	**One to five** elements identified by a bullet.
Expanded Problem Focused	**At least six** elements identified by a bullet.
Detailed	**At least two** elements identified by a bullet **from each of six areas/systems** or **at least 12** elements identified by a bullet **in two or more areas/systems**.
Comprehensive	**At least two** elements identified by a bullet **from each of nine areas/systems**.

* Content, or individual elements—At least ten organ systems must be reviewed. Those systems with positive or pertinent negative responses must be individually documented. For the remaining systems, a notation indicating all other systems are negative is permissible. In the absence of such a notation, at least ten systems must be individually documented.

SINGLE ORGAN SYSTEM EXAMINATIONS

The single organ system examinations recognized in the CPT codebook are described in detail in the single–organ-system examination tables in the CMS' 1997 Documentation Guidelines for Evaluation and Management Services. As an example, we have included one of the single organ system examination tables here. [See Table 2-5, Cardiovascular Examination.] Variations among these examinations in the organ systems and body areas identified in the left columns and in the elements of the examinations described in the right columns reflect differing emphases among specialties. To qualify for a given level of single organ system examination, the following content and documentation requirements should be met [Table 2.6].

- *Problem Focused Examination*—should include performance and documentation of one to five elements identified by a bullet (•), whether in a box with a shaded or unshaded border [in the single–organ-system examination tables beginning from page 19 in the CMS' *1997 Documentation Guidelines for Evaluation and Management Services*].

- *Expanded Problem Focused Examination*—should include performance and documentation of at least six elements identified by a bullet (•), whether in a box with a shaded or unshaded border [in the single–organ-system examination tables on pages 19-45 in the CMS' *1997 Documentation Guidelines for Evaluation and Management Services*].

- *Detailed Examination*—examinations other than the eye and psychiatric examinations should include performance and documentation of at least twelve elements identified by a bullet (•), whether in box with a shaded or unshaded border [in the single–organ-system examination tables on pages 19-45 in the CMS' *1997 Documentation Guidelines for Evaluation and Management Services*].

- *Comprehensive Examination*—should include performance of all elements identified by a bullet (•), whether in a shaded or unshaded box. Documentation of every element in each box with a shaded border and at least one element in each box with an unshaded border is expected [in the single–organ-system examination tables on pages 19-45 in the CMS' *1997 Documentation Guidelines for Evaluation and Management Services*].

TABLE 2-5. Cardiovascular Examination

System/Body Area	Elements of Examination
Constitutional	• Measurement of **any three of the following seven** vital signs: 1) sitting or standing blood pressure, 2) supine blood pressure, 3) pulse rate and regularity, 4) respiration, 5) temperature, 6) height, 7) weight (May be measured and recorded by ancillary staff) • General appearance of patient (eg, development, nutrition, body habitus deformities, attention to grooming)
Head and Face	
Eyes	• Inspection of conjunctivae and lids (eg, xanthelasma)
Ears, Nose, Mouth and Throat	• Inspection of teeth, gums, and palate • Inspection of oral mucosa with notation of presence of pallor or cyanosis
Neck	• Examination of jugular veins (eg, distension; a, v, or cannon a waves) • Examination of thyroid (eg, enlargement, tenderness, mass)
Respiratory	• Assessment of respiratory effort (eg, intercostal retractions, use of accessory muscles, diaphragmatic movement) • Auscultation of lungs (eg, breath sounds, adventitious sounds, rubs)
Cardiovascular	• Palpation of heart (eg, location, size, and forcefulness of the point of maximal impact; thrills; lifts; palpable S3 or S4) • Auscultation of heart including sounds, abnormal sounds, and murmurs • Measurement of blood pressure in two or more extremities when indicated (eg, aortic dissection, coarctation) Examination of: • Carotid arteries (eg, waveform, pulse amplitude, bruits, apical-carotid delay) • Abdominal aorta (eg, size, bruits) • Femoral arteries (eg, pulse amplitude, bruits) • Pedal pulses (eg, pulse amplitude) • Extremities for peripheral edema and/or varicosities
Chest (Breasts)	
Gastrointestinal (Abdomen)	• Examination of abdomen with notation of presence or masses or tenderness • Examination of liver and spleen • Obtain stool sample for occult blood from patients who are being considered for thrombolytic or anticoagulant therapy
Genitourinary (Abdomen)	
Lymphatic	
Musculoskeletal	• Examination of the back with notation of kyphosis or scoliosis • Examination of gait with notation of ability to undergo exercise testing and/or participation in exercise programs • Assessment of muscle strength and tone (eg, flaccid, cog wheel, spastic) with notation of any atrophy and abnormal movements

continued

TABLE 2-5. Cardiovascular Examination *(continued)*

System/ Body Area	Elements of Examination
Extremities	• Inspection and palpation of digits and nails (eg, clubbing, cyanosis, inflammation, petechiae, ischemia, infections, Osler's nodes)
Skin	• Inspection and/or palpation of skin and subcutaneous tissue (eg, stasis dermatitis, ulcers, scars, xanthomas)
Neurological/ Psychiatric	Brief assessment of mental status including: • Orientation to time, place, and person • Mood and affect (eg, depression, anxiety, agitation)

For the current *1997 Documentation Guidelines for Evaluation and Management Services,* go to: www.cms.gov/MLNProducts/Downloads/MASTER1.pdf. Accessed October 2011.

TABLE 2-6. Content* and Documentation Requirements: Cardiovascular System

Level of Exam	Perform and Document
Problem Focused	**One to five** elements identified by a bullet.
Expanded Problem Focused	**At least six** elements identified by a bullet.
Detailed	**At least 12** elements identified by a bullet.
Comprehensive	Perform **all** elements identified by a bullet; document every element in a shaded box and at least one element in an unshaded box.

* Content, or individual elements—All elements identified by a bullet (•) in Table 2-5 should be performed, unless specific directions limit the content of the examination

EDITOR'S NOTE For the purposes of this text, only the general multi-system and the cardiovascular system specialty examination tables are included. For a complete list of specialty examination tables, go to www.cms.gov/MLNProducts/Downloads/MASTER1.pdf.

DOCUMENTATION OF THE COMPLEXITY OF MEDICAL DECISION MAKING

The levels of E/M services recognize four types of medical decision making (straightforward, low complexity, moderate complexity, and high complexity). Medical decision making refers to the complexity of establishing a diagnosis and/or selecting a management option as measured by:

• the number of possible diagnoses and/or the number of management options that must be considered;

• the amount and/or complexity of medical records, diagnostic tests, and/or other information that must be obtained, reviewed and analyzed; and

• the risk of significant complications, morbidity and/or mortality, as well as comorbidities associated with the patient's presenting problem(s), the diagnostic procedure(s), and/or the possible management options.

[Table 2-7] shows the progression of the elements required for each level of medical decision making. To qualify for a given type of decision making, **two of the three elements in the table must be either met or exceeded.**

TABLE 2-7. Progression of Elements: Medical Decision Making

Number of Diagnoses or Management Options	Amount and/ or Complexity of Data to be Reviewed	Risk of Complications and/or Morbidity or Mortality	Type of Decision Making
Minimal	Minimal or none	Minimal	*Straightforward*
Limited	Limited	Low	*Low complexity*
Multiple	Moderate	Moderate	*Moderate complexity*
Extensive	Extensive	High	*High complexity*

From *1997 Documentation Guidelines for Evaluation and Management Services.* Available at: www.cms.gov/MLNProducts/Downloads/MASTER1.pdf. Accessed December 2010.

Each of the elements of medical decision making is described below.

Number of Diagnoses or Management Options

The number of possible diagnoses and/or the number of management options that must be considered is based on the number and types of problems addressed during the encounter, the complexity of establishing a diagnosis, and the management decisions that are made by the physician.

Generally, decision making with respect to a diagnosed problem is easier than that for an identified but undiagnosed problem. The number and type of diagnostic tests employed may be an indicator of the number of possible diagnoses. Problems that are improving or resolving are less complex than those that are worsening or failing to change as expected. The need to seek advice from others is another indicator of complexity of diagnostic or management problems.

- •DG: *For each encounter, an assessment, clinical impression, or diagnosis should be documented. It may be explicitly stated or implied in documented decisions regarding management plans and/or further evaluation.*

  - *For a presenting problem with an established diagnosis the record should reflect whether the problem is: a) improved, well controlled, resolving, or resolved; or, b) inadequately controlled, worsening, or failing to change as expected.*

  - *For a presenting problem without an established diagnosis, the assessment or clinical impression may be stated in the form of differential diagnoses or as a "possible," "probable," or "rule out" (R/O) diagnosis.*

- •DG: *The initiation of, or changes in, treatment should be documented. Treatment includes a wide range of management options including patient instructions, nursing instructions, therapies, and medications.*

- •DG: *If referrals are made, consultations requested, or advice sought, the record should indicate to whom or where the referral or consultation is made or from whom the advice is requested.*

Amount and/or Complexity of Data to Be Reviewed

The amount and complexity of data to be reviewed is based on the types of diagnostic testing ordered or reviewed. A decision to obtain and review old medical records and/or obtain history from sources other than the patient increases the amount and complexity of data to be reviewed.

Discussion of contradictory or unexpected test results with the physician who performed or interpreted the test is an indication of the complexity of data being reviewed. On occasion the physician who ordered a test may personally review the image, tracing, or specimen to supplement information from the physician who prepared the test report or interpretation; this is another indication of the complexity of data being reviewed.

- •DG: *If a diagnostic service (test or procedure) is ordered, planned, scheduled, or performed at the time of the E/M encounter, the type of service, eg, lab or x-ray, should be documented.*

- •DG: *The review of lab, radiology, and/or other diagnostic tests should be documented. A simple notation such as "WBC elevated" or "chest x-ray unremarkable" is acceptable. Alternatively, the review may be documented by initialing and dating the report containing the test results.*

- •DG: *A decision to obtain old records or a decision to obtain additional history from the family, caretaker, or other source to supplement that obtained from the patient should be documented.*

- •DG: *Relevant findings from the review of old records and/or the receipt of additional history from the family, caretaker, or other source to supplement that obtained from the patient should be documented. If there is no relevant information beyond that already obtained, that fact should be documented. A notation of "Old records reviewed" or "additional history obtained from family" without elaboration is insufficient.*

- •DG: *The results of discussion of laboratory, radiology, or other diagnostic tests with the physician who performed or interpreted the study should be documented.*

- •DG: *The direct visualization and independent interpretation of an image, tracing, or specimen previously or subsequently interpreted by another physician should be documented.*

Risk of Significant Complications, Morbidity, and/or Mortality

The risk of significant complications, morbidity, and/or mortality is based on the risks associated with the presenting problem(s), the diagnostic procedure(s), and the possible management options.

- •DG: *Comorbidities/underlying diseases or other factors that increase the complexity of medical decision making by increasing the risk of complications, morbidity, and/or mortality should be documented.*

- •DG: *If a surgical or invasive diagnostic procedure is ordered, planned, or scheduled at the time of the E/M encounter, the type of procedure, eg, laparoscopy, should be documented.*

- •DG: *If a surgical or invasive diagnostic procedure is performed at the time of the E/M encounter, the specific procedure should be documented.*

- •DG: *The referral for or decision to perform a surgical or invasive diagnostic procedure on an urgent basis should be documented or implied.*

[Table 2-8, Table of Risk] may be used to help determine whether the risk of significant complications, morbidity, and/or mortality is *minimal*, *low*, *moderate*, or *high*. Because the determination of risk is complex and not readily quantifiable, the table includes common clinical examples rather than absolute measures of risk. The assessment of risk of the presenting problem(s) is based on the risk related to the disease process anticipated between the present encounter and the next one. The assessment of risk of selecting diagnostic procedures and management options is based on the risk during and immediately following any procedures or treatment. **The highest level of risk in any one category (presenting problem(s), diagnostic procedure(s), or management options) determines the overall risk.**

Documentation of an Encounter Dominated by Counseling or CoOrdination of Care

In the case where counseling and/or coordination of care dominates (more than 50%) of the physician/patient and/or family encounter (face-to-face time in the office or other or outpatient setting, floor/unit time in the hospital or nursing facility), time is considered the key or controlling factor to qualify for a particular level of E/M services.

- •DG: *If the physician elects to report the level of service based on counseling and/or coordination of care, the total length of time of the encounter (face-to-face or floor time, as appropriate) should be documented, and the record should describe the counseling and/or activities to coordinate care.*

Selecting an E/M Code

The selection of the appropriate E/M code is based on the clinical content of the service provided. The 1997 AMA guidelines for E/M code selection include several topics, each of which is described in more detail below:

- The category and subcategory of service

- Reporting instructions for the selected category or subcategory

- Level of E/M service descriptors in the selected category or subcategory

- Appropriate E/M selection

THE CATEGORY AND SUBCATEGORY OF SERVICE

Table 2-9 describes clinical services by category and subcategory and provides the corresponding E/M codes.

> **CODING TIP** A new patient is one who has not received any professional services from the physician or another physician of the exact same specialty and subspecialty who belongs to the same group practice within the past 3 years. The CPT codebook defines professional services as face-to-face services rendered by a physician and reported by a specific CPT code(s). Medicare carriers define new patient services as services that have not been rendered face-to-face within the past 3 years.

REPORTING INSTRUCTIONS FOR THE SELECTED CATEGORY OR SUBCATEGORY

Many of the categories and subcategories of service have special guidelines or instructions unique to the specific category. Instructional notes must be read carefully and then compared with a particular insurance carrier's information on code coverage and use. The mere presence of a code does not guarantee reimbursement. For example, the codes for team conferences and telephone calls are rarely reimbursed because these services are considered bundled into other E/M services.

TABLE 2-8. Table of Risk

Level of Risk	Presenting Problem(s)	Diagnostic Procedure(s) Ordered	Management Options Selected
Minimal	■ One self-limited or minor problem, eg, cold, insect bite, tinea corpus	■ Laboratory tests requiring venipuncture ■ Chest x-rays ■ EKG/EEG Urinalysis ■ Ultrasound, eg, echocardiography ■ KOH prep	■ Rest Gargles ■ Elastic bandages ■ Superficial dressings
Low	■ Two or more self-limited or minor problems ■ One stable chronic illness, eg, well-controlled hypertension or non–insulin-dependent diabetes, cataract, BPH ■ Acute uncomplicated illness or injury, eg, cystitis, allergic rhinitis, simple sprain	■ Physiologic tests not under stress, eg, pulmonary function tests ■ Non-cardiovascular imaging studies with contrast, eg, barium enema ■ Superficial needle biopsies ■ Clinical laboratory tests requiring arterial puncture ■ Skin biopsies	■ Over-the-counter drugs ■ Minor surgery with no identified risk factors ■ Physical therapy ■ Occupational therapy ■ IV fluids without additives
Moderate	■ One or more chronic illnesses with mild exacerbation, progression, or side effects of treatment ■ Two or more stable chronic illnesses ■ Undiagnosed new problem with uncertain diagnosis, eg, lump in breast ■ Acute illness with systemic symptoms, eg, pyelonephritis, pneumonia, colitis ■ Acute complicated injury, eg, head injury with brief loss of consciousness	■ Physiologic tests under stress, eg, cardiac stress test, fetal contraction stress test ■ Diagnostic endoscopies with no identified risk factors ■ Deep needle or incisional biopsy ■ Cardiovascular imaging studies with contrast and no identified risk factors, eg, arteriogram, cardiac catheterization ■ Obtain fluid from body cavity, eg, lumbar puncture, thoracentesis, culdocentesis	■ Minor surgery with identified risk factors ■ Elective major surgery (open, percutaneous or endoscopic) with no identified risk factors ■ Prescription drug management ■ Therapeutic nuclear medicine ■ IV fluids with additives ■ Closed treatment of fracture or dislocation without manipulation

TABLE 2-8. Table of Risk *(continued)*

Level of Risk	Presenting Problem(s)	Diagnostic Procedure(s) Ordered	Management Options Selected
High	▪ One or more chronic illnesses with severe exacerbation, progression, or side effects of treatment ▪ Acute or chronic illnesses or injuries that pose a threat to life or bodily function, eg, multiple trauma, acute MI, pulmonary embolus, severe respiratory distress, progressive severe rheumatoid arthritis, psychiatric illness with potential threat to self or others, peritonitis, acute renal failure ▪ An abrupt change in neurologic status, eg, seizure, TIA, weakness, sensory loss	▪ Cardiovascular imaging studies with contrast with identified risk factors ▪ Cardiac electrophysiological tests ▪ Diagnostic endoscopies with identified risk factors ▪ Discography	▪ Elective major surgery (open, percutaneous or endoscopic) with identified risk factors ▪ Emergency major surgery (open, percutaneous or endoscopic) ▪ Parenteral controlled substances ▪ Drug therapy requiring intensive monitoring for toxicity ▪ Decision not to resuscitate or to de-escalate care because of poor prognosis

Abbreviations: BPH indicates benign prostatic hypertrophy; EEG, electroencephalogram; EKG, electrocardiogram; KOH, potassium hydroxide; IV, intravenous; MI, myocardial infarction; and TIA, transient ischemic attack.

The highest level of risk in any one category (presenting problem[s], diagnostic procedure[s], or management option[s]) determines the overall risk.

From *1997 Documentation Guidelines for Evaluation and Management Services.*
Available at: www.cms.gov/MLNProducts/Downloads/MASTER1.pdf. Accessed October 2011.

TABLE 2-9. Clinical Services by Category and Subcategory

Category/Subcategory	Code Numbers
Office or Other Outpatient Services	
New Patient	**99201-99205**
Established Patient	**99211-99215**
Hospital Observation Services	
Initial Hospital Observation Services	**99218-99220**
Subsequent Hospital Observation Services	**99224-99226**
Hospital Observation Discharge Services	**99217**
Hospital Inpatient Services	
Initial Hospital Care	**99221-99223**
Subsequent Hospital Care	**99231-99233**
Observation or Inpatient Care Services (Including Admission and Discharge Services)	**99234-99236**
Hospital Discharge Services	**99238-99239**

Category/Subcategory	Code Numbers
Consultations	
Office/Outpatient Consultations	**99241-99245**
Inpatient Consultations	**99251-99255**
Emergency Department Services	**99281-99288**
Critical Care Services	**99291-99292**
Nursing Facility Services	
Initial Nursing Facility Care	**99304-99306**
Subsequent Nursing Facility Care	**99307-99310**
Nursing Facility Discharge Services	**99315-99316**
Domiciliary, Rest Home, or Custodial Care Services	
New Patient	**99324-99328**
Established Patient	**99334-99337**
Domiciliary, Rest Home, or Home Care	
Plan Oversight Services	**99339-99340**

continued

CHAPTER 2

TABLE 2-9. Clinical Services by Category
and Subcategory *(continued)*

Category/Subcategory	Code Numbers
Home Services	
New Patient	99341-99345
Established Patient	99347-99350
Prolonged Services	
With Direct Patient Contact	99354-99357
Without Direct Patient Contact	99358-99359
Physician Standby Services	99360
Anticoagulation Services	99363-99364
Team Conferences	99366-99368
Care Plan Oversight Services	99374-99380
Preventive Medicine Services	
New Patient	99381-99387
Established Patient	99391-99397
Individual Counseling	99401-99404
Behavior Change Interventions	99406-99409
Group counseling	99411-99412
Other	99420-99429
Non–Face-to-Face Services	
Telephone Calls	99441-99443
Online Medical Evaluation	99444
Special Evaluation and Management Services	
Disability Evaluation Services	99450-99456
Newborn Care Services	
Newborn Care Services	99460-99463
Delivery/Birthing Room Attendance and Resuscitation Services	99464-99465
Inpatient Neonatal Intensive Care Services and Pediatric and Neonatal Critical Care Services	99466-99480
Other E/M Services	99499

CODING TIP The Centers for Medicare & Medicaid Services (CMS) released guidelines in 1995 and 1997 to assist physicians in documenting their services for the purpose of selecting the appropriate level of E/M code. The 1997 guidelines were intended to augment and further clarify fundamental terms used to define and describe the E/M components. However, physicians found difficulty with actual implementation. Until new documentation guidelines are implemented, physicians and staff have the option of using the 1995 or the 1997 guidelines, depending on which are most advantageous. For reference, the *1995 Documentation Guidelines for Evaluation and Management Services* are available on the CMS Web site at *www.cms.hhs.gov/MLNProducts/Downloads/1995dg.pdf.* The *1997 Documentation Guidelines for Evaluation and Management Services* is available at *www.cms.hhs.gov/MLNProducts/Downloads/MASTER1.pdf.*

LEVEL OF E/M SERVICE DESCRIPTORS IN THE SELECTED CATEGORY OR SUBCATEGORY

The E/M guidelines identify history, examination, and complexity of medical decision making as the three key components for determining code selection. Currently, each of these three key E/M components has four types, resulting in a total of 12 essential definitions.

The four types of each of the key E/M components are as follows:

Type of History

Problem focused—Chief complaint; brief history of present illness or problem.

Expanded problem focused—Chief complaint; brief history of present illness or problem; pertinent system review.

Detailed—Chief complaint; extended history of present illness; problem-pertinent system review extended to include a review of a limited number of additional systems; pertinent past, family, and/or social history directly related to the patient's problems.

Comprehensive—Chief complaint; extended history of present illness; review of systems that is directly related to the problem(s) identified in the history of present illness plus a review of all additional body systems; complete past, family, and social history.

CODING TIP A common weakness in medical records documentation is the absence of a chief complaint or the reason for the visit. Physicians should document a clear statement of chief complaint, alone or in the history of present illness.

Type of Physical Examination

Problem focused—An examination that is limited to a single body area or organ system.

Expanded problem focused—A limited examination of the affected body area or organ system and other symptomatic or related organ system(s).

Detailed—An extended examination of the affected body area(s) and other symptomatic or related organ system(s).

Comprehensive—A complete single-system specialty examination or a general multi-system examination.

Types of Medical Decision Making

The type of decision making is based on the complexity of establishing a diagnosis and/or selecting a management option. To qualify for a given type of decision making, at least two of the three elements listed in the definition must be present.

Straightforward—Number of diagnoses and/or management options is minimal; amount and/or complexity of data reviewed is minimal or nonexistent; risk of complications, morbidity, and/or mortality is minimal.

Low complexity—Number of diagnoses and/or management options is limited; amount and/or complexity of data reviewed is limited; risk of complications, morbidity, and/or mortality is low.

Moderate complexity—Number of diagnoses and/or management options is multiple; amount and/or complexity of data reviewed is moderate; risk of complications, morbidity, and/or mortality is moderate.

High complexity—Number of diagnoses and/or management options is extensive; amount and/or complexity of data reviewed is extensive; risk of complications, morbidity, and/or mortality is high.

Other Factors

There are additional components that help a physician decide on the appropriate level of service and provide the documentation necessary to support a higher level. Nature of presenting problem is considered one of the contributory components and is defined as problems that are weighed beyond the key components for code selection. The diagnostic aspect of this component certainly has an impact on coding. Diagnostic statements, including differential diagnoses, are an important aspect of medical record documentation. All physicians should be certain that documentation reflects not only what service(s) were provided, but also why.

Nature of Presenting Problem

This is the disease, condition, illness, injury, symptom, sign, finding, complaint, or other reason for the encounter, with or without an established diagnosis at the time of the encounter.

The E/M codes recognize five types of presenting problems that are defined as follows:

Minimal—Service for a problem that may not require the presence of the physician, but service is provided under the physician's supervision.

Self-limited or minor—A problem that runs a definite and prescribed course, is transient in nature, and is not likely to permanently alter health status OR has a good prognosis with management/compliance.

Low severity—A problem in which the risk of morbidity without treatment is low; there is little to no risk of mortality without treatment; full recovery without functional impairment is expected.

Moderate severity—A problem in which the risk of morbidity without treatment is moderate; there is moderate risk of mortality without treatment; uncertain prognosis OR increased probability of prolonged functional impairment.

High severity—A problem in which the risk of morbidity without treatment is high to extreme; there is moderate to high risk of mortality without treatment OR high probability of severe, prolonged functional impairment.

Counseling

This is a discussion with a patient and/or family member concerning one or more of the following areas:

- Diagnostic results, impressions, and/or recommended diagnostic studies

- Prognosis

- Risks and benefits of management (treatment) options

- Instructions for management (treatment) and/or follow-up

- Importance of compliance with chosen management (treatment) options

- Risk factor reduction

- Patient and family education

Coordination of Care

This factor is not used in defining the levels of E/M services. When counseling and/or coordination of care dominates (more than 50%) the physician-patient and/or family encounter (face-to-face time in the office or other outpatient setting or floor/unit time in the hospital or nursing facility), then time shall be considered the key or controlling factor to qualify for a particular level of E/M services. This includes time spent with parties who have assumed responsibility for the care of the patient or decision making whether or not they are family members (eg, foster parents, person acting in loco parentis, legal guardian). The extent of counseling and/or coordination of care must be documented in the medical record.

Time

Average physician encounter times are provided for each code to serve as a contributing factor in selecting the proper code. Encounter time is defined as face-to-face time for office visits and face-to-face plus floor time for hospital visits. Time is considered the key or controlling factor only when counseling and/or coordination of care takes more than half the time of the encounter. The total time of the visit and the nature of the counseling and/or coordination of care must be documented in the medical record.

> **CODING TIP** Misuse of the time component continues to contribute substantially to coding errors, because physicians frequently use time as a highly inaccurate shortcut to code selection.

APPROPRIATE E/M CODE SELECTION

Appropriate E/M code selection is based on the content of the service provided. The criteria for levels of service in subcategories of codes do not "cross over." For example, the key component criteria are greater for code **99203** (new patient, level 3) than for code **99213** (established patient, level 3). New patient office visits require all three of the key components to be met or exceeded, but only two of the three key components must be met or exceeded for established patient encounters.

The following tables were designed to aid physicians in selecting the appropriate E/M codes. They are not meant to substitute for the instructions found in the E/M section of the CPT codebook.

Office Visit—New Patient

When choosing a code for services to a new patient, *all three* key components* must be met or exceeded. (See Table 2-10.)

Office Visit—Established Patient

When choosing a code for services to an established patient, *two of the three* key components* must be met or exceeded. (See Table 2-11.)

Hospital Inpatient Visit—Initial

When choosing a code for initial service to an inpatient, *all three* key components* must be met or exceeded. (See Table 2-12.)

Hospital Inpatient Visit—Subsequent

When choosing a code for subsequent inpatient services, *two of the three* key components* must be met or exceeded. (See Table 2-13.)

Hospital Observation Care—Initial

When choosing a code for initial service for a patient in observation status, *all three* key components* must be met or exceeded. (See Table 2-14.)

Hospital Observation Care—Subsequent

When choosing a code for a subsequent service for a patient in observation status, *two of the three* key components* must be met or exceeded. (See Table 2-15.)

* History, examination, medical decision making.

CHAPTER 2

TABLE 2-10. Office Visit—New Patient

	KEY COMPONENTS			OTHER FACTORS	
CPT Code	History	Examination	Medical Decision Making	Nature of Problem	Average Time (min)
99201	Problem focused	Problem focused	Straightforward	Self-limiting or minor	10
99202	Expanded problem focused	Expanded problem focused	Straightforward	Low to moderate severity	20
99203	Detailed	Detailed	Low complexity	Moderate severity	30
99204	Comprehensive	Comprehensive	Moderate complexity	Moderate severity	45
99205	Comprehensive	Comprehensive	High complexity	Moderate to high severity	60

TABLE 2-11. Office Visit—Established Patient

	KEY COMPONENTS			OTHER FACTORS	
CPT Code	History	Examination	Medical Decision Making	Nature of Problem	Average Time (min)
99211	N/A	N/A	N/A	Minimal	5
99212	Problem focused	Problem focused	Straight forward	Self-limiting or minor	10
99213	Expanded problem focused	Expanded problem focused	Low complexity	Low to moderate severity	15
99214	Detailed	Detailed	Moderate complexity	Moderate to high severity	25
99215	Comprehensive	Comprehensive	High complexity	Moderate to high severity	40

N/A indicates not applicable.

TABLE 2-12. Hospital Inpatient Visit—Initial

	KEY COMPONENTS			OTHER FACTORS	
CPT Code	History	Examination	Medical Decision Making	Nature of Problem	Average Time (min)
99221	Comprehensive	Comprehensive	Straightforward or low complexity	Low severity	30
99222	Comprehensive	Comprehensive	Moderate complexity	Moderate severity	50
99223	Comprehensive	Comprehensive	High complexity	High severity	70

TABLE 2-13. Hospital Inpatient Visit—Subsequent

| CPT Code | KEY COMPONENTS | | | OTHER FACTORS | |
	History	Examination	Medical Decision Making	Nature of Problem	Average Time (min)
99231	Problem focused interval history	Problem focused	Straightforward or low complexity	Stable, recovering, or improving	15
99232	Expanded problem focused interval history	Expanded problem focused	Moderate complexity	Inadequate response or minor complication	25
99233	Detailed interval history	Detailed	High complexity	Unstable, significant complication, or significant new problem	35

TABLE 2-14. Hospital Observation Care—Initial

| CPT Code | KEY COMPONENTS | | | OTHER FACTORS | |
	History	Examination	Medical Decision Making	Nature of Problem	Average Time (min)
99218	Detailed/ Comprehensive	Detailed/Comprehensive	Straightforward or low complexity	Low severity	N/A
99219	Comprehensive	Comprehensive	Moderate complexity	Moderate severity	N/A
99220	Comprehensive	Comprehensive	High complexity	High severity	N/A

N/A indicates not applicable.

TABLE 2-15. Hospital Observation Care—Subsequent

| CPT Code | KEY COMPONENTS | | | OTHER FACTORS | |
	History	Examination	Medical Decision Making	Nature of Problem	Average Time (min)
99224	Problem-focused interval history	Problem focused	Straightforward or low complexity	Stable, recovering, or improving	15
99225	Expanded problem-focused interval history	Expanded problem focused	Moderate complexity	Inadequate response or minor complication	25
99226	Detailed interval history	Detailed	High complexity	Unstable, significant complication, or significant new problem	35

Observation or Inpatient Care Services (Including Admission and Discharge Services)

When choosing a code for the admission and discharge of a patient on the same date for observation or inpatient services, *all three* key components* must be met or exceeded. (See Table 2-16.)

Hospital Discharge Services

The hospital discharge day management codes include, as appropriate, final examination of the patient; discussion of the hospital stay; instructions for continuing care to all relevant caregivers; and preparation of discharge records, prescriptions, and referral forms, even if the time spent by the physician on that date is not continuous.

CPT Code	Average Time (min)
99238	30 minutes or less
99239	More than 30 minutes

CODING TIP For non-Medicare patients, services provided to a patient in follow-up to an inpatient consultation should be reported using the appropriate subsequent hospital or nursing facility codes.

Office or Other Outpatient Consultation—New or Established Patient

When choosing a code for outpatient consultations, *all three* key components* must be met or exceeded. (See Table 2-17.)

* History, examination, medical decision making.

TABLE 2-16. Observation or Inpatient Care Services (Including Admission and Discharge Services)

CPT Code	KEY COMPONENTS			OTHER FACTORS	
	History	Examination	Medical Decision Making	Nature of Problem	Average Time (min)
99234	Detailed or comprehensive	Detailed or comprehensive	Straightforward or low complexity	Low severity	N/A
99235	Comprehensive	Comprehensive	Moderate complexity	Moderate severity	N/A
99236	Comprehensive	Comprehensive	High complexity	High severity	N/A

N/A indicates not applicable.

TABLE 2-17. Office or Other Outpatient Consultation—New or Established Patient

CPT Code	KEY COMPONENTS			OTHER FACTORS	
	History	Examination	Medical Decision Making	Nature of Problem	Average Time (min)
99241	Problem focused	Problem focused	Straightforward	Self-limiting or minor	15
99242	Expanded problem focused	Expanded problem focused	Straightforward	Low severity	30
99243	Detailed	Detailed	Low	Moderate	40
99244	Comprehensive	Comprehensive	Moderate complexity	Moderate to high severity	60
99245	Comprehensive	Comprehensive	High complexity	Moderate to high severity	80

Inpatient Consultations—New or Established Patient

When choosing a code for initial inpatient consultations, *all three* key components* must be met or exceeded. (See Table 2-18.)

In 2010, Medicare discontinued payment for services reported with the codes for consultative services (**99241-99245, 99251-99255**). Medicare has instructed physicians performing services that meet the CPT definition of a consultation to report instead the appropriate E/M code from the new patient office/outpatient codes (**99201-99205**), the established patient office/outpatient codes (**99211-99215**), initial hospital care codes (**99221-99223**), or subsequent hospital care codes (**99231-99233**). For example, a consultation with a patient who is new to the practice (ie, he or she has not received any professional services from the physician or another physician of the same specialty who belongs to the same group practice within the last 3 years) would be coded with the appropriate code from the new patient office/outpatient series. A consultation with a patient who has been seen within the past 3 years by another physician of the same specialty within the practice must be reported with a code from the established patient office/outpatient code series. Note that Medicare does not recognize the cardiology subspecialties as distinct specialties. For example, if a general cardiologist refers a patient to an electrophysiologist within the same practice, the patient is considered an established patient for the electrophysiologist.

* History, examination, medical decision making.

In the past, only the physician who admitted a patient to the hospital could report the initial hospital visit codes (**99221-99223**). Medicare now instructs physicians to report an initial hospital visit code for services that were previously reported as inpatient consultations. The physician who admits the patient to the hospital should append the Medicare modifier AI to the claims to indicate that he or she is the admitting physician.

Most private payers have continued to pay for consultations according to CPT rules, but it is best to confirm a policy with a payer before proceeding further.

Specialty-Specific Examples

One educational element of the E/M coding system is the inclusion of specialty-specific clinical examples or vignettes to serve as a guide to selection of codes. These examples are meant only to provide additional guidance to physicians and are not intended to assign specific patient presentations to a given level of service. The three key components (history, examination, and medical decision making) must be met and documented to support a particular level of service.

See Appendix C in the *CPT 2012* codebook for a complete listing of clinical examples of the CPT codes for E/M services.

The following tables (Table 2-19–Table 2-25) include the AMA-validated, cardiology-specific examples.

TABLE 2-18. Inpatient Consultations—New or Established Patient

	KEY COMPONENTS			OTHER FACTORS	
CPT Code	History	Examination	Medical Decision Making	Nature of Problem	Average Time (min)
99251	Problem focused	Problem focused	Straightforward	Self-limiting or minor	15
99252	Expanded problem-focused	Expanded problem-focused	Straightforward	Low severity	30
99253	Detailed	Detailed	Low complexity	Moderate severity	40
99254	Comprehensive	Comprehensive	Moderate complexity	Moderate to high severity	60
99255	Comprehensive	Comprehensive	High complexity	Moderate to high severity	80

TABLE 2-19. Office and Other Outpatient Services—New or Established Patient

Code	Clinical Example
NEW PATIENT	
99201	Initial office visit for a 25-year-old out-of-town patient for refill of a topical prescription medication
99202	This is an initial office visit for a 42-year-old female patient with a history and rash consistent with poison ivy who is not responding to over-the-counter medication
99203	Initial office visit for a 63-year old female with hypertension presents for a pre-employment physical after moving to the area. Her blood pressure has been adequately controlled with her current medication and home blood pressure monitoring
99204	Office visit for initial evaluation of a 63-year-old male with chest pain on exertion
99205	Office visit for initial evaluation of a 65-year-old female with chest pain, intermittent claudication, syncope, and a murmur of aortic stenosis
ESTABLISHED PATIENT	
99211	Office visit for a 58-year-old male, established patient, presenting for a blood pressure check. The blood pressure is 130/83. His blood pressure is acceptable
99212	Office visit for a mildly symptomatic 20-year-old female, established patient, with upper respiratory complaints consistent with an upper respiratory tract infection
99213	Office visit for a 56-year-old male, established patient, with stable exertional angina who complains of new-onset calf pain while walking
99214	Office visit for a 68-year-old male with stable angina, 2 months post–myocardial infarction, who is not tolerating one of his medications. Outpatient visit for a 77-year-old male, established patient with hypertension, presenting with a 3-month history of episodic substernal chest pain on exertion
99215	Office visit for a 63-year-old male, established patient, with type II diabetes mellitus (with neuropathy and nephropathy), congestive heart failure, hyperlipidemia, and chronic anxiety. He presents with blurred vision, frequency of urination, high blood sugars, and left leg pain and swelling

TABLE 2-20. Hospital Inpatient Services—New or Established Patient and Subsequent Hospital Care

Code	Clinical Example
INITIAL HOSPITAL CARE—NEW OR ESTABLISHED PATIENT	
99221	Initial hospital visit for a 69-year-old female with controlled hypertension, scheduled for surgery
99222	Initial hospital visit for a 61-year-old male with history of myocardial infarction, who now complains of chest pain
99223	Hospital admission, examination, and initiation of treatment program for a previously unknown 58-year-old male who presents with acute chest pain
	Initial hospital visit for a 65-year-old male who presents with acute myocardial infarction, oliguria, hypotension, and altered state of consciousness
	Initial hospital visit for a 45-year-old female, who has a history of rheumatic fever as a child and now has anemia, fever, and congestive heart failure
	Initial hospital visit for a 50-year-old male with acute chest pain and diagnostic electrocardiographic changes of an acute anterior myocardial infarction
	Initial hospital visit for a 70-year-old male admitted with chest pain, complete heart block, and congestive heart failure
	Initial hospital visit for an 82-year-old male who presents with syncope, chest pain, and ventricular arrhythmias
	Initial hospital visit for a 52-year-old male with known rheumatic heart disease who presents with anasarca, hypertension, and history of alcohol abuse
	Initial hospital visit for a 55-year-old female with a history of congenital heart disease, now presents with cyanosis
	Initial hospital visit for a 62-year-old male with history of previous myocardial infarction who presents with recurrent, sustained ventricular tachycardia
	Initial hospital visit for a 1-day-old male with cyanosis, respiratory distress, and tachypnea
	Initial hospital visit for a 3-year-old female with recurrent tachycardia and syncope

CHAPTER 2

TABLE 2-20. Hospital Inpatient Services—New or Established Patient and Subsequent Hospital Care *(continued)*

Code	Clinical Example
SUBSEQUENT HOSPITAL CARE	
99231	Follow-up hospital visit for a 50-year-old male with uncomplicated myocardial infarction who is clinically stable and without chest pain
	Subsequent hospital visit for a 25-year-old male admitted for supraventricular tachycardia and converted on medical therapy
	Subsequent hospital visit for a 70-year-old male admitted with congestive heart failure who has responded to therapy
99232	Follow-up hospital visit for a 54-year-old male patient, post–myocardial infarction, who is out of the coronary care unit but is now having frequent premature ventricular contractions on telemetry
	Subsequent hospital visit for a 37-year-old female on day 5 of antibiotics for bacterial endocarditis, who still has a low-grade fever
99233	Subsequent hospital visit for a 65-year-old male with acute myocardial infarction who now demonstrates complete heart blockage and congestive heart failure
	Subsequent hospital visit for a 65-year-old male following an acute myocardial infarction who complains of shortness of breath and new chest pain
	Subsequent hospital care for a 50-year-old male, post–aortocoronary bypass surgery, who now develops hypotension and oliguria

TABLE 2-21. Office and Other Outpatient Consultations—New or Established Patient

Code	Clinical Example
99241	A 21-year-old female was seen for an office consultation for rectal bleeding. She has had prior sigmoidoscopy within 1 year, which showed only internal hemorrhoids. She has recently become constipated, and while straining, saw scant blood on the tissue
99242	A 30-year-old male is seen for an office consultation for heartburn. He is otherwise healthy but describes episodic burning substernal pain with typical provocative meals, eating late, or excessive coffee. He experiences relief with antacids and has no symptoms suggesting serious disease
99243	Office consultation for a 31-year-old female complaining of palpitations and chest pains, whose internist described a mild systolic click
99244	A 60-year-old female is seen for an office consultation for the evaluation of complaints of heart palpitations with occasional dizziness and abdominal pain. She has a past history of hypertension, osteoarthritis, and morbid obesity. Past medical history includes total abdominal hysterectomy 15 years previously for dysfunctional uterine bleeding. She has had no follow-up for 15 years
99245	Office consultation for a 58-year-old male with a history of myocardial infarction and congestive heart failure who complains of the recent onset of rest angina and shortness of breath; systolic blood pressure is 90 mm Hg, and patient is in New York Heart Association (NYHA) class IV heart failure
	Emergency room consultation for a 1-year-old male with a 3-day history of fever and increasing respiratory distress who is thought to have cardiac tamponade by the emergency physician

Some of the E/M codes do not have AMA-approved cardiology vignettes available. Members of the ACC's Coding Task Force offer the following example vignettes:

TABLE 2-22. Inpatient Consultations—New or Established Patient

Code	Clinical Example
99251	Initial inpatient consultation for a 45-year-old female admitted with unrelenting low back pain for 2 days. There is no significant past medical history and she is on no medications. The neurological exam is normal
99252	Initial inpatient preoperative consultation for a 43-year-old female with cholecystitis and well-controlled hypertension
99253	Initial inpatient consultation for a 75-year-old female with a status post right hip fracture with a history of hypertension and well-controlled type II diabetes mellitus. A consultation is requested for surgical clearance
99254	Initial inpatient consultation for a 75-year-old female admitted with cellulitis around a right great toe ulcer. She has a history of type II diabetes mellitus, ischemic cardiomyopathy, atherosclerotic peripheral vascular disease, hypertension, and chronic renal insufficiency. She is a widow living in a nursing home. She has developed a fever and a hot, swollen painful left knee
99255	Initial hospital consultation in the intensive care unit for a 70-year-old male who experienced a cardiac arrest during surgery and was resuscitated
	Initial hospital consultation for a 50-year-old male with a history of previous myocardial infarction who now presents with acute pulmonary edema and hypotension

TABLE 2-23. New Patient Office Visit

Code	Clinical Example
99203	Office visit for initial evaluation of a 35-year-old female with skipped heart beats (average patient encounter time, 30 min)

TABLE 2-24. New or Established Patient—Office and Other Outpatient Consultations

Code	Clinical Example
99244	Office consultation for a 63-year-old male with chest pain on exertion (average patient encounter time, 60 min)

TABLE 2-25. New or Established Patient— Inpatient Consultations

Code	Clinical Example
99253	Inpatient preoperative consultation for a 65-year-old male with a prior coronary artery bypass graft (average patient encounter time, 40 min)
99254	Inpatient consultation for a 72-year-old female with hypertension admitted for management of new-onset atrial fibrillation with a rapid ventricular response (average patient encounter time, 60 min)

Observation Care Services

CPT CODES **99217-99220, 99224-99226**

CPT codes **99217-99220** and **99224-99226** are used to report E/M services provided to patients designated/ admitted as "observation status" in a hospital. It is not necessary that the patient be located in an observation area designated by the hospital.

If such an area does exist in a hospital (eg, as a separate unit in the hospital, in the emergency department, etc), these codes are to be utilized if the patient is placed in such an area.

For definitions of key components and commonly used terms, please see **Evaluation and Management Services Guidelines.**

CPT codes **99218-99220** are used to report the encounter(s) by the supervising physician with the patient when designated as "observation status." This refers to the initiation of observation status, supervision of the care plan for observation, and performance of periodic reassessments. For observation encounters by other physicians, see Office or Other Outpatient Consultation codes (**99241-99245**) or Subsequent Observation Care codes (**99224-99226**) as appropriate.

To report services provided to a patient who is admitted to the hospital after receiving hospital observation care services on the same date, see the notes for initial hospital inpatient care (page 15 of the *CPT 2012 Professional Edition* codebook).

For observation care services on other than the initial or discharge date, see Subsequent Observation Services codes (**99224-99226**). For a patient admitted to the hospital on a date subsequent to the date of observation status, the hospital admission would be reported with the appropriate Initial Hospital Care code (**99221-99223**). For a patient admitted and discharged from observation or inpatient status on the same date, the services should be reported with codes **99234-99236** as appropriate. Do not report observation discharge (**99217**) in conjunction with a hospital admission.

When "observation status" is initiated in the course of an encounter in another site of service (eg, hospital emergency department, physician's office, nursing facility), all E/M services provided by the supervising physician in conjunction with initiating "observation status" are considered part of the initial observation care when performed on the same date. The observation care level of service reported by the supervising physician should include the services related to initiating "observation status" provided in the other sites of service as well as in the observation setting.

E/M services on the same date provided in sites that are related to initiating "observation status" should not be reported separately.

These codes may not be utilized for postoperative recovery if the procedure is considered part of the surgical "package." These codes apply to all evaluation and management services that are provided on the same date of initiating "observation status."

The great majority of cardiovascular services have a "zero day" global period that encompasses the day of the procedure.

Observation care discharge of a patient from "observation status" includes final examination of the patient, discussion of the hospital stay, instructions for continuing care, and preparation of discharge records. For observation or inpatient hospital care including the admission and discharge of the patient on the same date, see codes **99234-99236** as appropriate.

Code **99217** is reported only when the patient is discharged from observation status (not transferred to inpatient status) on a date other than the date of initial observation care.

SUBSEQUENT OBSERVATION CARE

All levels of subsequent observation care include reviewing the medical record and reviewing the results of diagnostic studies and changes in the patient's status (ie, changes in history, physical condition, and response to management) since the last assessment by the physician.

> **CODING TIP** Observation is an outpatient hospital service, even though CPT guidelines refer to "admitting" a patient to observation. Thus, the outpatient place of service should be noted accordingly.

Observation or Inpatient Care Services (Including Admission and Discharge Services)

CPT CODES **99234-99236**

Codes **99234-99236** are used to report observation or inpatient hospital care services provided to patients admitted and discharged on the same date of service. When a patient is admitted to the hospital from observation status on the same date, the physician should report only the initial hospital care code. The initial hospital care code reported by the admitting physician should include the services related to the observation status services he or she provided on the same date of inpatient admission.

When "observation status" is initiated in the course of an encounter in another site of service (eg, hospital emergency department, physician's office, nursing facility), all E/M services provided by the supervising physician in conjunction with initiating "observation status" are considered part of the initial observation care when performed on the same date. The observation care level of service should include the services related to initiating "observation status" provided in the other sites of service as well as in the observation setting when provided by the same physician.

For patients admitted to observation or inpatient care and discharged on a different date, see codes **99218-99220, 99224-99226, 99217,** or **99221-99223, 99238,** and **99239.**

PAYMENT POLICY ALERT Medicare will pay for hospital admission services (**99221-99223**) and hospital discharge services (**99238-99239**) when a patient is a hospital inpatient for 24 hours or more, as documented in the medical record. For stays of less than 8 hours, only the admission codes (**99221-99223** or **99218-99220**) will be paid on that day; the discharge is not separately billable. For stays (hospital inpatient or observation care) of more than 8 but less than 24 hours, the admission and discharge will be paid (**99234-99236**). The new policy allows payment for CPT codes **99234-99236** only for stays of at least 8 hours but less than 24 hours. The medical record must document the length of stay, that the billing physician was present and personally performed the services, and that the admission and discharge note were written by the billing physician. Codes **99218-99220** should be used if the patient is discharged on the same day as the admission for observation only, while observation care codes **99224-99226** and observation care discharge code **99217** may be used only on the second or subsequent days of observation care.

Critical Care Services

CPT CODES **99291-99292**

Critical care is the direct delivery by a physician(s) of medical care for a critically ill or critically injured patient. A critical illness or injury acutely impairs one or more vital organ systems such that there is a high probability of imminent or life-threatening deterioration in the patient's condition. Critical care involves high complexity decision making to assess, manipulate, and support vital system function(s) to treat single or multiple vital organ system failure and/or to prevent further life-threatening deterioration of the patient's condition. Examples of vital organ system failure include, but are not limited to: central nervous system failure; circulatory failure; shock; and renal, hepatic, metabolic, and/or respiratory failure. Although critical care typically requires interpretation of multiple physiologic parameters and/or application of advanced technology(s), critical care may be provided in life-threatening situations when these elements are not present. Critical care may be provided on multiple days, even if no changes are made in the treatment rendered to the patient, provided that the patient's condition continues to require the level of physician attention described above.

Providing medical care to a critically ill, injured, or postoperative patient qualifies as a critical care service only if both the illness or injury *and* the treatment being provided meet the above requirements. Critical care is usually, but not always, given in a critical care area, such as the coronary care unit (CCU), intensive care unit, pediatric intensive care unit, respiratory care unit, or the emergency care facility.

The presence of a patient in a CCU does not necessarily support the use of the critical care codes. Patients receiving critical care services need the constant attention of the physician (eg, to treat cardiac arrest, shock, bleeding, respiratory failure, postoperative complications).

The critical care codes **99291** and **99292** are used to report the total duration of time spent by a physician providing critical care services to a critically ill or critically injured patient, even if the time spent by the physician on that date is not continuous. For any given period of time spent providing critical care services, the physician must devote his or her full attention to the patient and, therefore, cannot provide services to any other patient during the same period of time.

Time spent with the individual patient should be recorded in the patient's record. The time that can be reported as critical care is the time spent engaged in work directly related to the individual patient's care whether that time was spent at the immediate bedside or elsewhere on the floor or unit. For example, time spent on the unit or at the nursing station on the floor reviewing test results or imaging studies, discussing the critically ill patient's care with other medical staff, or documenting critical care services in the medical record would be reported as critical care, even though it does not occur at the bedside. Also, when the patient is unable or clinically incompetent (lacks capacity) to participate in discussions, time spent on the floor or unit with family members or surrogate decision makers obtaining a medical history, reviewing the patient's condition or prognosis, or discussing treatment or limitation(s) of treatment may be reported as critical care, provided that the conversation bears directly on the management of the patient.

Time spent in activities that occur outside of the unit or off the floor (eg, telephone calls whether taken at home, in the office, or elsewhere in the hospital) may not be reported as critical care because the physician is not immediately available to the patient. Time spent in activities that do not directly contribute to the treatment of the patient may not be reported as critical care, even if they are performed in the critical care unit (eg, participation in administrative meetings or telephone calls to discuss other patients). Time spent performing separately reportable procedures or services should not be included in the time reported as critical care time. No physician may report remote real-time interactive video-conference critical care services (**0188T-0189T**) for the period in which any physician reports codes **99291-99292**.

The following services are included in reporting critical care when performed during the critical period by the physician(s) providing critical care: the interpretation of cardiac output measurements (**93561, 93562**); chest x-rays (**71010, 71015, 71020**); pulse oximetry (**94760, 94761, 94762**); blood gases and information data stored in computers (eg, ECGs, blood pressures, hematologic data [**99090**]); gastric intubation (**43752, 43753**); temporary transcutaneous pacing (**92953**); ventilator management (**94002-94004, 94660, 94662**); and vascular access procedures (**36000, 36410, 36415, 36591, 36600**). Any services performed that are not listed above should be reported separately.

An example of a procedure code that is not bundled into the critical care codes and can therefore be billed separately is placement of a Swan-Ganz catheter, code **93503**.

CODING TIP Critical care codes **99291** and **99292** should be reported for the physician's attendance during the transport of critically ill or critically injured patients older than 24 months of age to or from a facility or hospital. For physician transport services of critically ill or critically injured pediatric patients 24 months of age or younger, report codes **99466, 99467**. Critical care can be reported in addition to other E/M services provided by the physician on the same date of service. (See CPT codebook's definition of modifier 25.) The CPT codebook's introductory language for critical care services is excerpted above. Review of the complete guidelines for use of codes **99291-99292** is recommended.

Prolonged Services

CPT CODES **99354-99359**

CPT codes **99354-99359** are used to report prolonged services provided by physicians both with and without face-to-face patient contact. These codes are reported in addition to the appropriate E/M code for that patient encounter.

CPT CODES **99354-99357**

Codes **99354-99357** are used when a physician provides prolonged service involving direct (face-to-face) patient contact that is beyond the usual service in either the inpatient or outpatient setting. This service is reported in addition to the designated E/M services at any level and any other physician services provided at the same session as E/M services. Appropriate codes should be selected for supplies provided or procedures performed in the care of the patient during this period.

Codes **99354-99355** are used to report the total duration of face-to-face time spent by a physician on a given date providing prolonged service, even if the time spent by the physician on that date is not continuous. Codes **99356-99357** are used to report the total duration of unit time spent by a physician on a given date providing prolonged service to a patient, even if the time spent by the physician on that date is not continuous.

Code **99354** or **99356** is used to report the first hour of prolonged service on a given date, depending on the place of service. (See Table 2-26.)

Either code should be used only once per date, even if the time spent by the physician is not continuous on that date. Prolonged service of less than 30 minutes total duration on a given date is not separately reported because the work involved is included in the total work of the E/M codes.

Code **99355** or **99357** is used to report each additional 30 minutes beyond the first hour, depending on the place of service. Either code may also be used to report the final 15 to 30 minutes of prolonged service on a given date. Prolonged service of less than 15 minutes beyond the first hour or less than 15 minutes beyond the final 30 minutes is not reported separately.

Each additional 30 minutes of prolonged service beyond the first hour is reported using either code **99355** (outpatient) or **99357** (inpatient).

TABLE 2-26. E/M Services Provided and Reporting CPT Codes **99354-99357**

To Report Code	For	One of These E/M Services Must Be Provided:
99354	Prolonged physician service in the office or other outpatient setting; first hour	99201-99205 99212-99215 99241-99245 99324-99337 99341-99350 90809-90815
99355	Prolonged physician service in the office or other outpatient setting; each additional 30 minutes	99354 plus one of the E/M codes required for use with 99354
99356	Prolonged physician service in the inpatient setting; first hour	99218-99220 99221-99233 99251-99255 99304-99310 90822 90829
99357	Prolonged physician service in the inpatient setting; each additional 30 minutes	99356 plus one of the E/M codes required for use with 99356

CPT CODES **99358** AND **99359**

CPT codes **99358** and **99359** are used when a physician provides prolonged service not involving direct (face-to-face) care that is beyond the usual non–face-to-face component of physician service time.

This service is to be reported in relation to other physician services, including E/M services at any level. This prolonged service may be reported on a different date than the primary service to which it is related. For example, extensive record review may relate to a previous E/M service performed earlier and commences upon receipt of past records. However, it must relate to a service or patient in which direct (face-to-face) patient care has occurred or will occur and relate to ongoing patient management. A typical time for the primary service need not be established within the CPT code set.

Codes **99358** and **99359** are used to report the total duration of non–face-to-face time spent by a physician on a given date providing prolonged service, even if the time spent by the physician on that date is not continuous. Code **99358** is used to report the first hour of prolonged service on a given date regardless of the place of service. It should be used only once per date.

Prolonged service of less than 30 minutes total duration on a given date is not separately reported.

Code **99359** is used to report each additional 30 minutes beyond the first hour, regardless of the place of service. It may also be used to report the final 15 to 30 minutes of prolonged service on a given date.

These codes are also reported in addition to any other E/M services provided, without restriction to timed services.

CODING TIP As indicated, codes **99358** and **99359** describe prolonged services provided without direct patient contact. Cardiologists may be frequent providers of these services. For example, a cardiologist may be asked to review a complex patient history with another physician, including the evaluation of graphic data essential to evaluating the patient's current medical status. A patient may present with restenosis after angioplasty; a review of multiple previous angiograms is required to determine the most effective management strategy. Similarly, review of prior echocardiograms or stress echocardiograms may be required to provide a comprehensive assessment of a patient and to structure an appropriate management strategy. With complete documentation, such services might be considered as part of the next (face-to-face) E/M encounter and a level of service selected accordingly.

PAYMENT POLICY ALERT Medicare does not pay for prolonged services that do not involve direct patient contact (**99358-99359**).

Anticoagulant Management

CPT CODES **99363-99364**

Anticoagulant services are intended to describe the outpatient management of warfarin therapy, including ordering, review, and interpretation of International Normalized Ratio (INR) testing, communication with the patient, and dosage adjustments as appropriate.

When reporting these services, the work of anticoagulant management may not be used as a basis for reporting an evaluation and management (E/M) service or care plan oversight time during the reporting period. Do not report these services with **98966-98969**, **99441-99444** when telephone or online services address anticoagulation with warfarin management. If a significant, separately identifiable E/M service is performed, report the appropriate E/M service code using modifier 25.

These services are outpatient services only. When anticoagulation therapy is initiated or continued in the inpatient or observation setting, a new period begins after discharge and is reported with code **99364**. Do not report **99363-99364** with **99217-99239**, **99291-99292**, **99304-99318**, **99471-99480**, or other code(s) for physician review, interpretation, and patient management of home INR testing for a patient with mechanical heart valve(s).

Any period less than 60 continuous outpatient days is not reported. If less than the specified minimum number of services per period is performed, do not report the anticoagulant management services (**99363-99364**).

Code **99363** is reported for an initial 90 days of therapy and must include a minimum of nine INR measurements. Code **99364** is reported for each subsequent 90 days of therapy and must include a minimum of three INR measurements.

Do not report codes **99363-99364** with codes for observation care, hospital inpatient care, critical care services, discharge day management, or nursing home services (**99217-99239**, **99291-99292**, **99304-99318**, and **99471-99480**) or with other code(s) for physician review, interpretation, and patient management of home INR testing for a patient with mechanical heart valve(s). Any period of less than 60 continuous outpatient days is not reported. If less than the specified minimum number of services per period is performed, do not report the anticoagulant management services (**99363-99364**).

PAYMENT POLICY ALERT Medicare considers the services described in the anticoagulation management codes to be bundled into the E/M codes that physicians already report, meaning that physicians may not charge Medicare patients for these services. Some private payers recognize this service, so physicians are advised to check the payment policy for their local insurers.

Care Plan Oversight

CPT CODES **99374-99380**

CPT codes **99374-99380** allow physicians to report the total time spent in care plan oversight for a patient in a 30-day period. This category was revised and expanded in 1998 to reflect separate codes for home health, hospice, and nursing facility services. The codes also reflect service of 15 to 29 minutes and 30 minutes or more. Only one physician may report services for a given period.

PAYMENT POLICY ALERT Medicare does not pay for the aforementioned care plan oversight codes but does pay for two similar G codes for care plan oversight of patients under the care of a home health agency or a hospice if more than 30 minutes is spent in a month. **G0181** is used to report home health care plan oversight, and **G0182** is used to report hospice care plan oversight. The reporting physician must be overseeing the care plan of a patient served by a home health agency or hospice. Care plan oversight services for patients in nursing facilities (codes **99379** and **99380**) are not covered by Medicare. In addition to documenting the actual services provided, total time devoted to the service must be at least 30 minutes.

E/M Services and Procedures Performed by the Same Physician on the Same Day

The AMA's CPT consultation guidelines state: "A physician consultant may initiate diagnostic and/or therapeutic services at the same or subsequent visit." It should be noted that services that constitute transfer of care (ie, are provided for the management of the patient's entire care or for the care of a specific condition or problem) are reported with the appropriate new or established patient codes for office or other outpatient visits, domiciliary, rest home services, or home services, rather than with the consultation services codes 99241-99245. Transfer of care is the process whereby a physician who is providing management for some or all of a patient's problems relinquishes this responsibility to another physician who explicitly agrees to accept this responsibility and who, from the initial encounter, is not providing consultative services. At the initial consultation that does not constitute transfer of care, the physician consultant offers opinion or advice. After communicating this opinion or advice to the requesting physician, the physician consultant may initiate diagnostic or therapeutic services. The initial consultative visit is still considered a consultative visit.

This information also applies if a diagnostic or therapeutic procedure is performed on or after the date of the initial consultation. These separately performed procedures usually result from the decision-making component of the initial consultative visit. For example, if a cardiologist is asked to consult regarding a patient's diagnosis of unstable angina and, as a result of this consultative visit, the cardiologist determines that a diagnostic cardiac catheterization should be performed, this decision is a result of the decision-making component of the E/M service. Therefore, the appropriate level E/M code may be reported with modifier 25 appended. The use of the modifier communicates to the third-party payer that on the date the procedure was performed (ie, cardiac catheterization), the patient's condition required significant, separate E/M services, above and beyond the usual preoperative and postoperative care associated with the procedure that was performed.

Non–Face-to-Face Services

TELEPHONE SERVICES

CPT Codes 99441-99444

Telephone services are non–face-to-face evaluation and management (E/M) services provided by a physician to a patient using the telephone. These codes are used to report episodes of care by the physician initiated by an established patient or guardian of an established patient. If the telephone service ends with a decision to see the patient within 24 hours or next available urgent visit appointment, the code is not reported; rather the

encounter is considered part of the preservice work of the subsequent E/M service, procedure, and visit. Likewise, if the telephone call refers to an E/M service performed and reported by the physician within the previous 7 days (either physician requested or unsolicited patient follow-up) or within the postoperative period of the previously completed procedure, then the service(s) are considered part of that previous E/M service or procedure. (Do not report codes 99441-99443 if reporting codes 99441-99444 performed in the previous seven days.)

The telephone services codes are differentiated by the time spent on the phone with the patient as outlined in the code descriptors. As is the case with all time-based codes, it is important to document the time spent on the phone when reporting these codes.

99441	Telephone evaluation and management service provided by a physician to an established patient, parent, or guardian not originating from a related E/M service provided within the previous 7 days nor leading to an E/M service or procedure within the next 24 hours or soonest available appointment; 5-10 minutes of medical discussion
99442	11-20 minutes of medical discussion
99443	21-30 minutes of medical discussion

ONLINE MEDICAL EVALUATION

CPT Code 99444

An online electronic medical evaluation is a non–face-to-face evaluation and management (E/M) service provided by a physician to a patient using Internet resources in response to a patient's online inquiry. Reportable services involve the physician's personal timely response to the patient's inquiry and must involve permanent storage (electronic or hard copy) of the encounter. This service is reported only once for the same episode of care during a 7-day period, although multiple physicians could report their exchange with the same patient. If the online medical evaluation refers to an E/M service previously performed and reported by the physician within the previous 7 days (either physician requested or unsolicited patient follow-up) or within the postoperative period of the previously completed procedure, then the service(s) are considered covered by the previous E/M service or procedure. A reportable service encompasses the sum of communication (eg, related telephone calls, prescription provision, laboratory orders) pertaining to the online patient encounter.

CHAPTER 2

Code **99444** is used to report an online medical evaluation provided to a patient through electronic means. Like telephone service codes **99441-99443**, online medical evaluation reports an electronic communication that is a replacement for an E/M visit rather than a supplement to an E/M visit. The code is used to report an entire conversation, which includes related telephone calls, prescription provision, and laboratory orders, pertaining to the online patient encounter, rather than each time a communication takes place between the physician and patient, and/or each time a different message or instruction is communicated by the physician to the patient. As with the telephone services codes **99441-99443**, code **99444** may not be reported if an E/M service has been provided within the past 7 days, or if it leads to another E/M service within the next 24 hours or the next available urgent visit appointment. Code **99444** should not be reported during the same time period in which care plan oversight (**99339-99340, 99374-99380**) or anticoagulant management services (**99363-99364**) are reported.

99444   Online evaluation and management service provided by a physician to an established patient, guardian, or health care provider not originating from a related E/M service provided within the previous 7 days, using the Internet or similar electronic communications network

---

CODING TIP Code **99444** does not specify software requirements for online medical evaluation. However, documentation of the contents of the online medical evaluation should be maintained in the patient's medical record, and communication standards that comply with the Health Insurance Portability and Accountability Act (HIPAA) should be used. Standard e-mail protocol generally does not meet the privacy requirements of HIPAA.

PAYMENT POLICY ALERT Medicare does not cover telephone services (**99441-99443**) or online medical evaluation (**99444**). However, a growing number of commercial payers are covering these non–face-to-face services.

CHAPTER 3

Cardiology Basics

The Heart

The heart is a hollow, cone-shaped muscle located between the lungs and behind the sternum (breastbone). Two-thirds of the heart is located to the left of the midline of the body, and one-third is located to the right of midline. Its role is to pump oxygen- and nutrient-rich blood throughout the body and oxygen- and nutrient-poor blood to the lungs for replenishment.

The heart has three layers: (1) the endocardium, which is the smooth inside lining of the heart; (2) the myocardium, which is the middle layer of heart muscle; and (3) the pericardium, which is a fluid-filled sac that surrounds the myocardium.

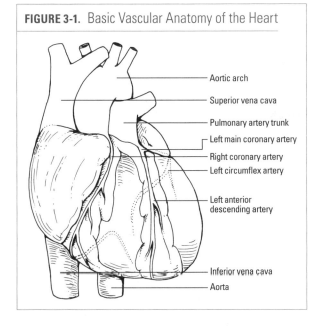

FIGURE 3-1. Basic Vascular Anatomy of the Heart

Aortic arch
Superior vena cava
Pulmonary artery trunk
Left main coronary artery
Right coronary artery
Left circumflex artery
Left anterior descending artery
Inferior vena cava
Aorta

CHAMBERS AND VALVES

The heart is divided into four chambers: (1) the *right atrium* (RA); (2) the *right ventricle* (RV); (3) the *left atrium* (LA); and (4) the *left ventricle* (LV). The atria are the receiving chambers for blood: the right atrium receives oxygen-poor blood from the body, and the left

atrium receives oxygen-rich blood from the lungs. The ventricles deliver blood: the right ventricle delivers blood to the lungs for oxygen and nutrient replenishment, and the left ventricle delivers oxygen- and nutrient-rich blood to the body.

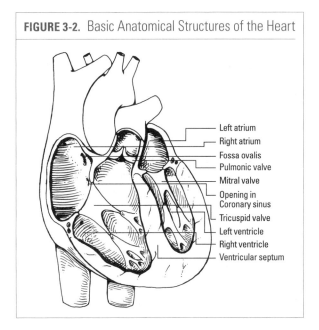

FIGURE 3-2. Basic Anatomical Structures of the Heart

Left atrium
Right atrium
Fossa ovalis
Pulmonic valve
Mitral valve
Opening in Coronary sinus
Tricuspid valve
Left ventricle
Right ventricle
Ventricular septum

Blood travels one way. Blood moves through the atria to the ventricles and exits the ventricles with the help of heart valves. Valves are one-way doors located in between each atrial and ventricular chamber and regulate the direction of blood flow. When it is finished contracting, the valve closes so that blood does not flow backward. There are four valves in the heart: (1) the *tricuspid valve*, which is at the exit of the right atrium; (2) the *pulmonary valve*, which is at the exit of the right ventricle; (3) the *mitral valve*, which is at the exit of the left atrium; and (4) the *aortic valve*, which is at the exit of the left ventricle.

When the heart muscle contracts or beats (systole), it pumps blood out of the heart. The heart contracts in two stages. In the first stage, the right and left atria contract at the same time, pumping blood to the right and left ventricles. Then the ventricles contract

FIGURE 3-3. Blood Flow Through the Heart and Lungs

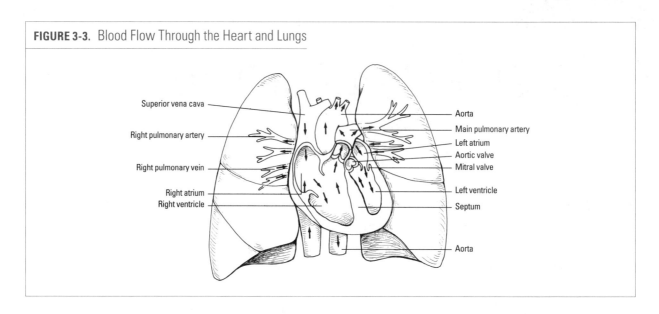

together to propel blood out of the heart. In the second stage, the heart muscle relaxes (diastole) before the next heartbeat. This allows blood to fill up the heart again.

The right and left sides of the heart have separate functions. The right side of the heart collects oxygen-poor blood from the body and pumps it to the lungs, where it picks up oxygen and releases carbon dioxide. The left side of the heart then collects oxygen-rich blood from the lungs and pumps it to the body.

Blood flow is as follows:

1. Oxygen-poor blood is delivered by the bloodstream to the right atrium.

2. The right atrium delivers blood to the right ventricle.

3. The right ventricle delivers blood to the lungs.

4. The lungs replenish blood with oxygen and nutrients and deliver it to the left atrium.

5. The left atrium delivers blood to the left ventricle.

6. The left ventricle delivers blood back into the bloodstream for nourishment throughout the body.

ANATOMY OF THE NORMAL CORONARY ARTERIES

The coronary arteries carry blood to the heart muscle. Because the heart muscle is continuously working (as opposed to other muscles of the body, which are often at rest), it has a very high requirement for oxygenated blood. The coronary arteries are vitally important for supplying that blood and allowing the heart to work normally.

Two major coronary arteries arise from the aorta: (1) the *right coronary artery* (RCA) and (2) the *left main artery* (LM). The left main artery quickly branches into two large arteries, the *left anterior descending artery* (LAD), which provides blood flow to the front of the heart, and the *circumflex artery* (Cx), which provides blood flow to the back of the heart. The right coronary artery usually provides blood flow to the right ventricle and the right side and bottom of the left ventricle. Occasionally, the right coronary artery is very small, and the circumflex artery will provide the majority of blood flow to the remaining heart muscle. Blockage in any of these major coronary arteries can damage large segments of heart muscle. Heart muscle death due to

FIGURE 3-4. Anterior View of the Heart Coronary Arteries

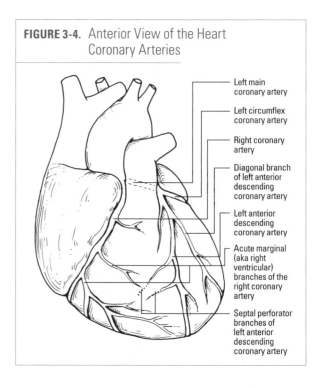

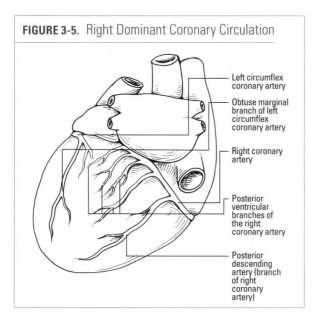

FIGURE 3-5. Right Dominant Coronary Circulation

Left circumflex
coronary artery

Obtuse marginal
branch of left
circumflex
coronary artery

Right coronary
artery

Posterior
ventricular
branches of
the right
coronary artery

Posterior
descending
artery (branch
of right
coronary
artery)

blockage in a coronary artery is referred to as a *myocardial infarction*, or heart attack.

Cardiovascular Surgery

Codes **33010-37799**, which are in the Cardiovascular System section of the CPT codebook, include most procedural codes used by cardiovascular surgeons. They identify diagnostic, therapeutic, and invasive cardiovascular procedures and are further organized into subsections: one for the heart and pericardium and a second for the arteries and veins. Nonetheless, a physician may use any CPT code in the book, provided it accurately represents a service that has been provided. The Surgery section of the CPT codebook includes codes **10000-69990**; many codes throughout this range can be used to report cardiovascular and related procedures.

Subsections of the Surgery section help physicians locate CPT codes more easily. They include:

- type of procedure, such as incision, excision, endoscopy, or shunting procedures;

- anatomy, such as aortic valve, mitral valve, sinus of Valsalva, or pulmonary artery;

- type of lesion, such as wounds of the heart or great vessels, septal defect, or truncus arteriosus; and

- miscellaneous, for codes that represent new technology or that have been recently added to the CPT code set.

Virtually all commonly performed surgical procedures can be found in the Surgery section. Exceptions are the rarest and newest surgical procedures. An unlisted procedure is reported using an "unlisted procedure" code (which typically end in 99). In such instances, a narrative description of the procedure must accompany the claim form. However, many payers question the use of unlisted procedure codes. Therefore, it is best to make every effort to find an appropriate listed code. Claims using an unlisted procedure code are also likely to be delayed in processing, especially if documentation is insufficient.

THE GLOBAL SURGERY PERIOD

The surgical procedures listed in the CPT codebook include the operation itself; local infiltration; metacarpal; digital block or topical anesthesia; and routine follow-up care. This concept is referred to as a "global surgical service" and is defined by a single, specific CPT code. Thus, routine preoperative care for the 24 hours before surgery, the operation itself, and routine care for a given period—usually 90 days following the operation—are part of the global surgical bundle. Certain services are excluded from the surgical bundle and may be reported separately. Examples include the following:

- The decision to perform surgery made by the surgeon on the day before or on the day of surgery. The appropriate Evaluation and Management (E/M) code for the visit during which that decision was made is reported with **modifier 57**.

- Other E/M services not related to preoperative care provided by the surgeon on the day before or the day of surgery. These should be reported using **modifier 25** and the appropriate *International Classification of Diseases, Ninth Revision, Clinical Modification* (ICD-9-CM) diagnosis code, designating why that service was needed.

- E/M services provided by the surgeon during postoperative days that are not part of the usual, uncomplicated care provided for that operation. These should be reported using **modifier 24**, again with the appropriate ICD-9-CM diagnosis code designating why that service was needed. (Refer to Chapter 6 for additional information related to the use of CPT modifiers.)

PAYMENT POLICY ALERT For Medicare, the pre-service time for the 90-day global procedures is the day before and the day of surgery. For the zero and 10-day global services, the global preservice period is for the day of the procedure only.

In addition, Medicare also makes the distinction that modifier 57 should be used to report E/M services that result in the decision to perform surgery for procedures with a 90-day global period, if the decision is made the day before or the day of the surgery. However, for zero and 10-day global procedures, if the decision to perform surgery is made the same day as the procedure, modifier 25 should be used to report any E/M services, not modifier 57. If the decision is made the day before, no modifier is required.

PERICARDIOCENTESIS (**33010, 33011**)

⊙**33010** Pericardiocentesis; initial

⊙**33011**   subsequent

TRANSMYOCARDIAL LASER REVASCULARIZATION (**33140, 33141**)

33140 Transmyocardial laser revascularization, by thoracotomy; (separate procedure)
CPT Assistant Nov 99:14, Nov 00:5, Apr 01:7; *CPT Changes: An Insider's View* 2000, 2001, 2002

+**33141**   performed at the time of other open cardiac procedure(s) (List separately in addition to code for primary procedure)
CPT Assistant Apr 01:7; *CPT Changes: An Insider's View* 2001

Transmyocardial laser revascularization (TMR) procedures are performed to create channels in the arterio-luminal sinusoids that connect directly with the left ventricular cavity, using a high-powered laser in order to increase blood supply to the myocardium. TMR may be performed "off" cardiopulmonary bypass (pump oxygenator). However, the majority of TMR procedures are performed "on pump," meaning the patient is placed on cardiopulmonary bypass (pump oxygenator). Therefore, it is appropriate to use code **33140** or **33141**, as appropriate, to report TMR performed either on pump or off pump.

Add-on code **33141** is reported when TMR is performed at the time of other open cardiac procedures, including the open coronary artery bypass graft procedures (**33510-33536**). Add-on code **33141** may also be reported when TMR is performed in addition to cardiac valve procedures reported by codes **33400-33496**.

Description of Service for Code 33140

A standard posterolateral thoracotomy skin incision is made. The pleural space is entered through the fourth intercostal space. Pleural adhesions are taken down as necessary, avoiding injury to the lung. The phrenic nerve is identified. An incision is made in the pericardium anterior to the phrenic nerve. Intrapericardial adhesions are taken down, as necessary, using sharp dissection to free up the lateral, posterior, and inferior walls of the left ventricle, avoiding injury to cardiac structures or patent bypass grafts. Pericardial retraction sutures are placed. The area to undergo laser revascularization is identified. The laser is used to create channels under echocardiographic guidance to avoid injury to the mitral valve apparatus. Channel production begins in the posterolateral wall in the circumflex coronary distribution and proceeds laterally and toward the apex. Channel production continues on the inferior wall in the distribution of the posterior descending artery. Approximately 30 laser sinusoids are created.

Bleeding is controlled from laser sites with a local hemostatic agent or fine suture. Temporary pacing wires are placed, if indicated. The wound is irrigated with saline (with or without antibiotics). A pleural chest tube is placed via a separate incision. The ribs are reapproximated with heavy pericostal sutures. Muscle fascias, subcutaneous tissues, and skin are closed with absorbable sutures.

Description of Service for Code +33141

A standard incision and exposure are made for the base cardiac procedure. The coronary arteries are assessed for operability. The region of proposed channeling for epicardial fat distribution is assessed for scarring. Initial determination of proposed channeling sites and potential traditional grafting sites is made. Bypass grafts (typical) with or without cardiac arrest are performed. Cardiopulmonary bypass (if used) is discontinued along with monitoring hemodynamics with arterial and pulmonary artery lines. When the patient is stable, protamine is administered to reverse anticoagulation. The laser is used to create channels under echocardiographic guidance to avoid injury to the mitral valve apparatus. Channel production begins in the posterolateral wall in the circumflex coronary distribution and proceeds laterally and toward the apex when this area cannot be revascularized by bypass surgery. Channel production continues on the inferior wall in the distribution of the posterior descending artery when this area cannot be revascularized by bypass surgery. Approximately 30 laser sinusoids are created. Bleeding from laser sites is controlled with a local hemostatic agent. Temporary pacing wires are placed if indicated. The wound is irrigated with saline (with or without antibiotics). After a final check for satisfactory hemostasis, incisional closure is performed in layers after the appropriate drainage tubes are placed.

PACEMAKER OR PACING CARDIOVERTER-DEFIBRILLATOR (**33202-33264**)

Intent and Use of Codes 33202-33264

The **33202-33264** series of codes refers to procedures involved with the actual implantation or revision of permanent pacemaker or cardioverter-defibrillator systems. The implantation of the system is to be distinguished from the electrophysiologic evaluation of newly implanted or replaced internal cardioverter-defibrillator lead(s) and/or pulse generator (**93640-93642**) during which arrhythmias are induced and defibrillation thresholds and sensing thresholds are determined. (Refer to Chapter 5 for additional information regarding electrophysiologic evaluation of implantable cardioverter-defibrillator lead[s] and/or pulse generator at the time of placement or subsequent electronic analyses and monitoring of pacers or defibrillators [**93279-93296**].)

As indicated in the CPT guidelines, a pacemaker system includes a pulse generator containing electronics, a battery, and one or more electrodes (leads). Pulse generators are placed in a subcutaneous "pocket" created in either a subclavicular site or underneath the abdominal muscles just below the ribcage. Electrodes may be inserted through a vein (transvenous) or they may be placed on the surface of the heart (epicardial). The epicardial location of electrodes requires a thoracotomy for electrode insertion.

A single-chamber pacemaker system includes a pulse generator and one electrode inserted in either the atrium or ventricle. A dual-chamber pacemaker system includes a pulse generator and one electrode inserted in the right atrium and one electrode inserted in the right ventricle. In certain circumstances, an additional electrode may be required to achieve pacing of the left ventricle (biventricular pacing). In this event, transvenous (cardiac vein) placement of the electrode should be separately reported using code **33224** or code **33225**. Epicardial placement of the electrode should be separately reported using code **33202** or code **33203**.

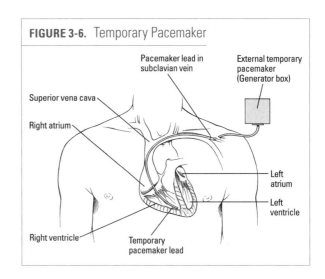

FIGURE 3-6. Temporary Pacemaker

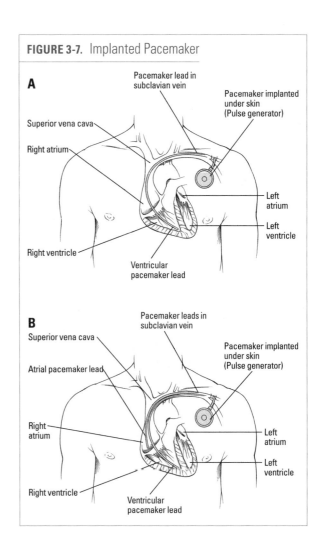

FIGURE 3-7. Implanted Pacemaker

FIGURE 3-8. Biventricular Pacing

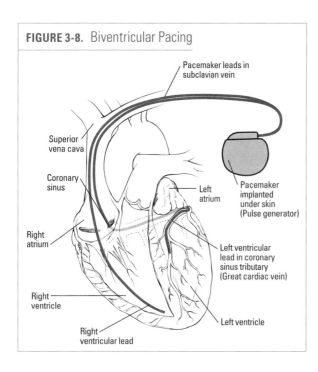

Like a pacemaker system, a pacing cardioverter-defibrillator (ICD) system includes a pulse generator and electrodes, although pacing cardioverter-defibrillators may require multiple leads, even when only a single chamber is being paced. A pacing cardioverter-defibrillator system may be inserted in a single chamber (eg, pacing in the ventricle) or in dual chambers (eg, pacing in atrium and ventricle). These devices use a combination of antitachycardia pacing, low-energy cardioversion, or defibrillating shocks to treat ventricular tachycardia or ventricular fibrillation.

Pacing cardioverter-defibrillator pulse generators may be implanted in a subcutaneous infraclavicular pocket or in an abdominal pocket. Removal of a pacing cardioverter-defibrillator pulse generator requires opening of the existing subcutaneous pocket and disconnection of the pulse generator from its electrode(s). A thoracotomy (or laparotomy in the case of abdominally placed pulse generators) is not required to remove the pulse generator.

The electrodes (leads) of a pacing cardioverter-defibrillator system are positioned in the heart via the venous system (transvenously) in most circumstances. In certain circumstances, an additional electrode may be required to achieve pacing of the left ventricle (biventricular pacing). In this event, transvenous (cardiac vein) placement of the electrode should be separately reported using code **33224** or code **33225**. Epicardial placement of the electrode should be separately reported using code **33202** or code **33203**.

Electrode positioning on the epicardial surface of the heart requires a thoracotomy, or thoracoscopic placement of the leads. Removal of electrode(s) may first be attempted by transvenous extraction (**33234**, **33235**, or **33244**). However, if transvenous extraction is unsuccessful, a thoracotomy may be required to remove the electrodes (**33238** or **33243**). Use code(s) **33212**, **33213**, **33221**, **33230**, **33231**, or **33240** as appropriate in addition to the thoracotomy or endoscopic epicardial lead placement codes (**33202** or **33203**) to report the insertion of the generator if done by the same physician during the same session. When the "battery" of a pacemaker or pacing cardioverter-defibrillator is changed, it is actually the pulse generator that is changed. Removal of pacemaker or pacing cardioverter-defibrillator pulse generator only is reported with code **33233** or **33241**. Removal of a pacemaker or pacing cardioverter-defibrillator pulse generator with insertion of a new pulse generator without any replacement or insertion of a lead(s) is reported with codes **33227-33229** and **33262-33264**. Insertion of a new pulse generator, when existing leads are already in place and when no prior pulse generator is removed, is reported with codes **33212**, **33213**, **33221**, **33230**, **33231**, and **33240**. When a pulse generator insertion involves the insertion or replacement of one or more lead(s), use the system codes **33206-33208** for pacemaker or **33249** for pacing cardioverter-defibrillator. Removal of a pulse generator (**33233** or **33241**) or extraction of transvenous leads (**33234**, **33235**, or **33244**) should be reported separately. An exception involves a pacemaker upgrade from single to dual system, which includes removal of pulse generator, replacement of new pulse generator, and insertion of new lead, reported with code **33214**.

Repositioning of a pacemaker electrode, pacing cardioverter-defibrillator electrode(s), or a left ventricular pacing electrode is reported using code **33215** or code **33226**, as appropriate.

The pacemaker and pacing cardioverter-defibrillator device evaluation codes **93279-93299** may not be reported in conjunction with pulse generator and lead insertion or revision codes **33206-33249**. Defibrillator threshold testing (DFT) during pacing cardioverter-defibrillator insertion or replacement may be separately reported using codes **93640**, **93641**.

Radiological supervision and interpretation related to the pacemaker or pacing cardioverter-defibrillator procedures is included in codes **33206-33249**. To report fluoroscopic guidance for diagnostic lead evaluation without lead insertion, replacement, or revision procedures, use code **76000**.

TABLE 3-1. Transvenous Procedure

Transvenous Procedure	SYSTEM	
	Pacemaker	Implantable Cardioverter-Defibrillator
Insert transvenous single lead only without pulse generator	33216	33216
Insert transvenous dual leads without pulse generator	33217	33217
Insert transvenous multiple leads without pulse generator	33217 + 33224	33217 + 33224
Initial pulse generator insertion only with existing single lead	33212	33240
Initial pulse generator insertion only with existing dual leads	33213	33230
Initial pulse generator insertion only with existing multiple leads	33221	33231
Initial pulse generator insertion or replacement plus insertion of transvenous single lead	33206 (atrial) or 33207 (ventricular)	33249
Initial pulse generator insertion or replacement plus insertion of transvenous dual leads	33208	33249
Initial pulse generator insertion or replacement plus insertion of transvenous multiple leads	33208 + 33225	33249 + 33225
Upgrade single chamber system to dual chamber system	33214 (includes removal of existing pulse generator)	33241 + 33249
Removal pulse generator only (without replacement)	33233	33241
Removal pulse generator with replacement pulse generator only single lead system (transvenous)	33227	33262
Removal pulse generator with replacement pulse generator only dual lead system (transvenous)	33228	33263
Removal pulse generator with replacement pulse generator only multiple lead system (transvenous)	33229	33264
Removal transvenous electrode only single lead system	33234	33244
Removal transvenous electrode only dual lead system	33235	33244
Removal and replacement of pulse generator and transvenous electrodes	33233 + (33234 or 33235) + (33206 or 33207 or 33208) and 33225, when appropriate	33241 + 33244 + 33249 and 33225, when appropriate

The following definitions apply to codes 33206-33249:

Single lead: A pacemaker or pacing cardioverter-defibrillator with pacing and sensing function in only one chamber of the heart.

Dual lead: A pacemaker or pacing cardioverter-defibrillator with pacing and sensing function in only two chambers of the heart.

Multiple lead: A pacemaker or pacing cardioverter-defibrillator with pacing and sensing function in three or more chambers of the heart.

CODING TIP For temporary transcutaneous pacing, see code **92953**.

...EMENT OF
... PACEMAKER

...; open
... sternotomy,

CPT Changes: An Insider's View 2007

33203 endoscopic approach (eg, thoracoscopy, pericardioscopy)
CPT Changes: An Insider's View 2007

⊙▲**33206** Insertion of new or replacement of permanent pacemaker with transvenous electrode(s); atrial
CPT Assistant Summer 94:10,17, Oct 96:9, Nov 99:15, Jun 08:14; *CPT Changes: An Insider's View* 2012

⊙▲**33207** ventricular
CPT Assistant Summer 94:10,17, Oct 96:9, Nov 99:15, Jun 08:14; *CPT Changes: An Insider's View* 2012

⊙▲**33208** atrial and ventricular
CPT Assistant Summer 94:10,17, Jul 96:10, Nov 99:15, Jun 08:14; *CPT Changes: An Insider's View* 2012

⊙**33210** Insertion or replacement of temporary transvenous single chamber cardiac electrode or pacemaker catheter (separate procedure)
CPT Assistant Summer 94:10,17, Mar 07:1

⊙**33211** Insertion or replacement of temporary transvenous dual chamber pacing electrodes (separate procedure)
CPT Assistant Summer 94:10,17, Mar 07:1

⊙▲**33212** Insertion of pacemaker pulse generator only; with existing single lead
CPT Assistant Summer 94:10,18, Fall 94:24, May 04:15, Jun 08:14; *CPT Changes: An Insider's View* 2012

⊙▲**33213** with existing dual leads
CPT Assistant Summer 94:10,18, Oct 96:10, Feb 98:11; *CPT Changes: An Insider's View* 2012

#⊙●**33221** with existing multiple leads
CPT Changes: An Insider's View 2012

Intent and Use of Codes 33202 and 33203

In current practice, the generator is often placed by a cardiologist at a session other than that of the electrode placement. Codes 33202 and 33203 separate the services of lead placement from generator placement. This allows reporting of lead placement in scenarios in which the cardiologist places the generator and one or more of the electrodes by a transvenous route and, for cases of biventricular generator placement, left ventricular lead placement is performed by another physician

at a different session. In these cases the surgeon is asked to place the additional leads via thoracotomy, median sternotomy, thoracoscopic approach, or subxiphoid approach. In addition, there are times when new leads are required via transthoracic placement, but no new pacemaker is required.

When epicardial lead placement is performed by the same physician at the same session as insertion of the generator, report codes 33202 and 33203 in conjunction with codes 33212 and 33213, as appropriate. Epicardial systems, though rarely implanted, are most typically used in pediatric cases for patients with mechanical tricuspid valve replacement or as adjuncts to other surgery such as coronary revascularization. In the last case, the procedure would be coded separately from the bypass surgery.

CODING TIP When epicardial lead placement is performed with insertion of the generator, report codes **33202**, **33203** in conjunction with codes **33212**, **33213**, **33221**, **33230**, **33231**, **33240**. When epicardial electrode placement is performed, report code **33224** in conjunction with codes **33202**, **33203**.

Description of Service for Code 33202

General endotracheal anesthesia is induced, and the patient is positioned, prepared, and draped for an anterior thoracotomy. The chest is entered at the level of the fourth interspace anteriorly, and the lung is retracted. The pericardium is opened and the heart examined. An area on the high lateral wall of the left ventricle is chosen, and the lead is attached using standard techniques. The lead is tested, and the pacing threshold parameters are found to be appropriate. The lead is brought through the upper aspect of the pericardial incision and out the thoracotomy incision where it is tunneled subcutaneously up the lateral chest wall toward the generator pocket. A chest tube is placed into the pericardium and brought out the chest wall below the thoracotomy incision. Several interrupted sutures are placed to approximate the pericardium. The thoracotomy incision is closed in the usual fashion. The generator and leads are again tested prior to completing the procedure.

Description of Service for Code 33203

In this case the patient requires a double lumen endotracheal tube for intubation and is positioned in a full lateral position. Following preparing and draping, the 2-cm initial port incision is made in the posterior axillary line at the level of the sixth interspace. The

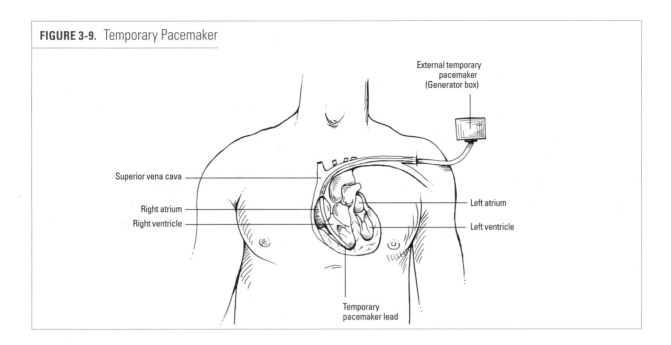

FIGURE 3-9. Temporary Pacemaker

port is inserted, and the camera positioned in the pleural cavity. Two additional ports are inserted in higher interspaces anterior and posterior to the first, and the pericardium is opened. The heart is examined, and a location for the electrode is found on the high lateral wall of the left ventricle. The electrode is placed using a standard epicardial screw-in device, and the lead is tested. A 2-cm counter incision is made several centimeters below the pacemaker generator pocket, and the lead is brought into this incision through the anterior chest wall. The ports are removed after placing a chest tube through the middle port incision, and the port incisions are closed. The lead is tunneled into the pocket, attached, and tested.

Intent and Use of Code ☉33206

Code 33206 refers to insertion of a new or replacement of a permanent pacemaker system using a transvenous atrial electrode.

Intent and Use of Code ☉33207

Code 33207 refers to insertion of a new or replacement of a permanent pacemaker system employing a ventricular electrode.

Intent and Use of Code ☉33208

Code 33208 refers to insertion of a new or replacement of a transvenous permanent pacemaker system employing both an atrial and a ventricular electrode.

CODING TIP Codes **33206-33208** refer to the insertion of a new or replacement of the entire system, including the lead(s) and pulse generator. If the pulse generator only is inserted or replaced, see code **33212** for single lead system or code **33213** for a dual lead system. If only lead(s) are inserted, see code **33216** for a single lead and code **33217** for two transvenous leads. Do not report codes **33206-33208** in conjunction with codes **33227-33229**. For removal and replacement of pacemaker pulse generator and transvenous electrode(s), use code **33233** in conjunction with either codes **33234** or **33235** and codes **33206-33208**.

When two physicians (ie, a surgeon and a cardiologist) act as co-surgeons in the implantation of a pacemaker, the use of **modifier 62** becomes necessary. Each physician reports his or her distinctive work by adding **modifier 62** to the single definitive procedure code to indicate both physicians were working together as the primary surgeon. For example, Physician A performs the surgical creation of the pocket for the pulse generator. Physician B inserts a permanent pacemaker with transvenous atrial and ventricular electrodes. Physician A reports code **33208 62** and Physician B reports code **33208 62**.

Intent and Use of Code ⊙ 33210

Code **33210** is used to report the insertion or replacement of a temporary transvenous pacemaker electrode.

Intent and Use of Code ⊙ 33211

Code **33211** applies if a dual-chamber temporary transvenous system is inserted.

> **CODING TIP** There is currently no code for the infrequently performed insertion of a transthoracic pacing electrode. Code **33999** (unlisted cardiac procedure) should be reported if this procedure is performed. For temporary transcutaneous pacing, see code **92953**.

Intent and Use of Code ⊙ 33212

Code **33212** represents the insertion of a pacemaker pulse generator only with an existing single lead. It is more typically used for pulse generator replacement (eg, at the end of the life of a generator). It may be applicable in the rare case of a primary insertion in which the permanent pacemaker leads have been placed without a generator during a previous procedure.

As indicated in the CPT guidelines, replacement of a pulse generator should be reported with a code for the removal of the pulse generator and another code for the insertion of a pulse generator. Removal of a permanent pacemaker pulse generator is reported with code 33233. Do not report codes 33212, 33213, or 33221 in conjunction with code 33233 for removal and replacement of the pacemaker pulse generator. Instead, use codes 33227-33229, as appropriate, when pulse generator replacement is indicated. Also, it would not be appropriate to report codes 33227-33229 in conjunction with code 33233, as the removal of the permanent pacemaker pulse generator is inherent in the replacement codes (33227-33229).

Use code **33234** for the extraction of a single (atrial or ventricular) transvenous pacemaker electrode and code **33235** for the extraction of dual transvenous electrodes.

> **CODING TIP** Many of the CPT codes for the implantation of pacemakers or defibrillators include the phrase "insertion or replacement." The term replacement is not intended to indicate that the work of removing an existing device is included. In those instances, report both the appropriate removal code and the insertion/replacement code. For removal and replacement of pacemaker pulse generator and transvenous electrode(s), use code **33233** in conjunction with either code **33234** or **33235** and codes **33206-33208**. For the removal and replacement of a pacing cardioverter-defibrillator system (pulse generator and electrodes), report code **33241** in conjunction with either code **33243** or **33244** and **33249**.

Description of Service for Code ⊙ 33212

The appropriate pectoral region is prepared and draped in a sterile manner. An incision is made in the subclavicular region and carried to the pectoralis fascia or the subpectoral region. A pocket for the pacemaker generator is created either in the plane of pectoralis fascia or underneath the pectoral muscles just above the ribcage. The existing lead is dissected free from fibrous tissue. Hemostasis is achieved. The lead is tested for sensing, capture threshold, and impedance. The pocket is irrigated. The pacing lead is connected to the new generator. The generator is inserted into the pocket. The pocket is closed with either suture alone or a combination of suture and staples or suture and tissue adhesive. Programming of the device is performed.

Intent and Use of Code ⊙ 33213

Code **33213** involves the insertion or replacement and programming of a dual-chamber pacemaker generator, including the disconnection, testing, and reconnection of two leads.

Description of Service for Code ⊙ 33213

The appropriate pectoral region is prepared and draped in a sterile manner. An incision is made in the subclavicular region and carried to the pectoralis fascia or the subpectoral region. A pocket for the pacemaker generator is created either in the plane of pectoralis fascia or underneath the pectoral muscles just above the ribcage. The existing leads are dissected free from fibrous tissue. Hemostasis is achieved. The leads are tested for sensing, capture threshold, and impedance. The pocket is irrigated. The pacing leads are connected to the new generator. The generator is inserted into the pocket. The pocket is closed with either suture alone or a combination of suture and staples or suture and tissue adhesive. Programming of the device is performed.

CODING TIP It is inappropriate to report the service of initial programming of temporary or permanent pacemakers at the time of implantation. Interrogation and programming codes in the **93279-93296** code series are for subsequent patient encounters separate from the initial insertion procedure.

UPGRADE, REPOSITIONING, REPAIR, OR REVISION OF PERMANENT SINGLE- OR DUAL-CHAMBER PACEMAKER SYSTEMS (**33214-33222**)

⊙**33214** Upgrade of implanted pacemaker system, conversion of single chamber system to dual chamber system (includes removal of previously placed pulse generator, testing of existing lead, insertion of new lead, insertion of new pulse generator)

     CPT Assistant Summer 94:10,18, Fall 94:24, Jun 08:14

33215 Repositioning of previously implanted transvenous pacemaker or pacing cardioverter-defibrillator (right atrial or right ventricular) electrode

     CPT Changes: An Insider's View 2003

⊙**33216** Insertion of a single transvenous electrode, permanent pacemaker or cardioverter-defibrillator

     CPT Assistant Summer 94:10,18, Jul 96:10, Nov 99:15-16; *CPT Changes: An Insider's View* 2000, 2003, 2010

⊙**33217** Insertion of 2 transvenous electrodes, permanent pacemaker or cardioverter-defibrillator

     CPT Assistant Summer 94:10,18, Jul 96:10, Nov 99:15-16, Jul 00:5, Apr 09:8; *CPT Changes: An Insider's View* 2000, 2010

⊙▲**33218** Repair of single transvenous electrode, permanent pacemaker or pacing cardioverter-defibrillator

     CPT Assistant Summer 94:10,19, Oct 96:9, Nov 99:15-16; *CPT Changes: An Insider's View* 2000, 2012

⊙▲**33220** Repair of 2 transvenous electrodes for permanent pacemaker or pacing cardioverter-defibrillator

     CPT Assistant Summer 94:10,19, Oct 96:9, Nov 99:15-16, Jun 08:14; *CPT Changes: An Insider's View* 2000, 2012

Code **33221** is out of numerical sequence. See **33202-33249**

⊙**33222** Revision or relocation of skin pocket for pacemaker

     CPT Assistant Spring 94:30, Summer 94:10, Nov 99:15-16, Jun 08:14; *CPT Changes: An Insider's View* 2000

Intent and Use of Code ⊙33214

Code **33214** is used to report an upgrade from a single-chamber to a dual-chamber system. This most commonly applies to conversion from a single-chamber ventricular pacer to a dual-chamber system under circumstances in which a dual-chamber pacing system has been deemed better suited for a patient after the original single-chamber pacing implant (eg, in a patient demonstrating pacemaker syndrome). This code includes removing the previous pulse generator, testing the existing lead (usually ventricular), and inserting a new pulse generator. Occasionally, a patient with an atrial demand pacemaker for sick sinus syndrome will subsequently demonstrate atrioventricular (AV) nodal conduction disease, which requires adding a ventricular pacing component. In this instance, code **33214** also applies.

CODING TIP Do not report code **33214** in conjunction with codes **33227-33229**.

Description of Service for Code ⊙33214

The risks and benefits of conversion from a single-chamber pacemaker to a dual-chamber system are discussed with the patient, and informed consent is obtained. The procedure is performed under ECG, blood pressure, and pulse oximetry monitoring. The patient is prepared and given moderate sedation, prophylactic IV antibiotics, and local anesthesia. The old pulse generator is removed by careful dissection to avoid lead damage. An adequate length of lead is freed from the fibrous capsule. The lead is disconnected from the pulse generator and tested with a pacing system analyzer to confirm adequate pacing, sensing, and impedance. The subclavian or cephalic vein is then cannulated and used to pass a new lead to the right heart. The lead is positioned and adequate sensing, pacing, and lead impedance are confirmed with a pacing system analyzer. Testing for phrenic nerve stimulation is performed, and the new lead is secured to the fibrous capsule with sutures. Both the previously implanted and newly implanted leads are then connected to a new pulse generator, which is programmed to the desired parameters. If necessary, the fibrous capsule is carefully enlarged, and the leads and pulse generator are reinserted. The incision is closed, and the wound is dressed. The physician documents these services, generates a report, and, as appropriate, communicates with the referring physician.

CODING TIP Surgical creation of a pocket for the pulse generator is included when the codes for pacemaker and pacing cardioverter-defibrillator procedures are reported and should not be reported separately. The CPT codes used for insertion of a pulse generator include codes from the **33206-33208** and **33212-33214** code series, and codes **33240** and **33249**. When the skin pocket is revised or relocated, report code **33222** for revising or relocating a pacemaker; report code **33223** for revising a skin pocket for the cardioverter-defibrillator.

Intent and Use of Code 33215

Code 33215 describes the repositioning of a previously placed right atrial or right ventricular electrode. Code 33215 applies to single- and dual-chamber pacemaker or pacing cardioverter-defibrillator systems.

Intent and Use of Codes ⊙33216 and ⊙33217

Codes 33216 and 33217 indicate the insertion of a single transvenous electrode (33216) or the insertion of two transvenous electrodes (33217). These codes apply to both permanent pacemakers and cardioverter-defibrillator systems. If transvenous removal of electrode(s) is performed at time of insertion, see codes 33234 or 33235 for a pacemaker system or code 33244 for a pacing cardioverter-defibrillator system.

CODING TIP Do not report codes **33216-33217** in conjunction with code **33214**.

Description of Service for Code ⊙33216

The risks and benefits of the insertion of a single-chamber transvenous electrode are discussed with the patient, and informed consent is obtained. The procedure is performed under ECG, blood pressure, and pulse oximetry monitoring. The patient is prepared and given moderate sedation, prophylactic IV antibiotics, and local anesthesia. Pacemaker-dependent patients may require the insertion of a temporary transvenous pacemaker (reported separately with code 33210). An incision is made, and the pulse generator is exposed by careful dissection to avoid lead damage. The pulse generator is removed, and an adequate length of lead is freed from the fibrous capsule. A new lead is inserted via cannulation of the subclavian or cephalic vein used to pass the lead to the right heart. The lead is positioned, and adequate pacing, sensing, and impedance are confirmed with a pacing system

analyzer. Phrenic nerve stimulation is tested; the lead is once again secured to the fibrous capsule with sutures and connected to the pulse generator, replacing the old lead, which is capped and anchored or extracted (reported separately with code 33234 or code 33235). The lead(s) and pulse generator are returned to the fibrous capsule, the incision is closed, and the wound is dressed. The physician documents these services, generates a report, and, as appropriate, communicates with the referring physician.

Intent and Use of Code ⊙33217

Code 33217 involves the insertion or replacement of two leads (atrial and ventricular) rather than one. This code applies to both permanent pacemakers and cardioverter-defibrillator systems. If transvenous removal of electrode(s) is performed at time of insertion, see code 33234 or code 33235 for a pacemaker system, or code 33244 for a pacing cardioverter-defibrillator system.

Intent and Use of Code ⊙33218

Code 33218 refers to the repair of a single transvenous pacing electrode, such as in splicing a fracture, modifying a terminal pin, or repairing an insulation defect. This code applies to both a permanent pacemaker and a pacing cardioverter-defibrillator system.

CODING TIP For repair of implantable cardioverter-defibrillator pulse generator and/or leads, see codes **33218, 33220**.

Description of Service for Code ⊙33218

The risks and benefits of, and the alternatives to, the repair of a transvenous pacemaker electrode are discussed with the patient, and informed consent is obtained. The procedure is performed under ECG, blood pressure, and pulse oximetry monitoring. The patient is prepared and given moderate sedation, prophylactic IV antibiotics, and local anesthesia. Pacemaker-dependent patients may require the insertion of a temporary transvenous pacemaker (reported separately with code 33210) prior to the repair procedure. An incision is made, and the pulse generator is exposed by careful dissection to avoid lead damage. The pulse generator is removed, and an adequate length of lead is freed from the fibrous capsule. The lead is disconnected from the pulse generator and visually inspected before being tested with the pacing system analyzer. A focal defect in the lead insulation is identified and repaired using a tubular piece of insulation, medical adhesive, and suture. Fractures in the lead conductor may require splicing techniques or terminal pin modifications. Repeat testing with the pacing system analyzer is performed before the lead is reconnected to the pulse generator. The system is placed back in the existing capsule, the pocket is closed with sutures, and the wound is dressed. The physician documents these services, generates a report, and communicates with the referring physician.

Intent and Use of Code ⊙33220

Code 33220 is used to report the repair of two transvenous pacing electrode(s) in a permanent pacemaker or pacing cardioverter-defibrillator system. For repair of two transvenous electrodes for permanent pacemaker or pacing cardioverter-defibrillator with replacement of pulse generator, use codes 33228, 33229 or 33263, 33264, and 33220.

Intent and Use of Code ⊙33221

Code 33221 describes insertion of a pacemaker pulse generator having multiple existing leads.

Description of Service for Code ⊙33221

The appropriate pectoral region is prepared and draped in a sterile manner. An incision is made in the subclavicular region and carried to the pectoralis fascia or the subpectoral region. A pocket for the pacemaker generator is created either in the plane of pectoralis fascia or underneath the pectoral muscles just above the ribcage. The existing leads are dissected free from fibrous tissue. Hemostasis is achieved. The leads are tested for sensing, capture threshold, and impedance. The pocket is irrigated. The pacing leads are connected to the new generator. The generator is inserted into the pocket. The pocket is closed with either suture alone or a combination of suture and staples or suture and tissue adhesive. Programming of the device is performed.

Intent and Use of Code ⊙33222

Code 33222 applies when the skin pocket of a pacer system must be revised or relocated, as in an incipient erosion.

Description of Service for Code ⊙33222

The risks and benefits of revising or relocating the pacemaker generator pocket are discussed with the patient, and informed consent is obtained. The procedure is performed under ECG, blood pressure, and pulse oximetry monitoring. The patient is prepared and given moderate sedation, prophylactic IV antibiotics,

and local anesthesia. Pacemaker-dependent patients may require the insertion of a temporary transvenous pacemaker (reported separately with code 33210) prior to the revision procedure. An incision is made, and the pulse generator is exposed by careful dissection to avoid lead damage. The pulse generator is removed, and an adequate length of lead is freed from the fibrous capsule. The lead is disconnected and tested with a pacing system analyzer to ensure adequate sensing and pacing. The capsule is inspected for evidence of erosion or infection. Under local anesthesia, a new pocket is made, and a subcutaneous tunnel is formed between the new pocket and the existing capsule. The existing lead is then reattached to the pulse generator with the use of a lead extension, if necessary. The pulse generator is placed in the new pocket, both pockets are closed, and both wounds are dressed. The physician documents these services, generates a report, and communicates with the referring physician.

BIVENTRICULAR PACING/CARDIAC RESYNCHRONIZATION: INSERTION OR REPOSITIONING (33224-33226)

▲33224 Insertion of pacing electrode, cardiac venous system, for left ventricular pacing, with attachment to previously placed pacemaker or pacing cardioverter-defibrillator pulse generator (including revision of pocket, removal, insertion, and/or replacement of existing generator
CPT Assistant Dec 07:16; CPT Changes: An Insider's View 2003, 2012

+▲33225 Insertion of pacing electrode, cardiac venous system, for left ventricular pacing, at time of insertion of pacing cardioverter-defibrillator or pacemaker pulse generator (including upgrade to dual chamber system and pocket revision) (List separately in addition to code for primary procedure)
CPT Assistant Dec 07:16; CPT Changes: An Insider's View 2003, 2012

▲33226 Repositioning of previously implanted cardiac venous system (left ventricular) electrode (including removal, insertion and/or replacement of generator)
CPT Changes: An Insider's View 2003, 2012

Intent and Use of Codes 33224-33226

Codes 33224, +33225, and 33226 represent placing or repositioning the left ventricular electrode in the cardiac venous system for biventricular pacing to achieve cardiac resynchronization. It is not appropriate to report code **35476** and code **75978 26** for the venous access en route to the coronary sinus, associated cardiac vein, and venography (including fluoroscopic guidance), as this is considered inherent (and not separately reportable) in the left ventricular pacing lead codes **33224**, **+33225**, and **33226**. Access to the cardiac veins may be complicated due to variations in cardiac vein anatomy. These differences may include anatomical variations in number, diameter, angulation, and tortuosity.

CODING TIP For insertion or replacement of a cardiac venous system lead, see codes **33224**, **33225**.

Intent and Use of Code 33224

The implant procedure for the biventricular pacing systems parallels that of a conventional pacemaker or intracardiac defibrillator with the addition of a left ventricular lead and its transvenous placement in a cardiac vein. Code **33224** is used to report the insertion of the left ventricular electrode with attachment to a previously placed pacemaker or pacing cardioverter-defibrillator generator. For example, placement of the left ventricular (LV) lead to an existing generator (eg, conversion of an existing single- or dual-chamber system to a biventricular system) or the removal of a nonfunctioning LV lead and the insertion of a new LV lead to the existing generator.

Intent and Use of Code +33225

Add-on code **33225** is used to report the insertion of the LV electrode at the time of insertion of a pacemaker or pacing cardioverter-defibrillator generator. This is an add-on code to be used with the base code for placing the generator. Use add-on code **33225** when a new generator and LV lead are placed for biventricular pacing. Add-on code **33225** is used in conjunction with codes **33206**, **33207**, **33208**, **33212**, **33213**, **33214**, **33216**, **33217**, **33221**, **33222**, **33230**, **33231**, **33233**, **33234**, **33235**, **33240**, **33249**.

Intent and Use of Code 33226

Code **33226** (as opposed to code **33215**) is used to report the repositioning of a previously implanted cardiac venous system (left ventricular) electrode.

REMOVAL OF PERMANENT PACEMAKER PULSE GENERATOR/ELECTRODE(S) (**33227-33229, 33233-33238**)

⊙▲**33233** Removal of permanent pacemaker pulse generator only
CPT Assistant Summer 94:10,19, Fall 94:24, Oct 96:10; *CPT Changes: An Insider's View* 2000, 2012

Code **33227** is out of numerical sequence. See 33202-33249

Code **33228** is out of numerical sequence. See 33202-33249

Code **33229** is out of numerical sequence. See 33202-33249

Code **33230** is out of numerical sequence. See 33202-33249

Code **33231** is out of numerical sequence. See 33202-33249

\#⊙●**33227** Removal of permanent pacemaker pulse generator with replacement of pacemaker pulse generator; single lead system
CPT Changes: An Insider's View 2012

\#⊙●**33228**   dual lead system
CPT Changes: An Insider's View 2012

\#⊙●**33229**   multiple lead system
CPT Changes: An Insider's View 2012

⊙**33234** Removal of transvenous pacemaker electrode(s); single lead system, atrial or ventricular
CPT Assistant Summer 94:10,19, Nov 99:16; *CPT Changes: An Insider's View* 2000

⊙**33235**   dual lead system
CPT Assistant Summer 94:10,19, Nov 99:16; *CPT Changes: An Insider's View* 2000

33236 Removal of permanent epicardial pacemaker and electrodes by thoracotomy; single lead system, atrial or ventricular
CPT Assistant Summer 94:10,19, Nov 99:16; *CPT Changes: An Insider's View* 2000

33237   dual lead system
CPT Assistant Summer 94:10,19, Nov 99:16; *CPT Changes: An Insider's View* 2000

33238 Removal of permanent transvenous electrode(s) by thoracotomy
CPT Assistant Summer 94:10,19, Nov 99:16; *CPT Changes: An Insider's View* 2000

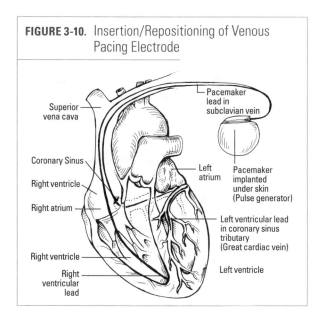

FIGURE 3-10. Insertion/Repositioning of Venous Pacing Electrode

Intent and Use of Code ⊙33227

Code 33227 describes removal of a permanent pacemaker pulse generator single lead system with replacement of the pacemaker pulse generator.

Description of Service for Code ⊙33227

The appropriate pectoral region is prepared and draped in a sterile manner. An incision is made of the existing generator and carried down to the level of the capsule surrounding the generator. The existing generator is dissected free, and the lead is freed from fibrous scar tissue. This must be performed in a manner preventing damage to the lead. Often extensive removal of scar tissue/capsule is required. During the procedure adequate hemostasis and sterility are maintained. The existing lead is tested to assess the adequacy, including capture threshold, sensing, and impedance. The pocket may need to be modified to accommodate the shape and size of the new generator. The pocket is copiously irrigated. The new generator is inserted in the pocket and attached to the existing lead. The pocket is closed with either suture alone or a combination of suture and staples or suture and tissue adhesive. Programming of the device is performed.

Intent and Use of Code ⊙33228

Code 33228 describes removal of a permanent pacemaker pulse generator dual lead system with replacement of the pacemaker pulse generator.

Description of Service for Code ⊙33228

The appropriate pectoral region is prepared and draped in a sterile manner. An incision is made of the existing generator and carried down to the level of the capsule surrounding the generator. The existing generator is dissected free, and the leads are freed from fibrous scar tissue. Often extensive removal of scar tissue/capsule is required. This must be performed in a manner preventing damage to the leads. During the procedure adequate hemostasis and sterility are maintained. The existing leads are tested to assess the adequacy, including capture threshold, sensing, and impedance. The pocket may need to be modified to accommodate the shape and size of the new generator. The pocket is copiously irrigated. The new generator is inserted in the pocket and attached to the existing leads. The pocket is closed with either suture alone or a combination of suture and staples or suture and tissue adhesive. Programming of the device is performed.

Intent and Use of Code ⊙33229

Code 33229 describes removal of a permanent pacemaker pulse generator multiple lead system with replacement of the pacemaker pulse generator.

Description of Service for Code ⊙33229

The appropriate pectoral region is prepared and draped in a sterile manner. An incision is made of the existing generator and carried down to the level of the capsule surrounding the generator. The existing generator is dissected free, and the leads are freed from fibrous scar tissue. Often extensive removal of scar tissue/capsule is required. This must be performed in a manner preventing damage to the leads. During the procedure adequate hemostasis and sterility are maintained. The existing leads are tested to assess the adequacy, including sensing, capture threshold, and impedance. The pocket may need to be modified to accommodate the shape and size of the new generator. The pocket is copiously irrigated. The new generator is inserted in the pocket and attached to the existing leads. The pocket is closed with either suture alone or a combination of suture and staples or suture and tissue adhesive. Programming of the device is performed.

Intent and Use of Code ⊙33233

Code 33233 is used to report the removal (without thoracotomy) of the pulse generator *only*. When performing removal of a pulse generator, it is not appropriate to report codes 33227-33229 in conjunction with code 33233.

CHAPTER 3

CODING TIP For pacemaker pulse generator replacement only, code **33233** is reported in addition to code **33212** for an existing single lead or code **33213** for existing dual leads. For pacemaker system upgrades or replacement procedures, code **33233** for pacemaker pulse generator removal and codes **33234** or **33235** for lead(s) removal may be reported in addition to codes **33206-33208** for insertion of new or replacement of permanent pacemaker electrode(s) or code **33214** for insertion of a pacemaker pulse generator only with multiple existing leads, as appropriate.

Description of Service for Code ⊙ 33233

The risks and benefits of removal of a permanent pacemaker generator are discussed with the patient, and informed consent is obtained. The procedure is performed under ECG, blood pressure, and pulse oximetry monitoring. The patient is prepared and given conscious sedation, prophylactic IV antibiotics, and local anesthesia. An incision is made, and the pulse generator is exposed and freed from the fibrous capsule. The capsule is inspected for evidence of infection. The lead is disconnected, capped, and returned to the capsule, if it is not to be reused. If the lead is to be used as part of a new pacing system (see codes 33206-33208 and 33212-33214, as appropriate), it is tested as described and attached to a new pulse generator. The pocket is closed, and the wound is dressed. The physician documents the service, generates a report, and, as appropriate, communicates with the referring physician.

Intent and Use of Code ⊙ 33234

Code 33234 is used to code for the extraction of a single (atrial or ventricular) transvenous pacemaker lead from a single lead system.

Description of Service for Code ⊙ 33234

The risks and benefits of removal of a single transvenous pacemaker lead are discussed with the patient, and informed consent is obtained. The procedure is performed under ECG, blood pressure, and pulse oximetry monitoring. The patient is prepared, placed under moderate sedation, and given prophylactic IV antibiotics. Femoral venous and arterial sheaths may be placed. A temporary transvenous pacemaker electrode may be passed into the right ventricular apex, especially if the patient is pacemaker dependent. With local anesthesia, an incision is made, and a pulse generator and lead are dissected free of scar tissue. Lead anchors or suture tie-downs are dissected free and removed. The lead is disconnected from the generator and cut

to expose its inner core. A locking stylet is inserted to the lead's tip, and gentle traction is applied. Once it is determined that the lead is adherent to the myocardium, an extension is applied to the locking stylet, and a plastic dilator is placed over the lead through the venous system to near the tip of the lead, thus dissecting it free from adhesions. Supplemental intravenous anesthesia is given as required. A counter traction is established by the dilator to the lead, which comes free and is removed. When a new lead is placed, that procedure (including lead placement only, connection to the generator, testing, and replacement of the existing generator in the pocket) is reported separately with codes 33216-33217. Hemostasis is achieved with direct pressure. The pocket is closed in layers, and the wound is dressed. The physician documents these services, generates a report, and, as appropriate, communicates with the referring physician.

Intent and Use of Code ⊙ 33235

Code 33235 is used to report the extraction of dual-chamber transvenous electrodes. The method of extraction is not specified and can be either by simple traction or with more elaborate snare or extraction devices. There is currently no separate code for reporting the removal of more than two pacemaker leads.

Description of Service for Code ⊙ 33235

This procedure, which involves removing multiple transvenous pacemaker leads, is the same service as described for code 33234 except that dual-lead system transvenous pacemaker leads are removed.

Intent and Use of Codes 33236-33238

Codes 33236-33238 are used to report the extraction of the pacer pulse generator via thoracotomy and pacing electrode(s) for an epicardial single-chamber system, epicardial dual-chamber system, and transvenous (single- or dual-chamber unspecified) pacer system, respectively.

Removal of an epicardial pacemaker lead(s) requires exposure of the heart. Removal of a single-lead system (code 33236) requires exposure of a small area of the heart. Removal of a dual-lead system (code 33237) usually requires more extensive exposure. The procedure described by code 33238 is used in cases in which an infected transvenous lead has to be removed but attempts to remove it via the usual mechanisms (ie, code 33234) are unsuccessful. For a "failed" attempt at transvenous extraction, it is appropriate to report code 33244 with **modifier 52** appended in addition to code 33238.

INSERTION, REPLACEMENT, OR REMOVAL OF PACING CARDIOVERTER-DEFIBRILLATOR SYSTEM (33223, 33230-33231, 33240, 33241, 33243, 33244, 33249, 33262-33264)

⊙**33223** Revision of skin pocket for cardioverter-defibrillator

CPT Assistant Summer 94:10,19, Nov 99:15-16, Jun 08:14; CPT Changes: An Insider's View 2000, 2010

⊙▲**33240** Insertion of pacing cardioverter-defibrillator pulse generator only; with existing single lead

CPT Assistant Summer 94:40, Jun 96:10, Nov 99:16-17, Jul 00:5, Apr 04:6, Jun 08:14; CPT Changes: An Insider's View 2000, 2012

Code **33230** is out of numerical sequence.

Code **33231** is out of numerical sequence.

#⊙●**33230** with existing dual leads

CPT Changes: An Insider's View 2012

#⊙●**33231** with existing multiple leads

CPT Changes: An Insider's View 2012

⊙▲**33241** Removal of pacing cardioverter-defibrillator pulse generator only

CPT Assistant Summer 94:40, Nov 99:16-17; CPT Changes: An Insider's View 2000, 2012

#⊙●**33262** Removal of pacing cardioverter-defibrillator pulse generator with replacement of pacing cardioverter-defibrillator pulse generator; single lead system

CPT Changes: An Insider's View 2012

#⊙●**33263** dual lead system

CPT Changes: An Insider's View 2012

#⊙●**33264** multiple lead system

CPT Changes: An Insider's View 2012

33243 Removal of single or dual chamber pacing cardioverter-defibrillator electrode(s); by thoracotomy

CPT Assistant Summer 94:40, Nov 99:16-17; CPT Changes: An Insider's View 2000

⊙**33244** by transvenous extraction

CPT Assistant Summer 94:40, Nov 99:16-17, Jul 00:5; CPT Changes: An Insider's View 2000, 2012

⊙▲**33249** Insertion or replacement of permanent pacing cardioverter-defibrillator system with transvenous lead(s), single or dual chamber

CPT Assistant Summer 94:21, Nov 99:16-17, Apr 04:6, May 08:14, Jun 08:14; CPT Changes: An Insider's View 2000, 2012

Intent and Use of Codes ⊙33223, ⊙33230, ⊙33231, ⊙33240, ⊙33241, 33243, ⊙33244, ⊙33249, and ⊙33262, ⊙33263, ⊙33264

Codes 33223, 33230, 33231, 33240, and 33241 are used to code placement of an implantable cardioverter-defibrillator pulse generator at the time of initial insertion, replacement of a previously implanted device, revision, removal, or removal with replacement. These codes refer only to the surgical component of the procedure and do not reflect defibrillator threshold testing performed at the time of pulse generator implant (see codes 93640-93641). If only the pacing cardioverter-defibrillator pulse generator is inserted, code 33240 should be used for insertion of a new pulse generator where an existing single lead had previously been in place. An additional code (33241) may be reported for the removal of the pulse generator only.

Code 32223 describes revision or relocation of a defibrillator generator skin pocket of a pacer system.

For removal of an existing implantable pacing cardioverter-defibrillator pulse generator system (pulse generator and electrodes), code 33241 should be reported in addition to code 33244 for transvenous lead removal. For removal and replacement of a pacing cardioverter-defibrillator pulse generator and electrode(s), use code 33241 in conjunction with either code 33243 or 33244, and code 33249.

Similarly, codes 33230 and 33231 represent insertion of a new pulse generator where existing dual or multiple leads, respectively, are in place, and the new pulse generator is inserted and attached to those existing leads. However, it would not be appropriate to report codes 33230, 33231, 33240 in conjunction with code 33241 for removal and replacement of the pacing cardioverter-defibrillator pulse generator. In this circumstance codes 33262-33264, as appropriate, should be reported when pulse generator removal and replacement are indicated.

Removal of a pulse generator does not require a thoracotomy, as the pulse generator is located outside of the thoracic cavity (ie, in a pocket under the abdominal muscles). With current technology, only the electrode system may need to be removed by thoracotomy. Both codes 33241 and 33243 should be reported for subcutaneous removal of a pulse generator (33241) and the electrode system by open thoracotomy (33243).

Removal of an electrode(s) is first attempted by transvenous extraction. However, if transvenous extraction is unsuccessful (code 33244), a thoracotomy is necessary to remove the electrodes (code 33243). For a failed attempt at transvenous extraction, it is appropriate to report code **33244** with **modifier 52** appended in addition to code **33243**.

> **CODING TIP** Use code **33240** in addition to the epicardial lead placement codes to report the insertion of the pulse generator when done by the same physician during the same session. When epicardial lead placement is performed with insertion of a pulse generator, code **33202** or **33203** should be reported in conjunction with code **33230**, **33231**, **or 33240**, as appropriate.

Description of Service for Code ⊙33223

The risks and benefits of revision or relocation of a pocket for an implantable cardioverter-defibrillator are discussed with the patient, and informed consent is obtained. The procedure is performed under ECG, blood pressure, and pulse oximetry monitoring. The patient is prepared and given moderate sedation, prophylactic IV antibiotics, and local anesthesia. An incision is made, and the pulse generator is exposed by careful dissection to avoid lead damage. The pulse generator is removed, and adequate lengths of leads are freed from the fibrous capsule. The capsule is inspected for evidence of erosion or infection. Under local anesthesia, a new pocket is made, and a tunnel is formed between the new pocket and the chronic capsule. The chronic leads are then reattached to the pulse generator with the use of lead extensions, as needed. The pulse generator is placed in the new pocket, both pockets are closed, and both wounds are dressed. The physician documents these services, generates a report, and communicates with the referring physician.

Description of Service for Code ⊙33230

The appropriate pectoral region is prepared and draped in a sterile manner. An incision is made in the subclavicular region and carried to the pectoralis fascia or the subpectoral region. A pocket for the pacemaker generator is created either in the plane of pectoralis fascia or underneath the pectoral muscles just above the ribcage. The existing leads are dissected free from fibrous tissue. Hemostasis is achieved. The leads are tested for sensing, capture threshold, and impedance. The pocket is irrigated. The pacing leads are connected to the new generator. The generator is inserted into the pocket. The pocket is closed with either suture alone or a combination of suture and staples or suture and tissue adhesive. Programming of the device is performed.

Description of Service for Code ⊙33231

The appropriate pectoral region is prepared and draped in a sterile manner. An incision is made in the subclavicular region and carried to the pectoralis fascia or the subpectoral region. A pocket for the pacemaker generator is created either in the plane of pectoralis fascia or underneath the pectoral muscles just above the ribcage. The existing leads are dissected free from fibrous tissue. Hemostasis is achieved. The leads are tested for sensing, capture threshold, and impedance. The pocket is irrigated. The pacing leads are connected to the new generator. The generator is inserted into the pocket. The pocket is closed with either suture alone or a combination of suture and staples or suture and tissue adhesive. Programming of the device is performed.

Description of Service for Code ⊙33240

The appropriate pectoral region is prepared and draped in a sterile manner. An incision is made in the subclavicular region and carried to the pectoralis fascia or the subpectoral region. A pocket for the pacemaker generator is created either in the plane of pectoralis fascia or underneath the pectoral muscles just above the ribcage. The existing lead is dissected free from fibrous tissue. Hemostasis is achieved. The lead is tested for sensing, capture threshold, and impedance. The pocket is irrigated. The pacing lead is connected to the new generator. The generator is inserted into the pocket. The pocket is closed with either suture alone or a combination of suture and staples or suture and tissue adhesive. Programming of the device is performed.

Description of Service for Code ⊙33241

The risks and benefits of removing a pacing cardioverter-defibrillator generator are discussed with the patient, and informed consent is obtained. The procedure is performed under ECG, blood pressure, and pulse oximetry monitoring. The patient is prepared and given moderate sedation, prophylactic IV antibiotics, and local anesthesia. An incision is made, and the pulse generator is exposed by careful dissection to avoid lead damage. The pocket is inspected for signs of infection or erosion. If the leads are not to be reused, they are disconnected, capped, and returned to the pocket. If the leads are to be used as a part of a new implantable cardioverter-defibrillator system, they are tested and attached to a new pulse generator. Lead and pulse generator testing is reported separately (code **93641**). The leads and pulse generator are returned to the pocket, which is closed with sutures. The wound is dressed. The physician documents these services, generates a report, and communicates with the referring physician.

Intent and Use of Codes 33243 and ⊙33244

Codes 33243-33244 are used to code the removal of a single- or dual-chamber pacing cardioverter-defibrillator electrode(s) by thoracotomy (33243) or by transvenous extraction (33244). For removal of electrode(s) by thoracotomy in conjunction with pulse generator removal or replacement, use code 33243 in conjunction with codes 33241, 33262-33264.

> **CODING TIP** Removal of an electrode(s) is first attempted by transvenous extraction. However, if transvenous extraction is unsuccessful (code **33244**), a thoracotomy is necessary to remove the electrodes (code **33243**). For a failed attempt at transvenous extraction, it is appropriate to report code **33244** with **modifier 52** appended in addition to code **33243**.

Description of Service for Code 33243

The risks and benefits of removing a pacing cardioverter-defibrillator lead by thoracotomy are discussed with the patient, and informed consent is obtained. The procedure is performed under ECG, blood pressure, and pulse oximetry monitoring. The patient is prepared and placed under general anesthesia. The thorax is opened through a median sternotomy or lateral thoracotomy. The pericardium is exposed by careful and extensive dissection of the retrosternal space. Removal of extrapericardial patches may require dissection into the plane between the heart and lung. Hemodynamic support with partial cardiopulmonary bypass may be used to more easily remove posterior patches in difficult cases. After removal of the patches and epicardial leads, the pulse generator pocket is opened. The pulse generator is removed and disconnected from the leads. The leads are dissected from the fibrous capsule and removed. Both incisions are closed, and the wounds are dressed. The physician documents these services, generates a report, and communicates with the referring physician.

Description of Service for Code ⊙33244

The risks and benefits of percutaneous removal of pacing cardioverter-defibrillator leads are discussed with the patient, and informed consent is obtained. The procedure is performed under ECG, blood pressure, and pulse oximetry monitoring. The patient is prepared and given moderate sedation and local anesthesia. General anesthesia and intra-arterial blood pressure monitoring may be warranted in selected cases. An incision is made, and the pulse generator is exposed and removed from the fibrous capsule. The leads, including suture

ties, are freed from the capsule. In patients with a periumbilical pulse generator, freeing the leads involves a second, infraclavicular incision. The leads are cut to expose their inner cores, which are sized with gauging pins. A locking stylet is passed through the inner core of one of the leads to its distal end, where it is engaged under gentle traction. A firm plastic sheath is passed over the stylet and lead, freeing the lead from intravascular adhesions as it is advanced toward the lead's distal end. Firm traction is applied to the locking stylet while counter traction is applied to the endocardial surface with the plastic sheath. This process is repeated for other transvenous leads in the implantable cardioverter-defibrillator system. Alternatively, leads can be extracted using a femoral approach. A large-bore sheath is inserted in the femoral vein and advanced to the cavo-atrial junction. A deflectable tip wire and a Dotter basket are passed through the sheath to the right atrium. Leads can be grasped with the wire and withdrawn into the basket, where they are ensnared. While applying traction to the lead, the sheath is passed over the wire, basket, and lead to the endocardial surface for counter traction. Once freed, a lead is withdrawn into the sheath, and both are removed from the vein, where pressure is applied until hemostasis is achieved. If a subcutaneous patch lead is a part of the implantable cardioverter-defibrillator system, an incision is made over the patch and extended to the surrounding capsule. The patch is then dissected free from the capsule, and the lead is removed. The wounds are closed and dressed. The physician documents these services, generates a report, and communicates with the referring physician.

Intent and Use of Code ⊙33249

Code 33249 refers to the implantation of a single- or dual-chamber pacing cardioverter-defibrillator system (lead[s] and pulse generator). For the removal and replacement of a pacing cardioverter-defibrillator system (pulse generator and electrodes), report codes 33241 and 33243 or codes 33244 and 33249.

Description of Service for Code ⊙33249

The risks and benefits of percutaneous implantation of a pacing cardioverter-defibrillator generator and leads are discussed with the patient, and informed consent is obtained. The procedure is performed under ECG, blood pressure, and pulse oximetry monitoring. The patient is prepared, given prophylactic IV antibiotics, and placed under general anesthesia. Access is gained to the subclavian or cephalic vein, through which the sensing, pacing, and defibrillation lead(s) is passed to the right heart using a peel-away sheath. The lead(s) is then tested as described in code 93641. When satisfactory lead function is confirmed, the lead(s) is sutured to the pectoralis fascia, and a pocket is formed in the pectoral or periumbilical region for the pulse generator. A subcutaneous tunnel is formed for the lead(s) when a periumbilical pocket is used. The lead(s) is then attached to the pulse generator, and the system is tested before it is placed in the pocket. The incision(s) is closed, and the wound(s) is dressed. The physician documents these services, generates a report, and communicates with the referring physician.

> **CODING TIP** Do not report codes **33262-33264** in conjunction with code **33241**.

Description of Service for Code ⊙33262

The appropriate pectoral region is prepared and draped in a sterile manner. An incision is made of the existing generator and carried down to the level of the capsule surrounding the generator. The existing generator is dissected free, and the lead is freed from fibrous scar tissue. This must be performed in a manner preventing damage to the lead. Often extensive removal of scar tissue/capsule is required. During the procedure adequate hemostasis and sterility are maintained. The existing lead is tested to assess the adequacy, including capture threshold, sensing, and impedance. The pocket may need to be modified to accommodate the shape and size of the new generator. The pocket is copiously irrigated. The new generator is inserted in the pocket and attached to the existing lead. The pocket is closed with either suture alone or a combination of suture and staples or suture and tissue adhesive. Programming of the device is performed.

Description of Service for Code ⊙33263

The appropriate pectoral region is prepared and draped in a sterile manner. An incision is made of the existing generator and carried down to the level of the capsule surrounding the generator. The existing generator is dissected free, and the leads are freed from fibrous scar tissue. Often extensive removal of scar tissue/capsule is required. This must be performed in a manner preventing damage to the leads. During the procedure adequate hemostasis and sterility are maintained. The existing leads are tested to assess the adequacy, including sensing, capture threshold, and impedance. The pocket may need to be modified to accommodate the shape and size of the new generator. The pocket is copiously irrigated. The new generator is inserted in the pocket and attached to the existing leads. The pocket is closed with either suture alone or a combination of suture and staples or suture and tissue adhesive. Programming of the device is performed.

Description of Service for Code ⊙33264

The appropriate pectoral region is prepared and draped in a sterile manner. An incision is made of the existing generator and carried down to the level of the capsule surrounding the generator. The existing generator is dissected free, and the leads are freed from fibrous scar tissue. Often extensive removal of scar tissue/capsule is required. This must be performed in a manner preventing damage to the leads. During the procedure adequate hemostasis and sterility are maintained. The existing leads are tested to assess the adequacy, including capture threshold, sensing, and impedance. The pocket may need to be modified to accommodate the shape and size of the new generator. The pocket is copiously irrigated. The new generator is inserted in the pocket and attached to the existing leads. The pocket is closed with either suture alone or a combination of suture and staples or suture and tissue adhesive. Programming of the device is performed.

ELECTROPHYSIOLOGIC OPERATIVE PROCEDURES (33250-33261 [ENDOSCOPY], 33265, 33266)

33250   Operative ablation of supraventricular arrhythmogenic focus or pathway (eg, Wolff-Parkinson-White, atrioventricular node re-entry), tract(s) and/or focus (foci); without cardiopulmonary bypass
CPT Assistant Summer 94:16, Nov 99:17-18; *CPT Changes: An Insider's View* 2000, 2002

33251   with cardiopulmonary bypass
CPT Assistant Summer 94:16, Nov 99:17-18; *CPT Changes: An Insider's View* 2000

33254   Operative tissue ablation and reconstruction of atria, limited (eg, modified maze procedure)
CPT Assistant Mar 07:1; *CPT Changes: An Insider's View* 2007

33255   Operative tissue ablation and reconstruction of atria, extensive (eg, maze procedure); without cardiopulmonary bypass
CPT Assistant Mar 07:1; *CPT Changes: An Insider's View* 2007

33256   with cardiopulmonary bypass
CPT Assistant Mar 07:1; *CPT Changes: An Insider's View* 2007

+33257 Operative tissue ablation and reconstruction of atria, performed at the time of other cardiac procedure(s), limited (eg, modified maze procedure) (List separately in addition to code for primary procedure)
CPT Changes: An Insider's View 2008

+33258 Operative tissue ablation and reconstruction of atria, performed at the time of other cardiac procedure(s), extensive (eg, maze procedure), without cardiopulmonary bypass (List separately in addition to code for primary procedure)
CPT Changes: An Insider's View 2008

+33259 Operative tissue ablation and reconstruction of atria, performed at the time of other cardiac procedure(s), extensive (eg, maze procedure), with cardiopulmonary bypass (List separately in addition to code for primary procedure)
CPT Changes: An Insider's View 2008

33261 Operative ablation of ventricular arrhythmogenic focus with cardiopulmonary bypass
CPT Assistant Summer 94:16

Code **33262** is out of numerical sequence. See **33202-33249**

Code **33263** is out of numerical sequence. See **33202-33249**

Code **33264** is out of numerical sequence. See **33202-33249**

Endoscopy

33265 Endoscopy, surgical; operative tissue ablation and reconstruction of atria, limited (eg, modified maze procedure), without cardiopulmonary bypass
CPT Assistant Mar 07:1; CPT Changes: An Insider's View 2007

33266 operative tissue ablation and reconstruction of atria, extensive (eg, maze procedure), without cardiopulmonary bypass
CPT Assistant Mar 07:1; CPT Changes: An Insider's View 2007

Intent and Use

According to CPT guidelines, the electrophysiologic operative procedures family of codes describes the surgical treatment of supraventricular dysrhythmias. Tissue ablation, disruption, and reconstruction can be accomplished by many methods including surgical incision or through the use of a variety of energy sources (eg, radiofrequency, cryotherapy, microwave, ultrasound, laser). If excision or isolation of the left atrial appendage by any method, including stapling, oversewing, ligation, or plication, is performed in conjunction with any of the atrial tissue ablation and reconstruction (maze) procedures (**33254-33259, 33265-33266**), it is considered part of the procedure. Codes

33254-33256 are only to be reported when there is no concurrently performed procedure that requires median sternotomy or cardiopulmonary bypass.

The appropriate atrial tissue ablation add-on code (**33257, 33258,** or **33259**) should be reported in addition to an open cardiac procedure requiring sternotomy or cardiopulmonary bypass if performed concurrently.

Definitions

Limited: Operative ablation and reconstruction that includes surgical isolation of triggers of supraventricular dysrhythmias by operative ablation that isolates the pulmonary veins or other anatomically defined triggers in the left or right atrium.

Extensive: Operative ablation and reconstruction that includes:

- the services included in "limited"; and

- additional ablation of atrial tissue to eliminate sustained supraventricular dysrhythmias. This must include operative ablation that involves the right atrium, the atrial septum, or the left atrium in continuity with the atrioventricular annulus.

Intent and Use of Codes 33250 and 33251

Supraventricular arrhythmias originate above the bundle of His. As indicated in the CPT guidelines, the newly established procedures describe combinations of surgical and electrophysiologic (eg, radiofrequency, cryotherapy, microwave, ultrasound, laser) techniques to place lesions that interrupt the intra-atrial reentrant pathways that support dysrhythmia (no rhythm) to create a mazelike pathway for sinus activation of the atria and the AV node. Any of the surgical methods described in the guidelines utilized to create the new impulse pathways, in which excision or isolation of the left atrial appendage is accomplished, including stapling, oversewing, ligation, or plication, are included and not separately reported.

Codes **33250** and **33251** are used to report the surgical ablation of arrhythmogenic foci for supraventricular arrhythmias without cardiopulmonary bypass (**33250**) or with cardiopulmonary bypass (**33251**).

Intent and Use of Codes 33254-33266

Codes **33254** and **33265** describe the limited (or modified) maze procedure. As defined in the CPT guidelines, these procedures include any method to isolate triggers of supraventricular dysrhythmias by operative ablation in the pulmonary veins or other anatomically defined trigger sites in the left or right atrium. Code **33254** describes a closed-heart operation for paroxysmal or short duration atrial fibrillation/flutter using atrial incision(s) and adjunctive ablation techniques that are limited to the left atrium or do not extend to the AV annulus.

Codes **33255**, **33256**, and **33266** are used to report atrial tissue ablation and reconstruction (maze) procedures. These codes are to be used only when there is no concurrently performed procedure that requires median sternotomy or cardiopulmonary bypass. When the procedures described by codes **33254-33256** are performed with a concurrent procedure that requires a median sternotomy or cardiopulmonary bypass, physicians should report the primary procedure and, in addition, use codes **33257-33259**. These codes are identical in description to codes **33254-33256** but are limited to use as add-on codes when another cardiac procedure is performed.

Codes **33255**, **33256**, and **33266** represent the unmodified maze procedure and are intended to report the more extensive variant of these procedures. As defined in the new CPT guidelines, extensive operative ablation and reconstruction comprise both services included in the limited service description and any additional ablation of atrial tissue to eliminate sustained supraventricular dysrhythmias. To be considered extensive, the procedure must include operative ablation that involves the right atrium, the atrial septum, or the left atrium in continuity with the AV annulus.

Code **33256** is only reported if cardiopulmonary bypass is performed in addition to the maze procedure.

Do not report codes **33265-33266** in conjunction with codes **32551**, **33210**, or **33211**.

Description of Service for Code 33254

Following induction of general anesthesia, a median sternotomy incision is performed. The pericardium is opened, and a pericardial cradle is created. The pulmonary veins are isolated by dissection behind them. A series of atrial lesions is created using an ablative energy source to isolate or redirect abnormal atrial depolarization site(s). The left atrial appendage is excised using a stapling device. The chest and pericardial tubes are placed, and the wound is closed in a standard manner with stainless steel sternal wires and absorbable suture.

Description of Service for Code 33255

Following induction of general anesthesia, a median sternotomy incision is performed. The pericardium

is opened, and a pericardial cradle is created. The pulmonary veins are isolated by dissection behind them. A series of atrial lesions is created using an ablative energy source to isolate or redirect abnormal atrial depolarization site(s), which involves creating an extensive set of lesions involving both atria or creating a conduction block involving the atrioventricular annulus. The left atrial appendage is excised using a stapling device. Chest and pericardial tubes are placed, and the wound is closed in a standard manner with stainless steel sternal wires and absorbable suture.

Description of Service for Code 33256

Following induction of general anesthesia, a median sternotomy incision is performed. The pericardium is opened, a pericardial cradle is created, and the pulmonary veins are isolated by dissection behind them. Aortic and atrial purse string sutures are placed. The patient is given systemic heparin. Cannulas for cardiopulmonary bypass are inserted and secured, and cardiopulmonary bypass is established. The patient is cooled to approximately 34 degrees Centigrade. The aorta is clamped, and the heart is arrested with cold blood cardioplegia. Additional doses of cardioplegia are given intermittently throughout the period of aortic clamping.

The left and right atria are opened. Both atrial appendages are excised and stapled or oversewn. An extensive lesion set is made using incisions or ablative techniques that involve both atria, or by creating a conduction block involving the atrioventricular annulus. The lesions encircle the pulmonary veins and extend to both the mitral and tricuspid annuli. The atria are closed with monofilament sutures.

The patient is warmed and weaned from cardiopulmonary bypass. The cannulas are removed, and the cannulation sites are oversewn. Protamine is administered, and a careful inspection for hemostasis is made. The chest and pericardial tubes are placed, and the wound is closed in a standard manner with stainless steel sternal wires and absorbable suture.

Description of Service for Code 33257

A series of atrial lesions is created using an ablative energy source to isolate or redirect any abnormal atrial depolarization sites. The creation of these lesions requires sharp and blunt dissection of the pulmonary veins from the pericardial reflections to ensure that the ablation energy is directed to the body of the left atrium rather than to the pulmonary veins. Special attention is given to ablative energy delivery to avoid injury to coronary arteries and the esophagus. The left atrial appendage is excised. Temporary atrial and ventricular pacing wires are placed.

Description of Service for Code 33258

Under general anesthesia and through median sternotomy on the beating, working heart, a series of atrial lesions is created using an ablative energy source to isolate or redirect any abnormal atrial depolarization sites. An extensive lesion set involving both atria is made, or a conduction block involving the atrioventricular annulus is created. Special attention is given to ablative energy delivery to avoid injury to coronary arteries or the esophagus. The left atrial appendage is excised. Temporary atrial and ventricular pacing wires are placed.

Description of Service for Code 33259

Under general anesthesia and on cardiopulmonary bypass, a series of atrial lesions is created using surgical incision and/or an ablative energy source to isolate or redirect any abnormal atrial depolarization sites. An extensive lesion set involving both atria is made, or a conduction block involving the atrioventricular annulus is created. Special attention is given to ablative energy delivery to avoid injury to coronary arteries and the esophagus. The left atrial appendage is excised. Temporary atrial and ventricular pacing wires are placed.

Intent and Use of Code 33261

Code **33261** is used to report the surgical ablation of other arrhythmogenic foci in a procedure that includes use of cardiopulmonary bypass. The number of supraventricular foci (eg, in the case of a patient with both Wolff-Parkinson-White syndrome and AV nodal reentry) is not specified.

Intent and Use of Code 33265

Code **33265** describes a closed-heart, endoscopic operation for paroxysmal or short-duration atrial fibrillation/flutter using atrial incision(s) and adjunctive ablation techniques that are limited to the left atrium or do not extend to the AV annulus.

Description of Service for Code 33265

Following induction of one-lung ventilation and general anesthesia, multiple ports are placed into the right and left side of chest. With thoracoscopic assistance, the pericardium is opened, the pulmonary veins are encircled, and a series of atrial lesions is created using an ablative energy source to isolate or redirect

abnormal atrial depolarization site(s). The left atrial appendage is excised using a stapling device. The chest and pericardial tubes are placed, and the multiple chest wounds are closed with absorbable sutures.

Intent and Use of Code 33266

Code **33266** describes a closed-heart endoscopic operation for chronic atrial fibrillation or flutter, Cox Maze III or variation, atrial incision(s), and adjunctive ablation techniques that include extensive lesion sets and annular lesions.

Description of Service for Code 33266

Following induction of one-lung ventilation and general anesthesia, multiple ports are placed into the right and left side of chest. With thoracoscopic assistance, the pericardium is opened, the pulmonary veins are encircled, and a series of atrial lesions is created using surgical incision and/or an ablative energy source to isolate or redirect abnormal atrial depolarization site(s). An extensive lesion set is made, involving both atria or creating a conduction block involving the AV annulus. The left and right atrial appendages are excised using stapling devices. Chest tubes and external pacing wires are placed, and the multiple chest wounds are closed with absorbable suture.

> **CODING TIP** Codes **33254**, **33255**, and **33256** should not be reported with codes for cardiac and intracardiac tumor removal, valve procedures, coronary artery repairs, coronary bypass graft procedures, and cardiac anomaly, aortic aneurysm, and pulmonary artery repairs. In addition, the insertion of temporary cardiac electrode or pacemaker catheters, thoracotomy, and thoracostomy are included in these procedures and not separately reported.

PATIENT-ACTIVATED EVENT RECORDER (33282, 33284)

33282   Implantation of patient-activated cardiac event recorder

CPT Assistant Nov 99:17-18, Jul 00:5, Jun 08:14; *CPT Changes: An Insider's View* 2000

33284   Removal of an implantable, patient-activated cardiac event recorder

CPT Assistant Nov 99:17-18, Jul 00:5; *CPT Changes: An Insider's View* 2000

Intent and Use of Codes 33282 and 33284

Codes **33282** and **33284** describe the implantation and removal of a patient-activated or auto-triggered implantable cardiac event recorder. The implantable loop recorder is a technology capable of extending the cardiac monitoring period sufficiently to address infrequent, recurrent symptoms. Implantable loop recorders are used for transient cardiac symptoms such as difficult-to-diagnose syncope that is infrequent, recurrent, and unexplained. In these cases, the physician seeks to document the heart rhythm coincident with the patient's symptoms. Implantable loop recorders may also be programmed to auto-trigger the recording of asymptomatic arrhythmias such as atrial fibrillation. Implanting and explanting an insertable loop recorder is very similar to the implantation of a pacemaker pulse generator, without leads, as medically necessary for patients requiring longer-term cardiac monitoring.

> **CODING TIP** Code **33282** includes the initial programming of the device. For subsequent or periodic electronic analysis, as well as any necessary reprogramming, use codes **93285**, **93291**, **93298**, and **93299**.

Description of Service for Code 33282

The patient is prepared for the procedure using standard, sterile technique, and the surgical site and surrounding area are cleaned with an antimicrobial agent. Drapes are placed to create a sterile field. The patient may require administration of moderate sedation. Local anesthetic is injected into the skin and subcutaneous tissue, and a 2-cm incision is made down to the subcutaneous fat. Additional local anesthetic is placed in the subcutaneous plane as needed for patient comfort during the procedure. Using blunt dissection, a subcutaneous pocket the size and shape of the recording device is created deeply enough to improve patient comfort and reduce the risk for skin erosion of the device. Hemostasis is maintained using standard techniques. The device is then inserted into the pocket. The ECG signal quality and amplitude are verified by placing the programmer head in a sterile sleeve over the recorder, establishing telemetry. The waveform is evaluated on the programmer screen, and the gain is adjusted to optimize waveform amplitude. The device may require repositioning or orientation within the pocket until adequate signal amplitude is achieved. Once the signal amplitude is satisfactory, the device is sutured to the adjacent underlying tissue using nonabsorbable sutures through the anchoring suture holes in the device to prevent rotation or migration following implantation. The incision is then closed with subcuticular absorbable sutures and a cutaneous nonabsorbable suture. The wound is dressed, the device is programmed using a pacemaker programmer, and record is initiated.

Description of Service for Code 33284

The patient is prepared for the procedure using standard, sterile technique. The surgical site and surrounding area are cleaned and prepared with an antimicrobial solution, and drapes are placed to create a sterile field. The patient may require moderate sedation. Local anesthetic is injected into the skin and subcutaneous fat, and the previously created pocket that contains the device is opened. The sutures anchoring the recorder to the subcutaneous tissue are cut, and the device is removed from the pocket. The pocket is then flushed with an antimicrobial solution and closed with subcuticular absorbable sutures and a subcutaneous nonabsorbable suture. The wound is dressed.

VENOUS GRAFTING ONLY FOR CORONARY ARTERY BYPASS (**33510-33516**)

33510 Coronary artery bypass, vein only; single coronary venous graft
CPT Assistant Fall 91:5, Winter 92:12, Jul 99:11, Apr 01:7, Feb 05:14, Jan 07:7, Mar 07:1

33511 2 coronary venous grafts
CPT Assistant Fall 91:5, Winter 92:12, Jul 99:11, Apr 01:7, Feb 05:14, Jan 07:7, Mar 07:1

33512 3 coronary venous grafts
CPT Assistant Fall 91:5, Winter 92:12, Apr 01:7, Feb 05:14, Jan 07:7, Mar 07:1

33513 4 coronary venous grafts
CPT Assistant Fall 91:5, Winter 92:12, Apr 01:7, Feb 05:14, Jan 07:7, Mar 07:1

33514 5 coronary venous grafts
CPT Assistant Fall 91:5, Winter 92:12, Apr 01:7, Feb 05:14, Jan 07:7, Mar 07:1

33516 6 or more coronary venous grafts
CPT Assistant Fall 91:5, Winter 92:12, Jul 99:11, Apr 01:7, Feb 05:14, Jan 07:7, Mar 07:1

Intent and Use of Codes 33510-33516

According to the CPT guidelines, codes **33510-33516** are used to report coronary artery bypass procedures using venous grafts only. These codes should not be used to report the performance of coronary artery bypass procedures using arterial grafts and venous

FIGURE 3-11. Coronary Artery Bypass—Venous Grafting Only

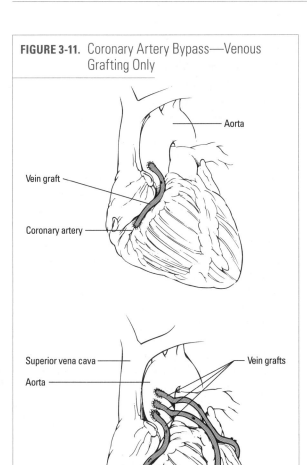

Aorta

Vein graft

Coronary artery

Superior vena cava

Aorta

Vein grafts

grafts during the same procedure. See codes **33517-33523** and codes **33533-33536** for reporting combined arterial venous grafts.

Procurement of the saphenous vein graft is included in the description of the work for codes **33510-33516** and should not be reported as a separate service or co-surgery. To report harvesting of an upper extremity vein, report code **35500** in addition to the bypass procedure. To report the harvesting of a femoropopliteal vein segment, report code **35572** in addition to the bypass procedure. When surgical assistant performs graft procurement, add **modifier 80** to codes **33510-33516**.

Some patients do not have a lower extremity vein available for harvest (such as the greater saphenous or lesser saphenous veins). To provide a graft long enough to use for the replacement, the patient may require that the physician perform either a multiple-site, autogenous vein harvest, or a single arm autogenous vein harvest procedure.

Codes **33510-33516** represent a bypass operation performed using *only saphenous veins* reported with a *single code* reflecting the number of grafts used. For example, triple bypass using only saphenous veins is reported with code **33512**.

Description of Service for Code 33510

A standard sternotomy skin incision is performed. The sternum is divided in the midline with the reciprocating saw. The sternal edges are assessed for hemostasis and cauterized; bone wax or Vancomycin paste is placed, if indicated. The pericardium is incised. Pericardial retraction sutures are placed. The aorta is inspected for signs of atherosclerosis with determination of the cannulation site. The appropriate cannulas are determined based on anatomy and patient body surface area. Systemic heparin is administered, and place purse string sutures are placed in the aorta and right atrium. Discussion with the anesthesiologist and/or perfusionist occurs regarding activated clotting time to assess level of heparinization. Cannulas are inserted for cardiopulmonary bypass in the aorta and the right atrium. Cardiopulmonary bypass is initiated with inspection of the aorta for signs of dissection. Systemic cooling is initiated. Antegrade and retrograde (if necessary) cardioplegia cannulas are placed if cardiac arrest is planned.

Cross-clamping of the aorta and administration of cardioplegia and topical hypothermia are performed. The vessel to be grafted is exposed with assessment of vessel quality. The location area for arteriotomy is identified based on knowledge of arteriogram and appearance of vessel. Coronary arteriotomy is performed. End-to-side vein graft anastomosis is performed to target coronary vessel using fine monofilament suture and optical magnification. The vein graft is perfused with cardioplegia solution checking that suture line is hemostatic. Measurement of the vein for appropriate length is performed, and the vein is cut. The aortic cross-clamp is removed taking care to avoid cerebral air embolus. Partial occlusion aortic clamp is applied. (This step may be omitted if proximal anastomosis is to be performed with the cross-clamp in place.) The area at which to perform proximal anastomosis is selected based on echocardiographic appearance of aorta and direct examination. A small aortotomy is performed. Aortotomy is enlarged with aortic punch. End-to-side proximal vein graft anastomosis is performed with fine monofilament suture and optical magnification. A small clamp is placed on the vein graft. The aortic clamp is removed, and the vein graft is de-aired. The vein graft clamp is also removed.

Resuscitation of the heart is performed by allowing it to beat while unloaded on cardiopulmonary bypass. Once all suture lines are hemostatic, which requires elevating the heart from the pericardium and placing additional sutures if there are anastomotic leaks, temporary pacing wires are placed, and atrial, atrioventricular, or ventricular pacing is started, if indicated. Cardiopulmonary bypass is discontinued by reducing arterial flow and retarding venous return to pump while hemodynamics are continuously monitored with arterial and pulmonary artery lines. The post-procedure, intra-operative echocardiogram is evaluated, with particular attention paid to ventricular function and regional wall motion abnormalities.

When the patient is stable, protamine is administered, and the arterial and venous cannulas are removed. The cannulation, vent, and cardioplegia sites are repaired with additional sutures. The wound is irrigated with saline with or without antibiotics. When hemostasis is adequate, the pericardial is placed and, if necessary, pleural drains are placed through separate small incisions. The sternum is re-approximated with multiple stainless steel wires twisted to "just tight." The fascia, subcutaneous tissues, and skin are closed in multiple layers with absorbable suture. The leg and arm incisions are closed in multiple layers with absorbable suture, and drains are inserted as needed through separate incisions.

Description of Service for Code 33511

A standard sternotomy skin incision is performed. The sternum is divided in the midline with the reciprocating saw. The sternal edges are assessed for hemostasis and cauterized; bone wax or Vancomycin paste is placed, if indicated. The pericardium is incised. Pericardial retraction sutures are placed. The aorta is inspected for signs of atherosclerosis with determination of the cannulation site. The appropriate cannulas are determined based on anatomy and patient body surface area. Systemic heparin is administered, and place purse string sutures are placed in the aorta and right atrium. Discussion with the anesthesiologist and/or perfusionist occurs regarding activated clotting time to assess level of heparinization. Cannulas are inserted for cardiopulmonary bypass in the aorta and the right atrium. Cardiopulmonary bypass is initiated with inspection of the aorta for signs of dissection. Systemic cooling is initiated. Antegrade and retrograde (if necessary) cardioplegia cannulas are placed if cardiac arrest is planned. Cross-clamping of the aorta and administration of cardioplegia and topical hypothermia are performed. The vessel to be grafted is exposed with assessment of vessel quality. The location area for arteriotomy is identified based on knowledge of arteriogram and appearance of vessel. Coronary arteriotomy is performed. End-to-side proximal vein graft anastomoses are performed using fine monofilament suture and optical magnification. A small clamp is placed on the vein grafts. The aortic clamp is removed, and the vein grafts is de-aired. The vein graft clamps are removed.

Resuscitation of the heart is performed by allowing it to beat while unloaded on cardiopulmonary bypass. Once all suture lines are hemostatic, which requires elevating the heart from the pericardium and placing additional sutures if there are anastomotic leaks, temporary pacing wires are placed, and atrial, atrioventricular, or ventricular pacing is started, if indicated. Cardiopulmonary bypass is discontinued by reducing arterial flow and retarding venous return to pump while hemodynamics are continuously monitored with arterial and pulmonary artery lines. The post-procedure, intra-operative echocardiogram is evaluated with particular attention paid to ventricular function and regional wall motion abnormalities.

When the patient is stable, protamine is administered, and the arterial and venous cannulas are removed. The cannulation, vent, and cardioplegia sites are repaired with additional sutures. The wound is irrigated with saline with or without antibiotics. When hemostasis is adequate, the pericardial is placed and, if necessary, pleural drains are placed through separate small incisions. The sternum is reapproximated with multiple stainless steel wires twisted to "just tight." The fascia, subcutaneous tissues, and skin are closed in multiple layers with absorbable suture and drains as needed inserted through separate incisions.

Description of Service for Code 33512

Same as for code **33511**, but with placement of 3 coronary venous grafts.

Description of Service for Code 33513

Same as for code **33511**, but with placement of 4 coronary venous grafts.

Description of Service for Code 33514

Same as for code **33511**, but with placement of 5 coronary venous grafts.

Description of Service for Code 33516

Same as for code **33511**, but with placement of 6 or more coronary venous grafts.

COMBINED ARTERIAL-VENOUS GRAFTING FOR CORONARY BYPASS (**+33517-+33530**)

+33517 Coronary artery bypass, using venous graft(s) and arterial graft(s); single vein graft (List separately in addition to code for primary procedure)

CPT Assistant Fall 91:5, Winter 92:13, Nov 99:18, Apr 01:7, Feb 05:14; *CPT Changes: An Insider's View* 2000, 2008

+33518 2 venous grafts (List separately in addition to code for primary procedure)

CPT Assistant Fall 91:5, Winter 92:13, Apr 01:7, Feb 05:14, Jan 07:7, Mar 07:1; *CPT Changes: An Insider's View* 2008

+33519 3 venous grafts (List separately in addition to code for primary procedure)

CPT Assistant Fall 91:5, Winter 92:13, Apr 01:7, Feb 05:14, Jan 07:7, Mar 07:1; *CPT Changes: An Insider's View* 2008

+33521 4 venous grafts (List separately in addition to code for primary procedure)

CPT Assistant Fall 91:5, Winter 92:13, Apr 01:7, Feb 05:14, Jan 07:7, Mar 07:1; *CPT Changes: An Insider's View* 2008

+33522 5 venous grafts (List separately in addition to code for primary procedure)

CPT Assistant Fall 91:5, Winter 92:13, Apr 01:7, Feb 05:14, Jan 07:7, Mar 07:1; *CPT Changes: An Insider's View* 2008

+33523 6 or more venous grafts (List separately in addition to code for primary procedure)

CPT Assistant Fall 91:5, Winter 92:13, Apr 01:7, Feb 05:14, Jan 07:7, Mar 07:1; *CPT Changes: An Insider's View* 2008

+33530 Reoperation, coronary artery bypass procedure or valve procedure, more than 1 month after original operation (List separately in addition to code for primary procedure)

CPT Assistant Winter 90:6, Fall 91:5, Winter 92:13, Apr 01:7, Jul 01:11, Feb 05:13-14, Jan 07:7

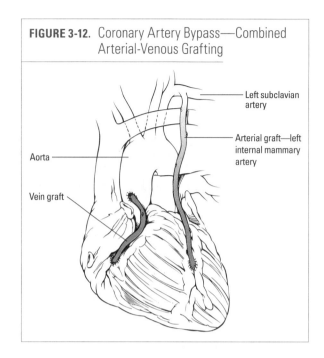

FIGURE 3-12. Coronary Artery Bypass—Combined Arterial-Venous Grafting

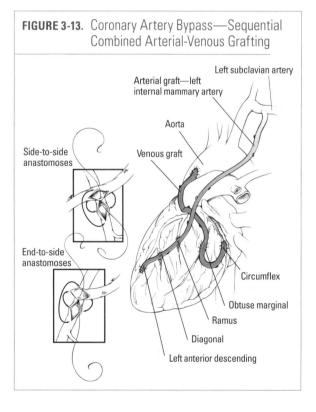

FIGURE 3-13. Coronary Artery Bypass—Sequential Combined Arterial-Venous Grafting

Intent and Use of Codes 33517-33530

According to CPT guidelines, the following codes are used to report coronary artery bypass procedures using venous grafts and arterial grafts during the same procedure. These codes may **not** be used alone.

To report combined arterial-venous grafts it is necessary to report two codes: (1) the appropriate combined arterial-venous graft code (**33517-33523**); and (2) the appropriate arterial graft code (**33533-33536**).

Procurement of the saphenous vein graft is included in the description of the work for codes **33517-33523** and should not be reported as a separate service or co-surgery. Procurement of the artery for grafting is included in the description of the work for codes **33533-33536** and should not be reported as a separate service or co-surgery, except when an upper extremity artery (eg, radial artery) is procured. To report harvesting of an upper extremity artery, report code **35600** in addition to the bypass procedure. To report harvesting of an upper extremity vein, report code **35500** in addition to the bypass procedure. To report harvesting of a femoro-popliteal vein segment, report code **35572** in addition to the bypass procedure. When a surgical assistant performs the arterial and/or venous graft procurement, add **modifier 80** to codes **33517-33523** and **33533-33536**, as appropriate.

The combined arterial-venous graft codes indicate that both arteries and veins were used and describe the number of venous anastomoses. To determine the number of bypass grafts in a coronary artery bypass, count the number of distal anastomoses (contact point[s]) where the bypass graft artery or vein is sutured to the diseased coronary artery(s).

For example, for a quadruple bypass using two saphenous veins, one internal mammary artery, and one gastroepiploic artery should be reported using codes **33518** and **33534**, *Coronary artery bypass, using arterial graft(s); 2 coronary arterial grafts*. Use of the combination code (**33518**) signals to the payer that both venous and arterial grafts were used and gives the number of vein grafts used. It also tells the payer that a second code has been entered, which will indicate the number of arterial grafts. Reporting of coronary bypass procedures must be done this way or the procedural coding will likely be rejected by certain third-party payers' computers.

Description of Service for Code +33517

Additional operative time is required to identify an additional coronary target vessel. Open the artery, tailor the vein end, and construct a hemostatic anastomosis. Probe the coronary/graft anastomosis to ensure patency. Perform a controlled aortotomy in an area of relatively normal aorta. Construct a hemostatic proximal aortograft anastomosis after tailoring the proximal end of the vein and ensuring that there will be appropriate graft length when the heart is full, beating, and working. Carefully inspect both proximal and distal anastomoses for hemostasis, and assess graft inflow and outflow characteristics before terminating cardiopulmonary bypass and before concluding the operation. Leg and incisions are closed with absorbable suture and drains as needed.

> **CODING TIP** When an upper extremity vein harvest is required, add-on code **35500** should be reported in addition to the coronary artery bypass graft procedure codes **33510-33536**.

Description of Service for Codes +33518-33523

Additional operative time is required to identify each additional coronary target vessel. Open each artery, tailor the vein end, and construct a hemostatic anastomosis. Probe the coronary/graft anastomosis to ensure patency. Perform a controlled aortotomy for each graft in an area of relatively normal aorta. Construct a hemostatic proximal aortograft anastomosis after tailoring the proximal end of each vein and ensuring that there will be appropriate graft lengths when the heart is full, beating, and working. Carefully inspect all proximal and distal anastomoses for hemostasis, and assess graft inflow and outflow characteristics before terminating cardiopulmonary bypass and before concluding the operation. Close the leg and incisions with absorbable suture and drains as needed.

Description of Service for Code +33530

Add-on code **33530** is reported in addition to the base procedure code (eg, coronary artery bypass graft or valve). Expose femoral vessels if indicated. Bring cardiopulmonary bypass lines onto field before the incision is made. Make a standard sternotomy skin incision. Divide the sternum in the midline with the oscillating saw.

Using cautery and sharp and blunt dissection, free adhesions from the chest wall. Isolate right ventricle, right atrium, and aorta from the surrounding adhesions. Take special care not to disturb the patent, but potentially diseased bypass grafts, or injure the cardiac structures. Cannulate in standard fashion or using femoral vessels if indicated. Complete the dissection after initiating cardiopulmonary bypass. Dissection may be accomplished with additional cardioplegic arrest when severe adhesions are present or if the old grafts are severely diseased. (Retrograde cardioplegia administration is standard.)

ARTERIAL GRAFTING FOR CORONARY ARTERY BYPASS (33533-33536)

33533   Coronary artery bypass, using arterial graft(s); single arterial graft
CPT Assistant Winter 92:12, Nov 99:18, Apr 01:7, Feb 05:14, Jan 07:7, Mar 07:1; *CPT Changes: An Insider's View* 2000

33534   2 coronary arterial grafts
CPT Assistant Winter 92:12, Apr 01:7, Feb 05:14, Jan 07:7, Mar 07:1

33535   3 coronary arterial grafts
CPT Assistant Winter 92:12, Apr 01:7, Feb 05:14, Jan 07:7, Mar 07:1

33536   4 or more coronary arterial grafts
CPT Assistant Winter 92:12, Apr 01:7, Feb 05:14, Jan 07:7, Mar 07:1

Intent and Use of Codes 33533-33536

According to CPT guidelines, the following codes are used to report coronary artery bypass procedures using either arterial grafts only or a combination of arterial-venous grafts. The codes include the use of the internal mammary artery, gastroepiploic artery, epigastric artery, radial artery, and arterial conduits procured from other sites.

To report combined arterial-venous grafts it is necessary to report two codes: (1) the appropriate arterial graft code (33533-33536); and (2) the appropriate combined arterial-venous graft code (33517-33523).

Procurement of the artery for grafting is included in the description of the work for codes 33533-33536 and should not be reported as a separate service or co-surgery, except when an upper extremity artery (eg, radial artery) is procured. To report harvesting of an upper extremity artery, report code 35600 in addition to the bypass procedure. To report harvesting of an upper extremity vein, report code 35500 in addition to the bypass procedure. To report harvesting of a femoro-popliteal vein segment, report code 35572 in addition to the bypass procedure. When a surgical assistant performs the arterial and/or venous graft procurement, add **modifier 80** to codes 33517-33523 and 33533-33536, as appropriate.

A bypass operation performed using only internal mammary arteries or other arteries should be reported with a single code, reflecting the number of grafts used. For example, for a double bypass using internal mammary arteries, code 33534 would be reported for the two-vessel bypass using arteries as the bypass conduit.

Description of Service for Code 33534

A standard sternotomy skin incision is made. The sternum is divided in the midline with the reciprocating saw. The sternal edges are assessed for hemostasis and cauterized with bone wax or Vancomycin paste, if indicated. The left side of the sternum is retracted for the planned left internal mammary artery (LIMA) harvest. The LIMA is assessed by palpation. Electrocautery is used to incise the endothoracic fascia and muscle on the chest wall creating a line 1.5 to 2.0 cm on each side of the LIMA. The LIMA is dissected using electrocautery, and clips are applied to the vessel branches on the LIMA. The LIMA integrity and presence of pulse are continually palpated and assessed. The left pleura is opened as necessary, with the lung retracted with a lap pad, if necessary. The proximal and distal extent of the LIMA dissection is assessed upon completion. Systemic heparin is administered. The chest wall is assessed for bleeding and cauterized as necessary. The LIMA is divided distally, the flow assessed, and the end of the LIMA clipped to allow continued pulsatile pressure within the lumen. The LIMA is wrapped in a papaverine-soaked sponge. The pericardium is incised. Pericardial retraction sutures are placed. The aorta is inspected for signs of atherosclerosis, and the cannulation site is determined. The appropriate cannulas to use are determined based on anatomy and patient body surface area. Purse string sutures are placed in the aorta and right atrium. The anesthesiologist and/or perfusionist is consulted regarding the activated clotting time value to assess level of heparinization. Cannulas for cardiopulmonary bypass are inserted in the aorta and the right atrium. The LIMA is prepared, and the flow reassessed. Cardiopulmonary bypass is initiated, and the aorta is inspected for signs of dissection. Systemic cooling is initiated. Initial inspection of target site on coronary artery is performed and marked with ink. Antegrade and retrograde (if necessary) cardioplegia cannulas are placed if cardiac arrest is planned. The aorta is cross-clamped, and cardioplegia and topical hypothermia are administered. The effectiveness of cardioplegia is assessed based on the arrest of the heart and the temperature probe in the ventricular septum. Septal temperature is maintained below 15 degrees Centigrade. Cardioplegia is repeated every 20 minutes or as necessary while the cross-clamp is in place. The vessel to be grafted is exposed. The vessel quality is assessed, and the area for the arteriotomy is located based on knowledge of the arteriogram and the appearance of the vessel. The coronary arteriotomy is performed. The pericardium is incised to allow the LIMA to reach the target vessel. An end-to-side LIMA anastomosis is performed to target the coronary vessel using fine monofilament suture and optical magnification. The cross-clamp is removed, taking care to avoid cerebral air embolus. Tacking sutures are placed to anchor the LIMA along the target vessel. The heart is resuscitated by allowing it to beat while unloaded on cardiopulmonary bypass. All suture lines are assessed to ensure they are hemostatic—this requires elevating the heart from the pericardium and placing additional sutures if there are anastomotic leaks. Temporary pacing wires are placed, and atrial, atrio-ventricular, or ventricular pacing is started, if indicated. Cardiopulmonary bypass is discontinued by reducing arterial flow and retarding venous return to pump while continuously monitoring hemodynamics with arterial and pulmonary artery lines. The post-procedure, intra-operative echocardiogram is evaluated, specifically examining for ventricular function and regional wall motion abnormalities. When the patient is stable, protamine is administered, and the arterial and venous cannulas are removed. The cannulation, vent, and cardioplegia sites are repaired with additional sutures. The wound is irrigated with saline with or without antibiotics. The pleural space(s) is checked for blood as appropriate, and the chest wall is assessed for bleeding at the LIMA site. When hemostasis is adequate, pericardial and, if necessary, pleural drains are placed through separate small incisions. The sternum is re-approximated with multiple stainless steel wires twisted to "just tight." The fascia, subcutaneous tissues, and skin are closed in multiple layers with absorbable suture.

Description of Service for Code 33535

A standard sternotomy skin incision is made. The sternum is divided in the midline with the reciprocating saw. The sternal edges are assessed for hemostasis and cauterized with bone wax or Vancomycin paste, if indicated. The left side of the sternum is retracted for the planned left internal mammary artery (LIMA) harvest. The LIMA is assessed by palpation. Electrocautery is used to incise the endothoracic fascia and muscle on the chest wall creating a line 1.5 to 2.0 cm on each side of the LIMA. The LIMA is dissected using electrocautery, and clips are applied to the vessel branches on the LIMA. The LIMA integrity and presence of pulse is continually palpated and assessed. The left pleura is opened as necessary, with the lung retracted with a lap pad, if necessary. The right side of the sternum is retracted for the planned right internal mammary artery (RIMA) harvest. The RIMA is assessed by

palpation. Electrocautery is used to incise the endothoracic fascia and muscle on the chest wall creating a line 1.5 to 2.0 cm on each side of the RIMA. The RIMA is dissected using electrocautery, and clips are applied to the vessel branches on the RIMA. RIMA integrity and presence of pulse is continually palpated and assessed. The right pleura is opened, as necessary, retracting the lung if necessary with a lap pad. The proximal and distal extent of the RIMA dissection is assessed when completed. The chest wall is assessed for bleeding and is cauterized as necessary. The RIMA is divided distally, flow assessed, and the end of the RIMA is clipped to allow continued pulsatile pressure within the lumen. The RIMA is wrapped in a papaverine-soaked sponge. The pericardium is incised. Pericardial retraction sutures are placed. The aorta is inspected for signs of atherosclerosis, and the cannulation site is determined. The appropriate cannulas are determined for use based on anatomy and patient body surface area. Purse string sutures are placed in the aorta and right atrium. The anesthesiologist and/or perfusionist is consulted regarding the activated clotting time value to assess the level of heparinization. Cannulas for cardiopulmonary bypass are inserted in the aorta and the right atrium. The LIMA is prepared and the flow is re-assessed. Cardiopulmonary bypass is initiated, and the aorta is inspected for signs of dissection. Systemic cooling is initiated. An initial inspection of the target sites on the coronary arteries is performed, and the sites are marked with ink. Antegrade and retrograde (if necessary) cardioplegia cannulas are placed if cardiac arrest is planned. The aorta is cross-clamped, and cardioplegia and topical hypothermia are administered. The effectiveness of the cardioplegia is assessed based on arrest of heart and temperature probe in ventricular septum. Septal temperature is maintained below 15 degrees Centigrade. Cardioplegia is repeated every 20 minutes or as necessary while the cross-clamp is in place. The vessel to be grafted is exposed. Vessel quality is assessed, and the area for arteriotomy is located based on knowledge of the arteriogram and the appearance of the vessel. Coronary arteriotomy is performed. The pericardium is incised to allow the LIMA to reach target vessel. An end-to-side LIMA anastomosis is performed to target the coronary vessel using fine monofilament suture and optical magnification. The additional vessel to be grafted is exposed. Vessel quality is assessed, and the area for arteriotomy is located based on knowledge of the arteriogram and the appearance of the vessel. Coronary arteriotomy is performed. The pericardium is incised to allow the RIMA to reach the target vessel. An end-to-side RIMA anastomosis is performed to the target coronary vessel using fine monofilament suture and optical magnification. The cross-clamp is removed taking care to avoid cerebral air embolus. Tacking sutures are placed to anchor the RIMA along the target vessel. The additional vessel to be grafted is exposed. Vessel quality is assessed, and the area for arteriotomy is assessed based on knowledge of the arteriogram and the appearance of the vessel. The coronary arteriotomy is performed. A side-to-side LIMA anastomosis is performed to target the coronary vessel using fine monofilament suture and optical magnification. The heart is resuscitated by allowing it to beat while unloaded on cardiopulmonary bypass. All suture lines are assessed to ensure they are hemostatic—this requires elevating the heart from the pericardium and placing additional sutures if there are anastomotic leaks. Temporary pacing wires are placed with onset of atrial, atrio-ventricular, or ventricular pacing if indicated. Cardiopulmonary bypass is discontinued by reducing arterial flow and retarding venous return to pump while continuously monitoring hemodynamics with arterial and pulmonary artery lines. The post-procedure, intra-operative echocardiogram is evaluated, specifically examining for ventricular function and regional wall motion abnormalities. When the patient is stable, protamine is administered, and the arterial and venous cannulas are removed. The cannulation, vent, and cardioplegia sites are repaired with additional sutures. The wound is irrigated with saline with or without antibiotics. The pleural space(s) is checked for blood as appropriate, and the chest wall is assessed for bleeding at the RIMA site. When hemostasis is adequate, pericardial and, if necessary, pleural drains are placed through separate small incisions. The sternum is re-approximated with multiple stainless steel wires twisted to "just tight." The fascia, subcutaneous tissues, and skin are closed in multiple layers with absorbable suture.

Description of Service for Code 33536

A standard sternotomy skin incision is made. The sternum is divided in the midline with the reciprocating saw. The sternal edges are assessed for hemostasis and cauterized with bone wax or Vancomycin paste, if indicated. The left side of the sternum is retracted for the planned left internal mammary artery (LIMA) harvest. The LIMA is assessed by palpation. Electrocautery is used to incise the endothoracic fascia and muscle on the chest wall creating a line of 1.5 to 2.0 cm on each side of the LIMA. The LIMA is dissected using electrocautery, and clips are applied to the vessel branches on the LIMA. The LIMA integrity and presence of pulse is continually palpated and assessed. The left pleura is opened as necessary, with the lung retracted, if necessary, with a lap pad. The right side of the sternum is retracted for the planned right internal mammary artery (RIMA) harvest. The RIMA is assessed by palpation. Electrocautery is used to incise the endothoracic fascia and muscle on the chest wall creating

a line 1.5 to 2.0 cm on each side of the RIMA. The RIMA is dissected using electrocautery, and clips are applied to the vessel branches on the RIMA. RIMA integrity and presence of pulse is continually palpated and assessed. The right pleura is opened, as necessary, retracting the lung if necessary with a lap pad. The proximal and distal extent of the RIMA dissection is assessed when completed. The chest wall is assessed for bleeding and is cauterized as necessary. The RIMA is divided distally, flow assessed, and the end of the RIMA is clipped to allow continued pulsatile pressure within the lumen. The RIMA is wrapped in a papaverine-soaked sponge. The pericardium is incised. Pericardial retraction sutures are placed. The aorta is inspected for signs of atherosclerosis, and the cannulation site is determined. The appropriate cannulas are determined for use based on anatomy and patient body surface area. Purse string sutures are placed in the aorta and right atrium. The anesthesiologist and/or perfusionist is consulted regarding the activated clotting time value to assess level of heparinization. Cannulas for cardiopulmonary bypass are inserted in the aorta and the right atrium. The LIMA is prepared and the flow re-assessed. Cardiopulmonary bypass is initiated, and the aorta is inspected for signs of dissection. Systemic cooling is initiated. An initial inspection of the target sites on the coronary arteries is performed, and the sites marked with ink. Antegrade and retrograde (if necessary) cardioplegia cannulas are placed if cardiac arrest is planned. The aorta is cross-clamped, and cardioplegia and topical hypothermia are administered. The effectiveness of cardioplegia is assessed based on arrest of heart and temperature probe in ventricular septum. Septal temperature is maintained below 15 degrees Centigrade. Cardioplegia is repeated every 20 minutes or as necessary while the cross-clamp is in place. The vessel to be grafted is exposed. Vessel quality is assessed, and the area for arteriotomy located based on knowledge of the arteriogram and the appearance of the vessel. Coronary arteriotomy is performed. The pericardium is incised to allow the LIMA to reach the target vessel. An end-to-side LIMA anastomosis is performed to target the coronary vessel using fine monofilament suture and optical magnification. The additional vessel to be grafted is exposed. Vessel quality is assessed, and the area for arteriotomy is located based on knowledge of the arteriogram and the appearance of the vessel. Coronary arteriotomy is performed. The pericardium is incised to allow the RIMA to reach the target vessel. An end-to-side RIMA anastomosis is performed to target the coronary vessel using fine monofilament suture and optical magnification. The cross-clamp is removed taking care to avoid cerebral air embolus. Tacking sutures are placed to anchor the RIMA along the target vessel. The additional vessel to be grafted is exposed. Vessel quality is assessed, and the area for arteriotomy is assessed based on knowledge of the arteriogram and the appearance of the vessel. The coronary arteriotomy is performed. A side-to-side RIMA anastomosis is performed to target the coronary vessel using fine monofilament suture and optical magnification. The heart is resuscitated by allowing it to beat while unloaded on cardiopulmonary bypass. All suture lines are assessed to ensure they are hemostatic—this requires elevating the heart from the pericardium and placing additional sutures if there are anastomotic leaks. Temporary pacing wires are placed with onset of atrial, atrio-ventricular, or ventricular pacing if indicated. Cardiopulmonary bypass is discontinued by reducing arterial flow and retarding venous return to pump while continuously monitoring hemodynamics with arterial and pulmonary artery lines. The post-procedure, intra-operative echocardiogram is evaluated, specifically examining for ventricular function and regional wall motion abnormalities. When the patient is stable, protamine is administered, and the arterial and venous cannulas are removed. The cannulation, vent, and cardioplegia sites are repaired with additional sutures. The wound is irrigated with saline with or without antibiotics. The pleural space(s) is checked for blood as appropriate, and the chest wall is assessed for bleeding at the RIMA site. When hemostasis is adequate, the pericardial and, if necessary, pleural drains are placed through separate small incisions. The sternum is re-approximated with multiple stainless steel wires twisted to "just tight." The fascia, subcutaneous tissues, and skin are closed in multiple layers with absorbable suture.

Complex Cardiac Anomalies

The CPT codes most often used by pediatric cardiologists include some that are commonly used by adult cardiologists as well as some that are unique to pediatric cardiology. In the last 15 years, a number of cardiology services codes designed to be used in reporting on the diagnosis and management of patients with congenital heart disease have been created. The code descriptions and related relative value unit (RVU) assignments are primarily based on the care of pediatric patients, but they may be applied to adults whose primary cardiovascular disease is related to congenital heart disease. Many insurance programs, both public (eg, Medicaid) and private, have adopted the relative value scale used by Medicare, necessitating re-evaluation of the RVU assignment for services provided to children as well as adults.

The work relative value units in the Resource-Based Relative Value Scale (RBRVS) are intended to reflect the typical patient treated by the typical doctor, based on the premise that while any specific patient may not be typical, such inequities are corrected by the broad experience of an individual physician's practice. Such an assumption creates obvious problems for the physician whose practice does not consist of typical adults. Therefore, appropriate valuation of the physician work effort involved in providing services for the typical pediatric patient requires different norms. In fact, physician work relative value units for many pediatric cardiology services have been demonstrated to be different from corresponding adult values. The American College of Cardiology is continuing efforts to obtain the appropriate recognition of all unique pediatric services. (Refer to Chapter 2 for additional information pertaining to pediatric cardiology E/M services.)

SINGLE VENTRICLE AND OTHER COMPLEX CARDIAC ANOMALIES (**33619-33622**)

33619 Repair of single ventricle with aortic outflow obstruction and aortic arch hypoplasia (hypoplastic left heart syndrome) (eg, Norwood procedure)
CPT Assistant Mar 07:1

33620 Application of right and left pulmonary artery bands (eg, hybrid approach stage 1)
CPT Assistant Apr 11:4, 6; *CPT Changes: An Insider's View* 2011

33621 Transthoracic insertion of catheter for stent placement with catheter removal and closure (eg, hybrid approach stage 1)
CPT Changes: An Insider's View 2011

33622 Reconstruction of complex cardiac anomaly (eg, single ventricle or hypoplastic left heart) with palliation of single ventricle with aortic outflow obstruction and aortic arch hypoplasia, creation of cavopulmonary anastomosis, and removal of right and left pulmonary bands (eg, hybrid approach stage 2, Norwood, bidirectional Glenn, pulmonary artery debanding)
CPT Changes: An Insider's View 2011

FIGURE 3-14. Hypoplastic Left Heart Syndrome

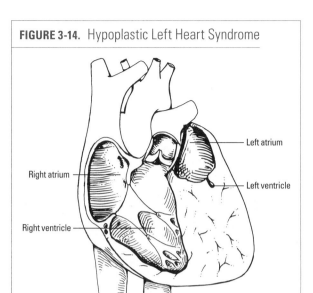

Right atrium

Left atrium

Left ventricle

Right ventricle

Intent and Use of Code 33619

In some cases, the extreme complexity of congenital anomalies cannot be described using standard ICD-9-CM diagnosis codes. Diagnosis coding is a crucial link in reporting complex congenital anomalies. In these cases, listing all applicable surgical and nonsurgical therapeutic procedure codes illustrates the complexity of the case. For example, there is no diagnostic code that describes a patient who has had a Norwood procedure, so this complex problem is best described by the methods used to treat it and the underlying defect. In this hypothetical case, reporting code **33619** for the Norwood procedure (ie, repair of single ventricle with aortic outflow obstruction, aortic arch hypoplasia), plus percutaneous balloon valvuloplasty for dilatation of pulmonary stenosis (**92990**) and/or aortic arch obstruction (**92986**) may adequately illustrate the complexity of the patient's disease and the high level of service required. The procedures performed will, of course, also be described in detail in the report that accompanies the claim. (Refer to Chapter 5 for additional information related to percutaneous therapeutic procedures.)

CODING TIP Do not report **modifier 63** in conjunction with code **33619**.

Description of Service for Code 33619

A skin incision is made via standard median sternotomy. The sternum is divided in the midline, and the pericardium is opened. Dissection of the pulmonary arteries and aortic arch brachiocephalic artery branches is performed. Cardiopulmonary bypass is initiated with occlusion of pulmonary arteries to prevent run-off into pulmonary circulation. The ductus arteriosus is ligated. Induction of deep hypothermia on bypass (ie, less than 20 degrees Centigrade) and induction of circulatory arrest and cardioplegic arrest of heart are performed. The main pulmonary artery is divided with oversewing of the distal orifice. Incision of the ascending aorta is made extending into the transverse arch and the descending aorta with excision of ductus arteriosus. The proximal main pulmonary artery is anastomosed to the aorta with patch augmentation of entire aortic arch and ascending aorta. A right atriotomy and atrial septectomy are performed. The heart is de-aired with reinstitution of cardiopulmonary bypass and rewarming. A right modified Blalock-Taussig shunt is constructed (see code **33750**). Atrial pressure monitoring catheters are inserted with institution of inotropic support. Atrial and ventricular pacing wires are placed. The patient is weaned from bypass with assessment of cardiac contraction and rhythm, blood pressure, atrial filling pressures, and oxygen saturations. The need for additional inotropic and/or vasoactive medications is assessed. Bypass cannulas are removed with repair of cannulation sites. Heparin is reversed by administering protamine. Chest tubes are placed. The cannulation, atriotomy, and ventriculotomy sites are inspected for bleeding; additional sutures are applied as necessary. The sternum is closed with wires if hemodynamically tolerated. The remaining layers are closed.

Intent and Use of Codes 33620-33622

A hybrid therapy or procedure is a mixture of therapies from different medical/surgical subspecialties. By definition, a hybrid cardiac procedure is a combination of surgical and catheter-based interventions to the heart combining the techniques of the interventional cardiologist with the cardiothoracic surgeon, electrophysiologists, echocardiographers, cardiac anesthesiologists, advanced-level nurse practitioners, physician assistants, cardiac catheterization lab nurses, operating room nurses, technicians, and perfusionists. The specialized hybrid cardiac operating suite is designed specifically for the cardiac surgical patient and can accommodate any cardiac surgical case, catheterization, or collaborative hybrid procedure.

Codes **33620-33622** represent operations that use a hybrid approach to treating neonates (Stage 1) and

10

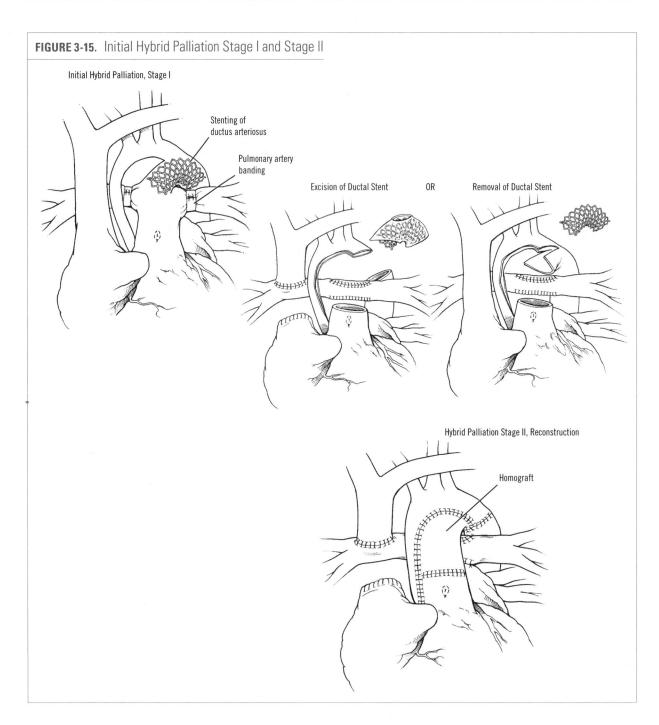

FIGURE 3-15. Initial Hybrid Palliation Stage I and Stage II

Initial Hybrid Palliation, Stage I

Stenting of
ductus arteriosus

Pulmonary artery
banding

Excision of Ductal Stent   OR   Removal of Ductal Stent

Hybrid Palliation Stage II, Reconstruction

Homograft

infants (Stage 2). All three procedures are generally performed on a patient but at different stages during the patient's development. Both aspects of the Stage 1 procedures (**33620, 33621**) represent techniques that are being used to treat congenital cardiac diseases. The techniques represented by codes **33620** and **33621** allow an alternate means of treatment of complex congenital anomalies, which includes various forms of single ventricle with obstruction to systemic blood flow.

The Stage 2 hybrid approach (**33622**) represents a procedure also reported using other individual codes

(**33619, 33767, 33822, 33840, 33845, 33851, 33853, 33917**). However, when these procedures are combined into a single session, the nature of the operation changes significantly due to the surgical complexity, surgical time, pre- and post-operative management, and risk for the patient. The combination of codes **33619, 33767,** and **33917** is representative of the work involved in the procedure when all three are performed in a single session. The complexity involved in this procedure is not accurately reflected by considering each of the components separately, given the magnitude of the operation and the associated technical challenges. Additional technical difficulties include the reoperative sternotomy and the removal of the stent from the arterial duct and the descending aorta.

> **CODING TIP** The hybrid procedures for the management of hypoplastic left heart syndrome should not be confused with "hybrid" coronary artery revascularization procedures (eg, coronary artery bypass graft and stenting).

Description of Service for Code 33620

Under general endotracheal anesthesia, in the supine position, the patient is prepared and draped in standard aseptic fashion. A skin incision is made via standard median sternotomy. The sternum is divided in the midline. A thymectomy is performed. The pericardium is opened, and the right and left branch pulmonary arteries are dissected and exposed. A band is placed around the left pulmonary artery, and then a second band is placed around the right pulmonary artery. Hemodynamic stability and oxygen saturation are assessed. Chest tubes and temporary pacing wires are placed. A pericardial substitute membrane is placed to aid in future median sternotomies. The sternum is closed with wires; the abdominal fascia, skin, and subcutaneous tissue are closed in layers. Sterile dressing is applied, and the patient is stabilized and transferred to the intensive care unit.

> **CODING TIP** For banding of the main pulmonary artery related to septal defect, code **33690** should be reported. Report both code **33620** and code **33621** if performed at the same session.

Description of Service for Code 33621

Under general endotracheal anesthesia, in the supine position, the patient is prepared and draped in standard aseptic fashion. A skin incision is made via standard median sternotomy. The sternum is divided in the midline. A thymectomy is performed. The pericardium is opened, and the anterior and ventricular surfaces at the ventricular outlet are dissected and exposed. Purse string sutures are placed in the anterior ventricular surface at the ventricular outlet. A catheter is placed through the purse string into the heart. Under fluoroscopic guidance, a guidewire is advanced through the catheter and the pulmonary valve into the patent ductus arteriosus. The surgeon stands by while the interventional cardiologist places the stent into the patent ductus arteriousus. Fluoroscopy is used to assess the adequacy of the stent position. Hemodynamic

stability and oxygen saturation are assessed and observed. Chest tubes and temporary pacing wires are placed. A pericardial substitute membrane is placed to aid in future median sternotomies. The sternum is closed with wires; the abdominal fascia, skin, and subcutaneous tissue are closed in layers. Sterile dressing is applied, and the patient is stabilized and transferred to the intensive care unit.

Description of Service for Code 33622

Under general endotracheal anesthesia, in the supine position, the patient is prepared and draped in standard aseptic fashion. A skin incision is made through the previous median sternotomy site. The sternum is divided in the midline. The old pericardial substitute membrane is removed. The right atrium, pulmonary artery, aortic arch, and ductus arteriosus are dissected and exposed. Cardiac cannulas are placed, and cardiopulmonary bypass is initiated. The ductus arteriosus is controlled, and the patient is cooled to 18° C for a period of 20 minutes on cardiopulmonary bypass. Tapes are placed around the superior vena cava and inferior vena cava while the patient is cooling. In addition, a complete dissection of the aortic arch, the innominate artery, the left carotid artery, the left subclavian artery, and the proximal descending thoracic aorta is performed preserving the left vagus, the left phrenic, and the left recurrent laryngeal nerves. The aorta is cross-clamped, and cold cardioplegic solution is infused into the aortic root. The right atrium is opened, and an atrial septectomy is performed. A vent is placed through the right atrium into the left atrium, and circulatory arrest is established. The ductal tissue is excised and the ductal stent removed. The main pulmonary artery distal to the pulmonary (neoaortic) valve is transected. The right and left branch pulmonary arteries are fully dissected and mobilized. The right pulmonary artery band is removed (PA debanding), and then the left pulmonary artery band is removed. The right pulmonary artery is opened where the superior cavopulmonary anastomosis will be created. The caliber of the branch pulmonary arteries is assessed, and they are probed. A patch pulmonary arteriolasty is performed, if necessary. The ascending to the descending aorta is opened, and the aortic arch is reconstructed. The ascending aorta is anastomosed to the proximal main pulmonary artery, and a neoaorta and "aortopulmonary amalgamation" is created. The aorta is recannulated, and cardiopulmonary bypass is reestablished. The atriotomy is now closed, air is evacuated from the cardiac chambers, and the cross-clamp is released. The patient is rewarmed to 28 degrees Centigrade. While rewarming, the superior vena cava is transected and oversewn at the cardiac end. The cranial end of the superior vena cava is anastomosed

CHAPTER 3

to the opening in the right pulmonary artery to create a superior cavopulmonary anastomosis. The patient is fully rewarmed and weaned from cardiopulmonary bypass. The cannulas are removed and the sites secured. Chest tubes and temporary pacing wires are placed. A pericardial substitute membrane is placed to aid in future median sternotomies. The sternum is closed with wires; the abdominal fascia, skin, and subcutaneous tissue are closed in layers. Sterile dressing is applied, and the patient is stabilized and transferred to the intensive care unit.

> **CODING TIP** Code **33622** may be reported with add-on code **33768** if a bilateral bidirectional Glenn is performed.

CATHETER- DELIVERED PROSTHETIC AORTIC VALVE REPLACEMENT (**0256T-0259T**)

0256T   Implantation of catheter-delivered prosthetic aortic heart valve; endovascular approach
CPT Changes: An Insider's View 2011

0257T   open thoracic approach (eg, transapical, transventricular)
CPT Changes: An Insider's View 2011

0258T   Transthoracic cardiac exposure (eg, sternotomy, thoracotomy, subxiphoid) for catheter-delivered aortic valve replacement; without cardiopulmonary bypass
CPT Changes: An Insider's View 2011

0259T   with cardiopulmonary bypass
CPT Changes: An Insider's View 2011

Intent and Use of Codes 0256T-0259T

Implantation of a catheter-delivered prosthetic aortic heart valve is represented by codes **0256T** and **0257T**. The endovascular approach is represented by code **0256T**. Code **0257T** describes the open thoracic approach. Other than diagnostic cardiac catheterization, codes **0256T** and **0257T** include all other catheterization(s), temporary pacing, intraprocedural contrast injection[s], fluoroscopic radiological supervision and interpretation, and imaging guidance, which are not reported separately when performed to complete the aortic valve procedure. When reporting code **0257T** for open thoracic implantation, transthoracic cardiac exposure is reported separately using code **0258T** or **0259T**, as appropriate.

The implantation of a prosthetic aortic heart valve through a transthoracic approach can be divided into an approach procedure and a therapeutic (valve implantation) procedure because two different physicians will often perform different parts of the procedure: a cardiothoracic surgeon to provide cardiac access and an interventional cardiologist to manipulate the wire and valve under fluoroscopy. Increasingly when peripheral access is inadequate, cardiac procedures involving the placement of an intracardiac prosthesis (ie, stent or valve) can be achieved though transthoracic cardiac exposure via a sternotomy, thoracotomy, or subxiphoid approach. Codes **0258T** and **0259T** for cardiac exposure facilitate the reporting of minimally invasive techniques that can be employed in the heart when peripheral access is not sufficient.

Codes **0258T** and **0259T** are used to report transthoracic cardiac exposure for the purpose of transcatheter-delivered aortic valve replacement. Code **0258T** describes the procedure without cardiopulmonary bypass. Code **0259T** describes the procedure with cardiopulmonary bypass.

> **CODING TIP** Codes **0256T** and **0257T** do not include cardiac catheterization (**93451-93572**) when performed at the time of the procedure for diagnostic purposes. Therefore, when performed, diagnostic cardiac catheterization should be reported separately using the appropriate code(s) from the **93451-93572** series.

Clinical Example for Code 0256T

A 75-year-old female with history of diabetes mellitus, chronic kidney disease, and chronic obstructive lung disease is on home oxygen. She has well-documented critical valvular aortic stenosis with estimated aortic valve orifice area of 0.5 cm². She has noted progressively worsening dyspnea on exertion despite stable lung disease. Of late she has become intermittently lightheaded when exerting herself and had one syncopal episode. Her cardiologist has recommended aortic valve replacement. She has been rejected for conventional open heart aortic valve replacement by two cardiovascular surgeons citing operative risks that outweigh the benefit. Implantation of catheter-delivered prosthetic aortic heart valve is performed using an endovascular approach.

Clinical Example for Code 0257T

A patient very similar to that described above for code 0256T has been rejected for conventional open heart surgery for aortic valve replacement by two cardiovascular surgeons citing operative risks that outweigh the benefit. Significant aortoiliac disease precludes transfemoral or transiliac vascular access. Implantation of catheter-delivered prosthetic aortic heart valve is performed using a transapical approach.

Clinical Example for Code 0258T

A patient very similar to that described above for code 0256T has been rejected for conventional open heart surgery for aortic valve replacement by two cardiovascular surgeons citing operative risks that outweigh the benefit. Significant aortoiliac disease precludes transfemoral or transiliac vascular access. Transthoracic cardiac exposure (0258T) is performed, which allows for implantation of catheter-delivered prosthetic aortic heart valve using a transapical approach (0257T).

Clinical Example for Code 0259T

A patient very similar to that described above for code 0256T has been rejected for conventional open heart surgery for aortic valve replacement by two cardiovascular surgeons citing operative risks that outweigh the benefit. Significant aortoiliac disease precludes transfemoral or transiliac vascular access. Transthoracic cardiac exposure with cardiopulmonary bypass (0259T) is performed, which allows for implantation of catheter-delivered prosthetic aortic heart valve using a transapical approach (0257T).

CARDIAC ASSIST—INTRA-AORTIC BALLOON ASSIST DEVICE (33967-33974)

33967   Insertion of intra-aortic balloon assist device, percutaneous
CPT Assistant Feb 02:2; *CPT Changes: An Insider's View* 2002

33968   Removal of intra-aortic balloon assist device, percutaneous
CPT Assistant Nov 99:19, Jan 00:10; *CPT Changes: An Insider's View* 2000

33970   Insertion of intra-aortic balloon assist device through the femoral artery, open approach
CPT Assistant Nov 99:19; *CPT Changes: An Insider's View* 2000

33971   Removal of intra-aortic balloon assist device including repair of femoral artery, with or without graft

33973   Insertion of intra-aortic balloon assist device through the ascending aorta

33974   Removal of intra-aortic balloon assist device from the ascending aorta, including repair of the ascending aorta, with or without graft

Intent and Use of Codes 33967-33974

Codes 33967-33974 represent procedures and approaches performed in association with insertion and removal of an intra-aortic balloon assist device (IABAD). An IABAD is intended to decrease the workload of the heart and increase blood flow to the heart and the rest of the body. The IABAD is used temporarily for emergency cardiac support conditions such as stabilization of patients with acute myocardial infarction referred for urgent cardiac surgery. Other uses include managing patients with refractory ventricular failure outside the setting of acute myocardial infarction, such as those with cardiomyopathy or severe myocardial damage associated with viral myocarditis; management of cardiogenic shock not rapidly reversed by pharmacological therapy; or stabilizing patients with refractory ventricular ectopy after myocardial infarction. Code 33967 should be reported when a physician inserts an IABAD by percutaneous technique.

It would be appropriate to report both the IABAD insertion and the intra-aortic balloon pump removal on the same day using codes 33967 and 33968. One indication would be an acute myocardial infarction (MI). Other indications could be the intent to do a left main coronary artery percutaneous coronary intervention. Most IABAD insertions for cardiogenic shock would not have removal in the same setting. Supporting a patient having an interventional cardiology procedure with an IABAD or some of the newer percutaneous assist devices is becoming the standard of care for some higher risk percutaneous coronary intervention patients.

CHAPTER 3

Description of Service for Code 33967

Preprocedure work includes patient evaluation and assessment and discussion of the reason for the procedure and its risks. The procedure may be performed in the cardiac catheterization laboratory, in the operating room, or at the bedside, depending on the clinical circumstances. Using sterile technique with local anesthetic and sedation, access to the femoral artery is accomplished, and a sheath is placed over a guidewire. The IABAD is placed under fluoroscopic control with its tip just distal to the left subclavian artery. In the absence of fluoroscopy, the catheter is placed over a long guidewire for a predetermined distance measured prior to insertion, using external landmarks. Following catheter placement, the physician supervises the initiation of balloon pumping, assuring that timing and augmentation are correct and effective. The IABAD is then secured in place and dressed.

Intent and Use of Code 33968

Code 33968 is used to report percutaneous removal of an intra-aortic balloon assist device.

Description of Service for Code 33968

The surgeon weans the patient off the IABAD by slowly decreasing the assistance of the balloon from a 1:1 ratio of pump-to-normal to a 1:3 ratio of pump-to-normal beat. Cardiac output is measured continuously after each change. When it is determined that the patient's heart is beating satisfactory on its own, the retaining sutures are cut, and the IABAD is carefully removed from the aorta and exited through the femoral artery incision site. The surgeon then administers compression on the large femoral artery puncture site for a period of time to assure hemostasis. Femoral artery and lower extremity pulse are checked for thrombosis and assure viable vascularization to the lower legs and feet.

Intent and Use of Code 33971

Code 33971 should be used to report the removal of an IABAD when a surgical repair of the artery is necessary.

Intent and Use of Code 33974

Code 33974 should be used to report the open removal of an IABAD from its prior placement in the ascending aorta when a surgical repair of the aorta is necessary.

CARDIAC ASSIST—INITIAL INSERTION OR REMOVAL OF A VENTRICULAR ASSIST DEVICE (33975-33980, 0048T, 0050T)

33975   Insertion of ventricular assist device; extracorporeal, single ventricle
CPT Assistant Feb 92:2, Jan 04:28, Nov 09:10, Jan 10:11, Apr 10:6; *CPT Changes: An Insider's View* 2002

33976   extracorporeal, biventricular
CPT Assistant Feb 02:2, Nov 09:10, Jan 10:11, Apr 10:6; *CPT Changes: An Insider's View* 2002

33977   Removal of ventricular assist device; extracorporeal, single ventricle
CPT Assistant Feb 02:2, Nov 09:10, Jan 10:11, Apr 10:6; *CPT Changes: An Insider's View* 2002

33978   extracorporeal, biventricular
CPT Assistant Feb 02:2, Nov 09:10, Jan 10:11, Apr 10:6; *CPT Changes: An Insider's View* 2002

33979   Insertion of ventricular assist device, implantable intracorporeal, single ventricle
CPT Assistant Feb 02:3, Jan 04:28, Nov 09:10, Jan 10:11, Apr 10:6; *CPT Changes: An Insider's View* 2002

33980   Removal of ventricular assist device, implantable intracorporeal, single ventricle
CPT Assistant Feb 02:3, Nov 09:10, Apr 10:6; *CPT Changes: An Insider's View* 2002

Category III

0048T   Implantation of a ventricular assist device, extracorporeal, percutaneous transseptal access, single or dual cannulation
CPT Assistant Jul 04:7-8, Jan 10:11, Apr 10:6; *CPT Changes: An Insider's View* 2004

0050T   Removal of a ventricular assist device, extracorporeal, percutaneous tarnsseptal access, single or dual cannulation
CPT Assistant Jul 04:7, Apr 10:6; *CPT Changes: An Insider's View* 2004

Initial Insertion and Removal

There are often multiple medical and/or surgical treatment options for cardiomyopathy, including coronary artery surgery or valve surgery. If heart failure worsens despite standard therapies, advanced treatment may be required to prolong survival. The next level of therapy is either a heart transplant (sometimes necessitating the use of a ventricular assist device [VAD] as a "bridge" to allow survival until a heart transplant is feasible) or a permanent VAD as definitive therapy. In some illnesses such as viral myocarditis, in which there is a significant chance of resolution of the dysfunction, a VAD may be used temporarily to support the circulation while the heart recovers. It is possible that differing types of VADs may be employed in the same patient, depending on the response to assist-device therapy. Prolonged complication-free patient survival has resulted in the need to change VAD devices and/or device components, as the device or component reaches the end of its functioning life.

Unlike a total artificial heart, a VAD doesn't replace the heart, but it increases heart output, thereby reducing some symptoms (eg, fatigue, shortness of breath); maintains or improves other organ function due to improved perfusion; and, at times through rest, allows the heart to recover.

Intent and Use of Codes 33975-33980

Initial VAD insertion procedures may occur during or independent of other cardiac surgery. To reflect the work for placing and the different types of devices, codes **33975-33976** specify the placement of *extracorporeal* (pump outside the body) devices, while code **33979** describes the placement of *intracorporeal* (pump inside the body) devices. For both types of VADs, there are inflow and outflow grafts or cannulas that are connected to a pump. Regardless of the type of intracorporeal or extracorporeal device placed, cardiopulmonary bypass (heart-lung machine) is typically required with each insertion procedure, and each device has to be connected to a controller console.

Implantable intracorporeal device insertion or removal (**33979, 33980, 33982, 33983**) refers to smaller VADs implanted inside the body, such as placement in an abdominal pocket (outside the abdominal cavity) with attachment to the appropriate ventricle, pulmonary artery or aorta, and driveline, exiting through the skin to an external computerized control unit.

Implantable extracorporeal device insertion or removal (**33975, 33976, 33977, 33978, 33981**) refers to technology that is partially implanted just below the heart (eg, with one end attached to the ventricle and the other attached to the aorta). A cannula (driveline) is passed through the skin and is connected to the external controller and power source. De-airing involves checking for and removal of air in the cannulas to prevent air emboli from entering the patient's circulation upon activation of the pump. The external part of the device is attached to a belt around the patient's waist or connected to a shoulder strap.

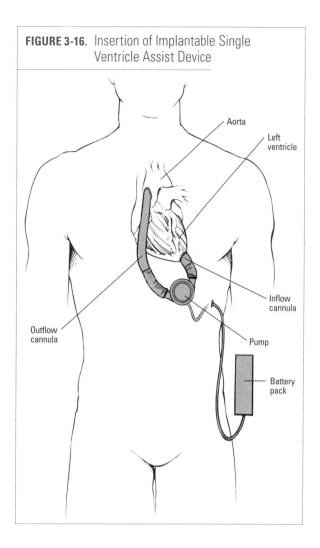

FIGURE 3-16. Insertion of Implantable Single Ventricle Assist Device

Aorta

Left ventricle

Inflow cannula

Outflow cannula

Pump

Battery pack

CHAPTER 3

Postoperative intracorporeal or extracorporeal VAD insertion care is reported using the appropriate critical care E/M code. It is not appropriate to report the prolonged extracorporeal circulation for cardiopulmoanry insufficiency codes (**33960, 33961**) for extracorporeal VAD care.

Category III code **0048T** differs from code **33975** or code **33979** because it describes services related to VAD implantation using a percutaneous transseptal approach for drainage of the left atrium and femoral artery cannulation for inflow function, which creates a left VAD. Implantation of this type of device may be performed in a cardiac catheterization laboratory. The cannulas are percutaneously placed, and the pump is extracorporeal; this device is intended for temporary support and can be removed at the bedside.

Category III code **0050T** describes removal of the entire device, including the cannula that was percutaneously placed. This type of removal may be performed at the patient's bedside.

Because interrogation and programming are considered inclusive in the initial insertion or replacement, it is not appropriate to report code **93750** in conjunction with codes **33975, 33976, 33979,** and **33981-33983.**

VAD programming and interrogation on a regular basis is necessary in longer-term VAD patients. Initially, these patients' conditions may not be stable, and the function of the VAD can be affected by minor changes in either exercise or activities of daily living. However, around the second month after the VAD insertion, patients typically tend to stabilize with less frequent interrogations. Code **93750** is used to report the work of the interrogation and programming of the device, which is similar, regardless of the condition of the patient.

The evaluation of the patient is not considered an inclusive component of code **93750.** Therefore, the level of E/M service provided will depend on the status of the patient and will vary throughout the course of the patient visits.

> **CODING TIP** The unlisted cardiac surgery code **33999** should be reported to describe pump replacement for an extracorporeal percutaneous transseptal access VAD when the pre-existing inflow and outflow cannulas are left in place. It is not appropriate to report either code **33976** or **33977** to describe this procedure, even though the percutaneous VAD is technically extracorporeal.

Intent and Use of Code 33975

Code **33975** represents the initial insertion of a single ventricle extracorporeal VAD by transthoracic approach.

Description of Service for Code 33975

Because these patients are so unstable, induction of anesthesia requires the presence of the surgeon in the operating room. The patient is positioned, prepared, and draped, and then placed on cardiopulmonary bypass. In the majority of these patients, reoperative median sternotomy is performed, as most of them have had a previous cardiac surgical procedure. The midline incision is extended to the umbilicus, and a pre-peritoneal pocket is created. The driveline is tunneled through the subcutaneous tissue, and then the heart is dissected, dividing the dense adhesions. At each step, care is taken to maintain meticulous hemostasis, as these sites will not be visible after the device is placed. The patient's aorta and right atrium are cannulated, and cardiopulmonary bypass is initiated. The apex

of the left ventricle is cored out, and a Silastic cuff is sewn to the edges of the cored ventricle. The inflow cannula of the left VAD (LVAD) is brought through an opening in the diaphragm and coupled with the Silastic cuff. Next, the outflow graft is measured, a partial occlusion clamp is applied to the aorta, and the graft is anasomosed to the aorta. The device is de-aired, and de-airing is confirmed by transesophageal cardiac ultrasound. The patient is then weaned from cardiopulmonary bypass. This requires, together with the anesthesia team, simultaneous management of the inotropes while assessing the heart, both visually and by transesophageal echocardiography. Following successful separation from bypass and decannulation, the incision is closed in layers.

> **CODING TIP** It would not be appropriate to report procedure code **33404** separately as it is a necessary component of the main procedure described by code **33975.**

Intent and Use of Code 33976

Code **33976** represents the initial insertion of a ventricular extracorporeal assist device by transthoracic approach.

Description of Service for Code 33976

Because these patients are so unstable, induction of anesthesia requires the presence of the surgeon in the operating room. The patient is positioned, prepared, and draped. In the majority of these patients, reoperative median sternotomy is performed, as most of them have had a previous cardiac surgical procedure. Patients with biventricular failure with resultant right ventricular enlargement may require exposure of the femoral vessels before the sternotomy is made. After the incisions, the patient is placed on cardiopulmonary bypass. The midline incision is extended to the umbilicus, and a pre-peritoneal pocket is created. The driveline is tunneled through the subcutaneous tissue, and the heart is dissected, dividing the dense adhesions. At each step, care is taken to maintain meticulous hemostasis, as these sites will not be visible after the device is placed. The patient's aorta and right atrium are cannulated, and cardipulmonary bypass is initiated. The apex of the left ventricle is cored out, and a Silastic cuff is sewn to the edges of the cored ventricle. The inflow cannula of the LVAD is brought through an opening in the diaphragm and coupled with the Silastic cuff. Next, the outflow graft is measured, a partial occlusion clamp is applied to the aorta, and the graft is anastomosed to the aorta. The device is de-aired, and de-airing is confirmed by transesophageal cardiac ultrasound. Attempts to wean the patient from cardiopulmonary bypass that are unsuccessful due to inadequate right ventricular function dictate the need for biventricular assist. The right VAD (RVAD) is placed, and the lines brought out through the skin. The patient is successfully weaned from cardiopulmonary bypass, albeit on high dose inotropes. This requires, together with the anesthesia team, simultaneous management of the inotropes while assessing the heart, both visually and by transesophageal echocardiography. Following successful separation from bypass and decannulation, the incision is closed in layers, but the sternum is left open. The patient is transported to the intensive care unit.

Intent and Use of Code 33977

Code 33977 describes an open-heart removal technique (requiring cardiopulmonary bypass) for removal of the entire device, including the cannulas, should the patient's condition warrant removal of the VAD without replacement at that particular session.

Description of Service for Code 33977

The patient is transferred from the cardiothoracic intensive care unit, intubated, and ventilated with all appropriate monitoring lines in-situ. The patient is placed supine on the operating room table and remains stable while general anesthesia is induced. The patient is prepared and draped in the usual sterile manner. The previous sternal incision is re-opened, and the pericardial cavity exposed. The chest is irrigated with warm saline, and the patient fully heparinized to achieve an activated coagulation time of greater than 400. The LVAD is then weaned with initial hemodynamic stability. However, the pulmonary artery and right ventricle begin to dilate with increasing left-sided failure. It appears as if the inflow cannula is obstructing the mitral valve as the transesophageal echocardiography reveals good ventricular contractility despite the worsening hemodynamics. Nitric oxide therapy is instituted while complete LVAD support is resumed. An attempt is made to wean the patient from the device once again with 20 ppm of nitric oxide support. Unfortunately, the right side fails again. Therefore, the ascending aorta and the right atrium are cannulated, and the patient is placed on cardiopulmonary bypass.

After achieving full flow, the LVAD outflow graft is divided with a vascular stapling device and the suture line oversewn with a 4-0 Prolene suture. The inflow cannula is then removed from the apex of the left ventricle and the purse string sutures secured. The apex is inspected for hemostasis, and the patient is weaned from cardiopulmonary bypass. This time the patient

weans easily from bypass with excellent hemodynamics. Transesophageal echocardiography reveals good biventricular function. Protamine is administered to reverse anticoagulation. The patient is decannulated. The chest is irrigated once again with warm saline and then closed after a final inspection for hemostasis. Stainless steel wires are employed to approximate the sternum, and absorbable sutures are used to close the pectoralis fascia, the subcutaneous tissue, and the skin. Three chest drains are left in the chest: a #36 French anterior mediastinal, and #32 French left and right pleural tubes. Temporary right atrial and right ventricular pacing wires are also placed prior to sternal closure. The patient tolerates the procedure well and is transferred to the cardiothoracic intensive care unit in stable condition.

Intent and Use of Code 33978

Code 33978 describes an open-heart removal technique (requiring cardiopulmonary bypass) for removal of the entire extracorporeal biventricular device, including the cannulas should the patient's condition warrant removal of the VAD without replacement at that particular session.

Intent and Use of Code 33979

Code 33979 represents the initial insertion of a single ventricle intracorporeal assist VAD by transthoracic approach.

Description of Service for Code 33979

Under general endotracheal anesthesia, in the supine position, the patient is prepared and draped in standard aseptic fashion. The previous midline incision is re-entered. The device pocket is created with electrocautery. The inferior phrenic vessels on the diaphragm are identified and ligated. The driveline egress site is created in the right upper abdomen. The LVAD is brought onto the field and placed into the pocket. The driveline is tunneled out from the right upper quadrant incision. Preparation for cardiopulmonary bypass includes activated clotting time–guided heparinization, cannulation of the aorta (3-0 Prolene purse string suture, Sarns 8.0 mm), and cannulation of the superior vena cava (3-0 Prolene purse string suture, 28 DLP) and inferior vena cava (3-0 Prolene purse string suture, 28 DLP). A Bentley cardioplegia needle is secured in the ascending aorta with a 4-0 Prolene suture. An apical left ventricular vent is placed, and the patient is cooled to 32 degrees Centigrade. The patient's pressure is temporarily reduced to 50 mm Hg. The aortic cross-clamp is applied, and 4:1 blood cardioplegia, 1000 mL, is given antegrade. The left atriotomy is re-opened and the left atrium inspected with findings described above. A large thrombus is removed, and a confirmation is made that no residual thrombus remains. The atriotomy is closed with running 3-0 Prolene suture. The patient is de-aired in standard fashion, and the atriotomy is tied shut. The aortic pressure is temporarily reduced to 50 mm Hg. The aortic cross-clamp is removed, and the patient is ventilated and de-aired once again. The apex is cored, and the left ventricle and tract are cleared of thrombus. The inflow cuff is attached to the apex of the left ventricle using pledgeted 2-0 Tevdek sutures in a mattress fashion. The cuff is attached to the LVAD and secured with #2 Tevdek tie as well as two umbilical tapes.

A partial occluding clamp is placed on the greater curvature of the ascending aorta. The outflow graft length is measured, and the graft is sewn to an eliptico-longitudinal aortotomy using semi-continuous running 3-0 Prolene sutures buttressed with a Teflon felt strip washer. The pressure is decreased to 50 mm Hg, aortic root suction applied, and the clamp released. The device is allowed to fill with blood, and the outflow graft is subsequently attached. A de-airing hole is made in the outflow graft, and the device is slowly de-aired.

The patient is weaned from cardiopulmonary bypass with norepinephrine, milrinone, dobutamine, and vasopressin. LVAD flows are 5.5 to 7 L/min. After protamine administration and decannulation, hemostasis is satisfactory. Two right ventricular and two right atrial pacing wires, a #36 anterior mediastinal chest tube, and a #32 left pleural chest tube are placed. Two large Jackson-Pratt drains are placed in the abdominal pocket. The sternum is closed with seven wires, the abdominal fascia is closed with #2 Prolene, and the skin and subcutaneous tissue are closed in layers of 0, 2-0, and 4-0 Vicryl. The patient is subsequently transported to the open heart recovery room in guarded condition.

Intent and Use of Code 33980

Code **33980** describes an open-heart removal technique (requiring cardiopulmonary bypass) for removal of the entire intracorporeal, single ventricle device, including the cannulas should the patient's condition warrant removal of the VAD without replacement at that particular session.

Description of Service for Code 33980

Under general endotracheal anesthesia, in the supine position, the patient is prepared and draped in standard aseptic fashion. Median sternotomy is completed carefully, and the LVAD pocket is opened. The

pericardial space contains moderate adhesions. The heart is evaluated by transesophageal echocardiography, with an ejection fraction estimated as 65% without inotropes. No left ventricular thrombus or purulent material is found in the LVAD pocket. Some serous material in the pocket is cultured. The heart is carefully dissected, and a pericardial well is created with 2-0 silk. Preparation for cardiopulmonary bypass includes activated clotting time–guided heparinization. The LVAD outflow graft is cannulated (3-0 Prolene purse string sutures, Sarns 6.5mm). Cannulation of the right atrium (3-0 Prolene purse string sutures, 36/51) is completed. Intraoperatively the patient has decreased blood pressure after aprotinin administration requiring epinephrine, norepinephrine, and vasopressin. In addition, the patient has increased bleeding requiring multiple transfusions of blood products. Cardiopulmonary bypass is initiated, and the dissection of the heart is completed. The patient remains at 36 degrees Centigrade. The inflow to the LVAD is freed and separated from the LVAD. The driveline is dissected free, and the device is removed from the field. The inflow cuff is removed. The cored hole at the apex is closed with double 2-0 Prolene purse string sutures and 3-0 Prolene mattress-type sutures buttressed with Dacron graft materials. When the purse string suture is tied down, de-airing maneuver is completed.

The patient is weaned from cardiopulmonary bypass with norepinephrine and vasopressin. After protamine and decannulation, the outflow graft is stapled close to the aorta and the stump oversewn using a 4-0 Prolene running suture. Hemostasis is unsatisfactory even with a large amount of protamine administration, requiring blood product transfusion. Satisfactory hemostasis is obtained after a lengthy and meticulous hemostatic procedure. Two right ventricular and two right atrial pacing wires are placed. A #36 (anterior mediastinal) chest tube and a #32 (left pleural) chest tube are placed. A large Jackson-Pratt drain is placed in the abdominal pocket. The sternum is closed with wire, and the skin closed in layers with 0, 3-0, and 4-0 Dexon sutures. The patient is transferred to the intensive care unit and subsequently extubated and transferred to the cardiac care unit. The patient continues to recover and is transferred to the floor where he or she continues to recover.

REPLACEMENT OF A VENTRICULAR ASSIST DEVICE (VAD) (**33981-33983**)

33981   Replacement of extracorporeal ventricular assist device, single or biventricular, pump(s), single or each pump
CPT Changes: An Insider's View 2010

33982   Replacement of ventricular assist device pump(s);
implantable intracorporeal, single ventricle,
without cardiopulmonary bypass
CPT Changes: An Insider's View 2010

33983   implantable intracorporeal, single ventricle,
with cardiopulmonary bypass
CPT Changes: An Insider's View 2010

Intent and Use of Codes 33981-33983

While implantable LVADs have been used primarily as bridges to cardiac transplantation, some patients have been maintained long term on these devices, thus allowing certain patients who have recovered to be weaned from the devices. They are also used as so-called "destination therapy" when transplantation or recovery may not be anticipated, but survival would be unlikely without the VAD.

Longer VAD support time creates the need for device replacement. Replacement of a VAD pump includes the removal of the old pump and insertion of a new pump with connection, de-airing, and initiation of the new pump performed at the same session. De-airing involves checking for and removal of air in the cannulas to prevent air emboli from entering the patient's circulation upon activation of the pump. Removal of the VAD system being replaced is not reported separately.

As with the insertion codes **33975**, **33976**, and **33979**, VAD replacement involves open-heart surgery (ie, sternotomy, chest tubes). Cardiopulmonary bypass may be required, depending on the patient's tolerance of being weaned from the VAD during pump replacement. In this instance, besides the existing inflow and outflow cannulae, the patient may also be cannulated for cardiopulmonary bypass to support circulation during the VAD replacement.

Transesophageal echocardiography (TEE) may be used to confirm placement prior to pump activation, or to check for air (de-airing) in the aortic root, graft, left ventricle, left atrium, or pulmonary veins. TEE is typically performed by the anesthesiologist and is reported in addition to the anesthesia service using code **93318**.

> **CODING TIP** The work of VAD pump replacement is described by codes **33981-33983**, regardless of whether the device pocket site is the same or newly created in a different anatomic site. It would not be appropriate to append **modifier 22** in the event the prior pocket site is closed and a new pocket site is created.

Intent and Use of Code 33981

Code **33981** describes the replacement of a single or biventricular pump of an extracorporeal VAD and is reported for each pump replaced.

Description of Service for Code 33981

Inflow and outflow cannulas are clamped. The VAD pump is removed and inspected. A new VAD pump is physically connected to the inflow and outflow cannulas. The pump is primed and de-aired to prevent gas embolization. The device is activated to support the circulation and its flow characteristics varied to ensure that adequate flow rates are achievable and that there is unobstructed inflow and outflow. During the process of VAD initiation, the patient's intravascular volume and vasoactive drug therapy are adjusted to achieve satisfactory, stable cardiovascular function and end-organ perfusion.

Intent and Use of Code 33982

Code **33982** describes replacement of single ventricle pump of an implantable, intracorporeal VAD. The procedure described by code **33982** is performed without the use of cardiopulmonary bypass.

Description of Service of Code 33982

A reoperative median sternotomy is performed, and the patient is fully anticoagulated. The implanted VAD is dissected free from surrounding scar tissue, avoiding injury to vital structures. The dissection is extended to permit ready access to the great vessels and the right heart for urgent cannulation to institute cardiopulmonary bypass should it be necessary. VAD flow rates are gradually reduced, and the patient is carefully weaned from its assistance with adjustment of intravascular volume and inotropic agents. Inflow and outflow cannulas are clamped, and the assist device pump is removed and inspected. A new VAD is physically connected to the inflow and outflow cannulas. The device is primed and de-aired to prevent gas embolization. The device pump is activated to support the circulation and its flow characteristics varied to ensure that adequate flow rates are achievable and that there is unobstructed inflow and outflow. During the process of VAD initiation, the patient's intravascular volume and vasoactive drug therapy are adjusted to achieve satisfactory, stable cardiovascular function and end-organ perfusion. Hemostasis is achieved, and the sternotomy is closed over drains.

CHAPTER 3

Intent and Use of Code 33983

Code **33983** describes the same procedure as code **33982**; however, the procedure is performed with cardiopulmonary bypass. The cross-reference note following the new guidelines has been revised to direct the user to the appropriate codes for implantation, removal, and replacement of an extracorporeal VAD with percutaneous transseptal access.

Description of Service for Code 33983

A reoperative median sternotomy is performed, and the patient is fully anticoagulated. The implanted VAD is dissected free from surrounding scar tissue, avoiding injury to vital structures. The dissection is extended to permit ready access to the great vessels and the right heart. (The patient does not tolerate weaning from the VAD and is therefore cannulated for cardiopulmonary bypass.) Cardiopulmonary bypass is initiated, the inflow and outflow VAD cannulas are clamped, and the assist device is removed and inspected. A new VAD pump is physically connected to the inflow and outflow cannulas. The pump is primed and de-aired to prevent gas embolization. The device is activated to support the circulation and its flow characteristics varied to ensure that adequate flow rates are achievable and that there is unobstructed inflow and outflow. During the process of VAD initiation, the patient's intravascular volume and vasoactive drug therapy are adjusted to achieve satisfactory, stable cardiovascular function and end-organ perfusion. Hemostasis is achieved. The sternotomy is closed over drains.

VAD Physician Follow-Up

Intent and Use

Typically, both the cardiothoracic surgeon and the cardiologist follow and monitor the patient after a VAD insertion. Either the cardiac surgeon or the cardiologist will provide the service to the patient on any given visit. With code **93750** being reportable on a per service basis, the physician reporting the service must provide detailed documentation to report his or her findings. Reporting the appropriate level E/M code is predicated on the physician meeting or exceeding the key components for reporting the E/M service, as reflected in the medical record.

While care of these complex patients is highly individualized, a typical pattern of care is illustrated as follows for a patient after being discharged from the hospital in an outpatient setting during the first year postinsertion:

- **First month:** The patient is seen weekly for evaluation and VAD interrogation and programming.
- **Second month:** The patient is seen every other week for evaluation and VAD interrogation and programming.
- **Third month to 1 year:** The patient is seen monthly for evaluation and VAD interrogation and programming.

The frequency and number of visits must be customized to the clinical needs of the specific patient's condition.

Peripheral Interventions

Increasingly, interventional cardiologists are finding it medically appropriate to image peripheral vessels during the same session as a cardiac catheterization. Because coding for cardiac interventional procedures is different from that of noncoronary vessels, appropriate coding for these simultaneous procedures often presents a conundrum for the coder.

Unlike cardiac catheterization and coronary intervention codes, which are bundled to include catheter placement as well as radiological supervision and interpretation (RS&I) services, peripheral interventions are almost universally reported using component codes. Multiple codes may be needed to accurately report peripheral vascular procedures.

An important principle of noncoronary interventions is that correct coding of these arterial procedures requires knowledge of the arterial access puncture site, the catheter movement, and the final position of the catheter. In addition, one must know which angiograms were taken and at what location during the catheter manipulation process contrast injections were performed. Finally, one must know both the specific intervention(s) performed and the location(s) in the arterial system where the intervention(s) was done. Multiple interventional procedures such as angioplasty, atherectomy, and stent placement are coded separately.

There are five vascular systems: (1) arterial; (2) venous; (3) pulmonary; (4) portal; and (5) lymphatic. Within each of these systems, there are numerous vascular families. Each family is defined by a primary branch of the vessel punctured, together with the more selective branches that arise from the primary vessel.

Noncoronary catheterizations are reported using either selective or nonselective catheter placement codes.

Nonselective placement means that the catheter or needle is placed directly into the major arterial conduit and not moved or manipulated further. An example of a nonselective arterial code is **36200**, *Introduction of catheter, aorta.*

If the catheter is moved from the original vessel and guided to or into another part of the arterial system other than the aorta or the vessel punctured, the selective catheter placement codes should be used. The exact code(s) used depends on how many branches the catheter must be guided through before it reaches its most distal or final destination. There are numerous vascular families that arise from the central aortic system. One such family is composed of the carotid and brachiocephalic arteries and the thoracic aorta. Another vascular family, in this case arising from the visceral abdominal aorta, is the iliac, femoral, and peripheral arterial branch family.

Within each of these vascular "families" only the most highly selective vessel catheterized within each vascular family is the determining factor for the level of coding. This vessel may or may not be the most distal in absolute distance from the puncture site or the origin of the primary vessel. Lesser-order branches of the same vascular family are not coded additionally. If multiple selective catheterizations are performed in different vascular families, then the highest level of selectivity is reported for each vascular family. The specific selective catheter placement arterial codes include the following vascular families:

- **36215:** First-order selective vessel, brachiocephalic and thoracic aorta

- **36216:** Second-order brachiocephalic and thoracic aorta

- **36217:** Third-order or higher branch, brachiocephalic and thoracic aorta

- **36218:** Additional second-order, third-order, or beyond

- **36245:** First-order abdominal aorta and branches

- **36246:** Second-order vessel, abdominal aorta and branches

- **36247:** Third-order or higher, abdominal aorta and branches

- **36248:** Additional second-order, third-order, or beyond

- **36251:** Main and accessory branches renal artery(s), unilateral

- **36252:** Main and accessory branches renal artery(s), bilateral

- **36253:** Superselective main and accessory branches renal artery(s), unilateral

- **36254:** Superselective main and accessory branches renal artery(s), bilateral

The first-order vessel is defined as selective catheterization of the first major branch off the main vessel (the aorta). A second-order vessel is defined as a catheterization of the first major branch off a first-order vessel. Likewise, a third-order branch is the catheterization of a first major branch off a second-order vessel. All **30000** series codes indicate the services for catheter placement only.

In addition to selective and/or nonselective catheter placement codes, codes **75600-75790** from the radiology imaging series are used to report the angiography as well as supervision and interpretation of the arterial injection. Unlike the more generic catheter placement codes, these RS&I codes are specific for the arterial system injected (ie, carotid, renal, iliac, femoral, popliteal).

EXAMPLE: Bilateral selective renal angiography.

Coding (Medicare and Non-Medicare Patient): Use these codes to report the procedures performed.

36252 26 Selective catheter placement (first-order), main renal artery and any accessory renal artery(s) for renal angiography, including arterial puncture and catheter placement(s), fluoroscopy, contrast injection(s), image postprocessing, permanent recording of images, and radiological supervision and interpretation, including pressure gradient measurements when performed, and flush aortogram when performed; bilateral

(See Chapter 4 and Appendix B for further information regarding the use of the HCPCS Level II, the **TC modifier**, and CPT **modifier 26**.)

Rationale: If therapeutic transcatheter procedures are performed, such as angioplasty, stenting, and/or atherectomy, the radiologic imaging may not be additionally reportable as it is considered inherent in the peripheral vessel therapeutic intervention. Radiologic imaging codes **75962-75968** are used in addition to the specific noncoronary intervention codes **35450, 35452, 35458,** and **35460** for open peripheral vessel angioplasty of the renal or other visceral artery, aorta, brachiocephalic trunk or branch, and vein, respectively.

Radiological supervision and interpretation (RS&I) code **75978** may be reported in addition to percutaneous angioplasty of the renal or other visceral artery, aorta, brachiocephalic trunk or branch, and vein, respectively (**35471, 35472, 35475, 35476**).

Coding Examples: Peripheral Arterial Procedures and Cardiac Procedures

PAYMENT POLICY ALERT Modifier application may vary by payer. For Medicare, **modifier 26** is used for codes with a technical component–professional component (TC/PC) split, if the service is performed in the facility setting. (Refer to Chapter 4 and Appendix B for additional information related to the TC/PC.)

EXAMPLE 1: The right femoral artery is entered, and a catheter is advanced to the left ventricle. An injection of contrast is made in the left ventricle. The ventricular catheter is withdrawn and exchanged for a coronary catheter and selective angiograms are made of the right coronary artery and the left coronary arteries. The coronary catheter is withdrawn and exchanged for a catheter that is *selectively* positioned in the left renal artery for injection of contrast. This catheter is then selectively repositioned in the right renal artery, and a contrast injection is made for the right renal angiogram. The catheter is removed, and hemostasis is achieved.

Coding Solution (Medicare and Non-Medicare Patient): Use the following codes to report the procedures performed.

⊙**93458** Catheter placement in coronary artery(s) for coronary angioplasty, including intraprocedural injection(s) for coronary angiography, imaging supervision and interpretation; with left heart catheterization including intraprocedural injection(s) for left ventriculography, when performed

⊙●**36252** Selective catheter placement (first-order), main renal artery and any accessory renal artery(s) for renal angiography, including arterial puncture and catheter placement(s), fluoroscopy, contrast injection(s), image postprocessing, permanent recording of images, and radiologic supervision and interpretation, including pressure gradient measurements

when performed, and flush aortogram when performed; bilateral

Rationale: As instructed by CMS, selective renal angiography performed at the time of cardiac catheterization should be reported in the standard way.

PAYMENT POLICY ALERT The Centers for Medicare & Medicaid Services (CMS) required the use of G-codes for iliac angiograms and renal angiograms performed at the time of cardiac catheterization for Medicare patients. Initially, these codes were mandated for both selective and nonselective injection of bilateral renal arteries at the time of catheterization; however, this has been modified and clarified to include only nonselective catheter placement with aortography at the level of the renal and iliac arteries. Selective renal angiography performed at the time of cardiac catheterization should be reported in the standard way (see Example 1). For *nonselective* catheter placement and aortography with nonselective renal artery angiography at the time of cardiac catheterization, the G-code should be used. G-code **G0275** should be used as an add-on code to report *nonselective* renal angiography performed at the time of cardiac catheterization. This includes the catheter placement at the level of the renal artery, injection of dye, aortogram, radiologic supervision and interpretation, and production of images.

For iliac angiography performed at the time of cardiac catheterization to assess for hemostatic closure devices, the G-code **G0278** should be used as an add-on code. This reports the iliac artery angiography performed at the time of cardiac catheterization, including the catheter placement in the iliac artery, injection of dye, radiologic supervision and interpretation, and production of images.

CODING TIP See Chapter 5 for further information regarding the reporting of cardiac catheterization and iliac and renal angiography (**G0275** and **G0278**).

EXAMPLE 2: The right brachial artery is entered, and a coronary catheter is advanced to the aortic root. Selective angiograms are made of the right coronary artery and the left coronary arteries. The coronary catheter is withdrawn and exchanged for a catheter that is then *nonselectively* positioned in the infrarenal aorta for injection of contrast for aortography and bilateral iliofemoral angiograms with runoff films. The catheter is removed, and hemostasis is achieved.

Coding Solution(s) (Non-Medicare Patient):
Use the following codes to report the procedures performed.

⊙**93454** Catheter placement in coronary artery(s) for coronary angiography, including intraprocedural injection(s) for coronary angiography, imaging supervision and interpretation

75630 Aortography, abdominal plus bilateral iliofemoral lower extremity, catheter, by serialography, radiological supervision and interpretation

Coding Solution(s) (Medicare Patient): Use the following codes to report the procedures performed.

⊙**93454** Catheter placement in coronary artery(s) for coronary angiography, including intraprocedural injection(s) for coronary angiography, imaging supervision and interpretation

G0278 Iliac and/or femoral artery angiography, non-selective, bilateral or ipsilateral to catheter insertion, performed at the same time as cardiac catheterization and/or coronary angiography, includes positioning or placement of the catheter in the distal aorta or ipsilateral femoral or iliac artery, injection of dye, production of permanent images, and radiologic supervision and interpretation (List separately in addition to primary procedure)

Rationale: CMS requires the use of G-codes for iliac angiograms and renal angiograms performed at the time of cardiac catheterization to include ONLY nonselective catheter placement with aortography at the level of the renal and iliac arteries. HCPCS Level II code **G0278** is used to report iliac and/or femoral artery angiography, *nonselective*, bilateral or ipsilateral to catheter insertion. This procedure is performed at the same time as cardiac catheterization and/or coronary angiography, includes positioning or placement of the catheter in the distal aorta or ipsilateral femoral or iliac artery, injection of dye, production of permanent images, and radiologic supervision and interpretation. (List each separately in addition to primary procedure.) CPT codes should be utilized if a *selective* study is performed.

EXAMPLE 3: Left heart catheterization from femoral artery, coronary angiography, descending aorta arteriography to visualize renal arteries.

Coding Solution(s) (Non-Medicare Patient):
Use the following codes to report the procedures performed.

⊙**93458** Catheter placement in coronary artery(s) for coronary angiography, including intraprocedural injection(s) for coronary angiography, imaging supervision and interpretation; with left heart catheterization including intraprocedural injection(s) for left ventriculography, when performed

75625 Aortography, abdominal, by serialography, radiological supervision and interpretation

Coding Solution(s) (Medicare Patient): Use the following codes to report the procedures performed.

⊙**93458** Catheter placement in coronary artery(s) for coronary angiography, including intraprocedural injection(s) for coronary angiography, imaging supervision and interpretation; with left heart catheterization including intraprocedural injection(s) for left ventriculography, when performed

G0275 Renal angiography, non-selective, one or both kidneys, performed at the same time as cardiac catheterization and/or coronary angiography, includes positioning or placement of any catheter in the abdominal aorta at or near the origins (ostia) of the renal arteries, injection of dye, flush aortogram, production of permanent images, and radiologic supervision and interpretation (list separately in addition to primary procedure)

Rationale: CMS requires the use of G-codes for iliac angiograms and renal angiograms performed at the time of cardiac catheterization to include ONLY nonselective catheter placement with aortography at the level of the renal and iliac arteries. HCPCS Level II code **G0275** is used to report renal artery angiography, nonselective, one or both kidneys, performed at the time of cardiac catheterization and/or coronary angiography. This procedure includes positioning or placement of any catheter in the abdominal aorta at or near the origins (ostia) of the renal arteries, injection of dye, flush aortography, production of permanent images, and radiologic supervision and interpretation. (List each separately in addition to the primary procedure.) CPT codes should be utilized if a *selective* study is performed.

EXAMPLE 4: The right femoral artery is entered, and a catheter is advanced to the left ventricle. An injection of contrast is made in the left ventricle. The ventricular catheter is withdrawn and exchanged for a coronary catheter and selective angiograms are made of the right coronary artery and the left coronary arteries. The coronary catheter is withdrawn and exchanged for a catheter that is positioned in

CHAPTER 3

the left iliac artery for injection of contrast. This catheter is then exchanged for a balloon catheter for angioplasty of the iliac artery. After angiographic evaluation of the angioplasty result, a stent is placed in the dilated segment of the iliac artery. The catheter is removed, and hemostasis is achieved.

Coding Solution(s) (Non-Medicare or Medicare Patient): Use the following codes to report the procedures performed.

- ⊙93458 Catheter placement in coronary artery(s) for coronary angiography, including intraprocedural injection(s) for coronary angiography, imaging supervision and interpretation; with left heart catheterization including intraprocedural injection(s) for left ventriculography, when performed

- ⊙37221 Revascularization, endovascular, open or percutaneous, iliac artery, unilateral, initial vessel; with transluminal stent placement(s), includes angioplasty within same vessel, when performed

Rationale: The work of accessing and selectively catheterizing the left iliac artery and traversing the lesion is considered an inclusive service of code **37221**. Therefore, code **36245** should not be reported in addition to code **37221**. The radiological supervision and interpretation directly related to the intervention(s) performed and imaging performed to document completion of the intervention in addition to the intervention(s), are also inclusive services.

PAYMENT POLICY ALERT When peripheral angiography is reported together with cardiac angiography, Medicare carriers will invoke the "multiple surgical procedures" rule, in which the highest valued surgical procedure code is reimbursed at 100%, while each additional surgical code is reimbursed at 50%. Imaging codes are not affected by the "multiple surgical procedures" rule.

CODING TIP More information on coding for peripheral vascular procedures can be obtained by ordering the *Interventional Radiology Coding Users' Guide* from the Society of Interventional Radiology at (888) 695-9733 or at the Society of Interventional Radiology Web site at www.sirweb.org.

BALLOON ANGIOPLASTY/ATHERECTOMY/STENT PLACEMENT—PERIPHERAL ARTERIES (**35450-35460, 35471-35476**)

35450	Transluminal balloon angioplasty, open; renal or other visceral artery *CPT Assistant* Feb 97:2-3
35452	aortic *CPT Assistant* Feb 97:2-3
35458	brachiocephalic trunk or branches, each vessel *CPT Assistant* Feb 97:2-3, May 01:11
35460	venous *CPT Assistant* Feb 97:2-3
⊙35471	Transluminal balloon angioplasty, percutaneous; renal or visceral artery *CPT Assistant* Aug 96:3, Feb 97:2-3; *CPT Changes: An Insider's View* 2011
⊙35472	aortic *CPT Assistant* Aug 96:3, Feb 97:2-3
⊙35475	brachiocephalic trunk or branches, each vessel *CPT Assistant* Aug 96:3, Feb 97:2-3, May 01:4, Sep 08:10
⊙35476	venous *CPT Assistant* Aug 96:3, Feb 97:2-3, May 01:4, Dec 03:2; *Clinical Examples in Radiology* Spring 05:8-10, Spring 07:1-3

Intent and Use

If a therapeutic procedure such as a peripheral vessel open or percutaneous angioplasty and/or stent placement occurs during the same session as diagnostic angiography, the code for both the diagnostic angiogram and the intervention (angioplasty and stenting) would be appropriate (eg, code **35471**).

Codes **35450, 35452, 35458,** and **35460** describe open peripheral vessel angioplasty of the renal or other visceral artery, aorta, brachiocephalic trunk or branch, and vein, respectively. Codes **35471, 35472, 35475,** and **35476** should be reported for percutaneous angioplasty of the renal or other visceral artery, aorta, brachiocephalic trunk or branch, and vein, respectively.

SELECTIVE/SUPERSELECTIVE CATHETERIZATION OF RENAL ARTERY FOR RENAL ANGIOGRAPHY (36251-36254)

⊙●**36251** Selective catheter placement (first-order), main renal artery and any accessory renal artery(s) for renal angiography, including arterial puncture and catheter placement(s), fluoroscopy, contrast injection(s), image postprocessing, permanent recording of images, and radiologic supervision and interpretation, including pressure gradient measurements when performed, and flush aortogram when performed; unilateral
CPT Changes: An Insider's View 2012

⊙●**36252** bilateral
CPT Changes: An Insider's View 2012

⊙●**36253** Superselective catheter placement (one or more second order or higher renal artery branches) renal artery and any accessory renal artery(s) for renal angiography, including arterial puncture, catheterization, fluoroscopy, contrast injection(s), image postprocessing, permanent recording of images, and radiologic supervision and interpretation, including pressure gradient measurements when performed, and flush aortogram when performed; unilateral
CPT Changes: An Insider's View 2012

⊙●**36254** bilateral
CPT Changes: An Insider's View 2012

Intent and Use of Codes ⊙●36251-⊙●36254

Codes 36251-36254 include arterial puncture and catheter placement(s), fluoroscopy, contrast injection(s), image postprocessing, permanent recording of images, and radiological supervision and interpretation. Pressure gradient measurements and flush aortogram are also included, when performed. Moderate sedation is an inclusive component of the procedures, which is indicated with the Moderate Sedation (⊙) symbol

Codes 36251 and 36252 describe first-order selective catheter placement in the main renal artery and any accessory renal artery(s) for renal angiography. Code 36251 describes a unilateral procedure, and code 36252 describes a bilateral procedure. Codes 36253 and 36254 describe superselective catheter placement. Code 36253 describes a unilateral procedure, and code 36254 describes a bilateral procedure.

Description of Service for Code ⊙●36251

Administer or supervise administration of moderate sedation. The access vessel is palpated, and local anesthesia is administered. Using Seldinger technique, the vessel is punctured, a guidewire is passed, and a flush catheter and guidewire are manipulated into the aorta. After forming the catheter, a small amount of contrast is injected to confirm appropriate and safe position. Digital subtraction angiography (DSA) imaging of the aorta and renal ostia is performed. After the non-selective imaging portion of the procedure is performed, the catheter is exchanged over guidewire for appropriate selective catheter, which is manipulated under fluoroscopic guidance and formed in the aorta. The origin of the renal artery is probed for and ultimately engaged with the catheter advanced into the main renal. Sterile saline flush and test injection of contrast are performed to ensure intraluminal and safe position of catheter. Selective DSA imaging with injection of contrast or CO_2 is performed in multiple projections. If appropriate, pressure measurements are performed with withdrawal of catheter across the vessel origin. Several minutes of time may be dedicated to monitoring of pressure measurements and wave forms with subsequent interpretation. The selective catheter is unformed under fluoroscopic observation in the thoracic aorta and subsequently removed. Manual compression or closure device is utilized for closure of the arteriotomy to achieve hemostasis.

Description of Service for Code ⊙●36252

Administer or supervise administration of moderate sedation. The access vessel is palpated, and local anesthesia is administered. Using Seldinger technique, the vessel is punctured, a guidewire is passed, and a flush catheter and guidewire are manipulated into the aorta. After forming the catheter, a small amount of contrast is injected to confirm appropriate and safe position. Digital subtraction angiography (DSA) imaging of the aorta and renal ostia is performed. After the non-selective imaging portion of the procedure is performed, the catheter is exchanged over guidewire for appropriate selective catheter, which is manipulated under fluoroscopic guidance and formed in the aorta. The origin of the renal artery is probed for and ultimately engaged. Sterile saline flush and test injection of contrast are performed to ensure intraluminal and safe position of catheter. Selective DSA imaging with injection of contrast or CO_2 is performed in multiple projections. If appropriate, pressure measurements are performed with withdrawal of catheter across the vessel origin. Several minutes of time may be dedicated to monitoring of pressure measurements and wave forms with subsequent interpretation. The selective catheter is advanced out of the renal artery and the contralateral renal artery is probed for and ultimately selected. Repeat test injection, DSA imaging, and pressure measurements are performed as described on the initial side. The selective catheter is unformed under fluoroscopic observation in the thoracic aorta and subsequently removed. Manual compression or closure device are utilized for closure of the arteriotomy to achieve hemostasis.

Description of Service for Code ⊙●36253

Administer or supervise administration of moderate sedation. The access vessel is palpated, and local anesthesia is administered. Using Seldinger technique, the vessel is punctured, a guidewire is passed, and a flush catheter and guidewire are manipulated into the aorta. After forming the catheter, a small amount of contrast is injected to confirm appropriate and safe position. Digital subtraction angiography (DSA) imaging of the aorta and renal ostia is performed. After the non-selective imaging portion of the procedure is performed, the catheter is exchanged over guidewire for appropriate selective catheter, which is manipulated under fluoroscopic guidance and formed in the aorta. The origin of the renal artery is probed for and ultimately engaged. Sterile saline flush and test injection of contrast are performed to ensure intraluminal and safe position of catheter. Selective DSA imaging with injection of contrast or CO_2 is performed in multiple projections. A second microcatheter is prepared on the back sterile table with assistant. Through the base catheter, this microcatheter and wire are introduced into the base catheter with sterile pressurized heparin flush connected and infused. Using careful fluoroscopic guidance, alternating wire and catheter maneuvers are performed, and the microcatheter is advance into the second or third order branch vessel of the renal artery. Magnification DSA imaging using contrast or CO_2 is performed in multiple projections. The microcatheter is withdrawn, and the base catheter is unformed under fluoroscopic observation in the thoracic aorta and subsequently removed. Manual compression or closure device are utilized for closure of the arteriotomy to achieve hemostasis.

Description of Service for Code ⊙●36254

Administer or supervise administration of moderate sedation. The access vessel is palpated, and local anesthesia is administered. Using Seldinger technique, the vessel is punctured, a guidewire is passed, and a flush catheter and guidewire are manipulated into the aorta. After forming the catheter, a small amount of contrast is injected to confirm appropriate and safe position. Digital subtraction angiography (DSA)

imaging of the aorta and renal ostia is performed. After the non-selective imaging portion of the procedure is performed, the catheter is exchanged over guidewire for appropriate selective catheter, which is manipulated under fluoroscopic guidance and formed in the aorta. The origin of the renal artery is probed for and ultimately engaged. Sterile saline flush and test injection of contrast are performed to ensure intraluminal and safe position of catheter. Selective DSA imaging with injection of contrast or CO_2 is performed in multiple projections. If appropriate, pressure measurements are performed with withdrawal of catheter across the vessel origin. Several minutes of time may be dedicated to monitoring of pressure measurements and wave forms with subsequent interpretation. A second microcatheter is prepared on the back sterile table with assistant. Through the base catheter, this microcatheter and wire are introduced into the base catheter with sterile pressurized heparin flush connected and infused. Using careful fluoroscopic guidance, alternating wire and catheter maneuvers are performed, and the microcatheter is advance into the second or third order branch vessel of the renal artery. Magnification DSA imaging using contrast or CO_2 is performed in multiple projections. The microcatheter is withdrawn, and the selective catheter is advanced out of the renal artery and the contralateral renal artery is probed for and ultimately selected. Repeat test injection, DSA imaging, and pressure measurements are performed as described on the initial side. The microcatheter is prepped and re-advanced through the base catheter, and using guidance, the contralateral second or third order branches are selected with repeat magnification imaging performed as indicated. The base catheter is unformed under fluoroscopic observation in the thoracic aorta and subsequently removed. Manual compression or closure device are utilized for closure of the arteriotomy to achieve hemostasis.

LOWER EXTREMITY REVASCULARIZATION— OPEN OR PERCUTANEOUS (37220-37235)

⊙37220   Revascularization, endovascular, open or percutaneous, iliac artery, unilateral, initial vessel; with transluminal angioplasty
CPT Changes: An Insider's View 2011

⊙37221   with transluminal stent placement(s), includes angioplasty within same vessel, when performed
CPT Changes: An Insider's View 2011

⊙+37222   Revascularization, endovascular, open or percutaneous, iliac artery, each additional ipsilateral iliac vessel; with transluminal

angioplasty (List separately in addition to code for primary procedure)
CPT Changes: An Insider's View 2011

⊙+37223   with transluminal stent placement(s), includes angioplasty within the same vessel, when performed (List separately in addition to code for primary procedure)
CPT Changes: An Insider's View 2011

⊙37224 Revascularization, endovascular, open or percutaneous, femoral/popliteal artery(s), unilateral; with transluminal angioplasty
CPT Changes: An Insider's View 2011

⊙37225   with atherectomy, includes angioplasty within the same vessel, when performed
CPT Changes: An Insider's View 2011

⊙37226   with transluminal stent placement(s), includes angioplasty within the same vessel, when performed
CPT Changes: An Insider's View 2011

⊙37227   with transluminal stent placement(s) and atherectomy, includes angioplasty within the same vessel, when performed
CPT Changes: An Insider's View 2011

⊙37228 Revascularization, endovascular, open or percutaneous, tibial/peroneal artery, unilateral, initial vessel; with transluminal angioplasty
CPT Changes: An Insider's View 2011

⊙37229   with atherectomy, includes angioplasty within the same vessel, when performed
CPT Changes: An Insider's View 2011

⊙37230   with transluminal stent placement(s), includes angioplasty within the same vessel, when performed
CPT Changes: An Insider's View 2011

⊙37231   with transluminal stent placement(s) and atherectomy, includes angioplasty within the same vessel, when performed
CPT Changes: An Insider's View 2011

⊙+37232 Revascularization, endovascular, open or percutaneous, tibial/peroneal artery, unilateral, each additional vessel; with transluminal angioplasty (List separately in addition to code for primary procedure)
CPT Changes: An Insider's View 2011

⊙+37233   with atherectomy, includes angioplasty within the same vessel, when performed (List separately in addition to code for primary procedure)
CPT Changes: An Insider's View 2011

⊙+37234   with transluminal stent placement(s), includes angioplasty within the same vessel, when performed (List separately in addition to code for primary procedure)
CPT Changes: An Insider's View 2011

⊙+37235   with transluminal stent placement(s) and atherectomy, includes angioplasty within the same vessel, when performed (List separately in addition to code for primary procedure)
CPT Changes: An Insider's View 2011

Codes 37220-37235 describe lower extremity endovascular revascularization services performed for occlusive disease. These lower extremity codes are built on progressive hierarchies with more intensive services inclusive of lesser intensive services.

Codes 37220-37235 should be reported for open or percutaneous peripheral vessel angioplasty of the iliac, femoral/popliteal, or tibial/peroneal arteries, respectively, when performed. Codes 37205 and 37206 should be reported for percutaneous transcatheter placement of intravascular stent(s) (except coronary, carotid, vertebral, iliac, and lower extremity arteries). Codes 37207 and 37208 should be reported for open stent(s) placement (except coronary, carotid, vertebral, iliac, and lower extremity arteries).

Codes 37221, 37223, 37226, 37227, 37230, 37231, 37234, and 37235 should be reported for open or percutaneous stent placement in the iliac, femoral, popliteal, or tibial/peroneal arteries. Codes 37225 and 37227 should be reported for open or percutaneous peripheral vessel atherectomy of the femoral/popliteal artery(s). Codes 37229, 37231, 37233, and 37235 should be reported for open or percutaneous peripheral vessel atherectomy of a tibial/peroneal artery.

Category III codes 0234T-0238T are used for open or percutaneous peripheral vessel atherectomy of a renal artery, a visceral artery, abdominal aorta, a brachiocephalic artery, and an iliac artery, respectively.

According to CPT guidelines, codes 37220-37235 are to be used to describe lower extremity endovascular revascularization services performed for occlusive disease. These lower extremity codes are built on progressive hierarchies with more intensive services inclusive of lesser intensive services. The code inclusive of all of the services provided for that vessel should be reported (ie, use the code inclusive of the most intensive services provided). Only one code from this family (37220-37235) should be reported for each lower extremity vessel treated.

FIGURE 3-17. Balloon Catheter in Iliac Artery

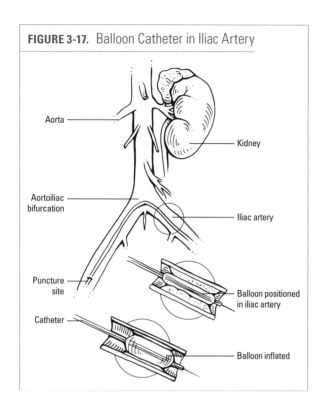

FIGURE 3-18. Iliac and Lower Extremity Arterial Anatomy Territory

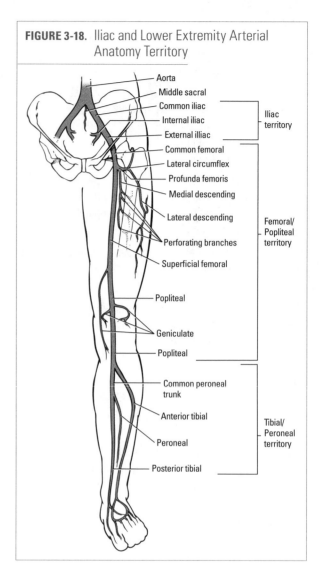

These lower extremity endovascular revascularization codes all include the work of accessing and selectively catheterizing the vessel, traversing the lesion, RSI directly related to the intervention(s) performed, embolic protection if used, closure of the arteriotomy by pressure and application of an arterial closure device or standard closure of the puncture by suture, and imaging performed to document completion of the intervention in addition to the intervention(s) performed. Extensive repair or replacement of an artery may be additionally reported (eg, code **35226** or **35286**). These codes describe endovascular procedures performed percutaneously and/or through an open surgical exposure. These codes include balloon angioplasty (eg, low-profile, cutting balloon, cryoplasty), atherectomy (eg, directional, rotational, laser), and stenting (eg, balloon-expandable, self-expanding, bare metal, covered, drug-eluting). Each code in this family (**37220-37235**) includes balloon angioplasty, when performed.

These codes describe endovascular procedures performed percutaneously and/or through an open surgical exposure. These codes include balloon angioplasty (eg, low-profile, cutting balloon, cryoplasty); atherectomy (eg, directional, rotational, laser); and stenting (eg, balloon-expandable, self-expanding, bare metal, covered, drug eluting). Each code in this family (**37220-37235**) includes balloon angioplasty, when performed. These codes describe revascularization therapies (ie, transluminal angioplasty, atherectomy, and stent placement)

provided in three arterial vascular territories: (1) iliac; (2) femoral/popliteal; and (3) tibial/peroneal.

- **Iliac Vascular Territory**: The iliac territory is divided into three vessels: (1) common iliac; (2) internal iliac; and (3) external iliac.

A single primary code is used for the initial iliac artery treated in each leg (**37220**, **37221**). If other iliac vessels are also treated in that leg, these interventions are reported with the appropriate add-on code(s) (**37222**, **37223**). Up to two add-on codes can be used in a unilateral iliac vascular territory, as there are three vessels that could be treated. Add-on codes are used for different vessels, not distinct lesions within the same vessel.

- **Femoral/Popliteal Vascular Territory**: The entire femoral/popliteal territory in one lower extremity is considered a single vessel for CPT reporting, specifically for the endovascular lower extremity revascularization codes **37224-37227**.

A single interventional code is used no matter what combination of angioplasty/stent/atherectomy is applied to all segments, including the common, deep, and superficial femoral arteries as well as the popliteal artery (37224, 37225, 37226, or 37227). There are no add-on codes for additional vessels treated within the femoral/popliteal territory. Because only one service is reported when two lesions are treated in this territory, report the most complex service (eg, use code 37227 if a stent is placed for one lesion and an atherectomy is performed on a second lesion).

- **Tibial/Peroneal Territory**: The tibial/peroneal territory is divided into three vessels: (1) anterior tibial; (2) posterior tibial; and (3) peroneal arteries. There are specific coding guidelines for each of the three vascular territories.

A single primary code is used for the initial tibial/peroneal artery treated in each leg (37228, 37229, 37230, or 37231). If other tibial/peroneal vessels are also treated in the same leg, these interventions are reported with the appropriate add-on code(s) (37232-37235). Up to two add-on codes could be used to describe services provided in a single leg, as there are three tibial/peroneal vessels that could be treated. Add-on codes are used for different vessels, not distinct lesions within the same vessel. The common tibio-peroneal trunk is considered part of the tibial/peroneal territory but is not considered a separate, fourth segment of vessel in the tibio-peroneal family for CPT reporting of endovascular lower extremity interventions. For instance, if lesions in the common tibio-peroneal trunk are treated in conjunction with lesions in the posterior tibial artery, a single code would be reported for treatment of this segment.

When treating multiple territories in the same leg, one primary lower extremity revascularization code is used for each territory treated. When second or third vessel(s) are treated in the iliac and/or tibial/peroneal territories, add-on code(s) are used to report the additional service(s).

When more than one stent is placed in the same vessel, the code should be reported only once. When multiple vessels in multiple territories in a single leg are treated at the same setting, the primary code for the treatment in the initial vessel in each vascular territory is reported. Add-on code(s) are reported when second and third iliac or tibial/peroneal arteries are treated in addition to the initial vessel in that vascular territory.

If a lesion extends across the margins of one vessel vascular territory into another but can be opened with a single therapy, this intervention should be reported with a single code despite treating more than one vessel and/or vascular territory. For instance, if a stenosis extends from the common iliac artery into the proximal external iliac artery and a single stent is placed to open the entire lesion, this therapy should be coded as a single stent placement in the iliac artery (37221). In this example, a code for an additional vessel treatment would not be used. (Do not report both code 37221 and code 37223.)

For bifurcation lesions distal to the common iliac origins that require therapy of two distinct branches of the iliac or tibial/peroneal vascular territories, a primary code and an add-on code would be used to describe the intervention. In the femoral/popliteal territory, all branches are included in the primary code, so treatment of a bifurcation lesion would be reported as a single code.

When the same territory(ies) of both legs is treated in the same session, modifiers may be required to describe the interventions. Use **modifier 59** to denote that different legs are being treated, even if the mode of therapy is different.

Mechanical thrombectomy and/or thrombolysis in the lower extremity vessels are sometimes necessary to aid in restoring flow to areas of occlusive disease and are reported separately.

CODING TIP Sometimes thrombus may be present in the target lesion initially, and treatment of that thrombus with an atherectomy device or device that removes both thrombus and plaque is inherent to the atherectomy procedure and not additionally reported as a separate procedure. However, if the clot removed is in a different vascular territory, downstream of the primary lesion being treated, secondary mechanical thrombectomy is reported using add-on code **37186** in addition to the appropriate atherectomy code (**37225, 37227, 37229, 37231, 37233, 37235**).

How to Use

To fully understand how to report these services, it is key to recognize:

1. The definitions of the vessels and vascular territories as specifically defined for this family of CPT codes;

2. Each leg is reported independently;

3. Interventions are reported per vessel, not per lesion, and the code inclusive of all of the services provided

for that vessel should be reported (ie, use the code inclusive of the most intensive services provided);

4. Only one primary code from this family (37220-37235) should be reported for each lower extremity vessel treated; and

5. These codes pertain to interventions performed percutaneously and/or through an open surgical exposure.

Inclusive Services

The inclusive services of each code in the 37220-37235 series include:

- the work of accessing and selectively catheterizing the vessel and traversing the lesion;

- radiological supervision and interpretation directly related to the intervention(s) performed;

- embolic protection, if used;

- closure of the arteriotomy by any method;

- imaging performed to document completion of the intervention in addition to the intervention(s) performed;

- balloon angioplasty (eg, low-profile, cutting balloon, cryoplasty);

- atherectomy (eg, directional, rotational, laser) including balloon angioplasty, when performed; and

- stenting (eg, balloon-expandable, self-expanding, bare metal, covered, drug eluting) including balloon angioplasty, when performed.

Except in very specific circumstances, the following codes would **not** be reported separately for lower extremity transluminal angioplasty, atherectomy, and/or stent procedures as they are considered inherent in each code in the 37220-37235 series when performed through the same access site:

36140	Introduction of needle or intracatheter; extremity artery
⊙▲36200	Introduction of catheter, aorta
⊙▲36245	Selective catheter placement, arterial system; each first order abdominal, pelvic, or lower extremity artery branch, within a vascular family
⊙▲36246	initial second order abdominal, pelvic, or lower extremity artery branch, within a vascular family

⊙▲36247	initial third order or more selective abdominal, pelvic, or lower extremity artery branch, within a vascular family
⊙▲36248	additional second order, third order, and beyond, abdominal, pelvic, or lower extremity artery branch, within a vascular family (List in addition to code for initial second or third order vessel as appropriate)
76000	Fluoroscopy (separate procedure), up to one hour physician time, other than **71023** or **71034** (eg, cardiac fluoroscopy)
75960	Transcatheter introduction of intravascular stent(s) (except coronary, carotid, vertebral, iliac, and lower extremity artery), percutaneous and/or open, radiological supervision and interpretation, each vessel
75962	Transluminal balloon angioplasty, peripheral artery other than cervical carotid, renal or other visceral artery, iliac or lower extremity, radiological supervision and interpretation
75964	Transluminal balloon angioplasty, each additional peripheral artery other than cervical carotid, renal or other visceral artery, iliac and lower extremity, radiological supervision and interpretation (List separately in addition to code for primary procedure)

Description of Service for Code ⊙▲36200

Administer or supervise administration of conscious sedation. The access vessel is palpated and local anesthesia is administered. Using Seldinger technique, the vessel is punctured, a guidewire is passed, and a vascular sheath is introduced into the artery. This is then flushed with sterile saline. Over guidewire, catheter and guidewire are manipulated into the diseased iliac vessels, and then ultimately into the diseased aorta. Sterile saline flush and test injection of contrast are performed to ensure intraluminal and safe position of catheter. Depending on imaging portion of procedure, the catheter may be repositioned or exchanged over appropriate guidewire for different caliber or shaped catheter to facilitate imaging and pressure measurement. Following the imaging portion of the procedure (performed and reported separately), manual compression or closure device are utilized for closure of the arteriotomy to achieve hemostasis.

Description of Service for Code ⊙▲36246

Administer or supervise administration of conscious sedation. Access vessel is palpated and local anesthesia is administered. Using Seldinger technique, the vessel is punctured, a guidewire is passed, and a catheter and guidewire are manipulated into the diseased aorta. After the nonselective imaging portion of the procedure is performed (separately), the catheter is exchanged over guidewire for appropriate selective catheter, which is manipulated under fluoroscopic guidance into the ori-gin of the chosen branch vessel. Sterile saline flush and test injection of contrast are performed to ensure intraluminal and safe position of catheter. Using guide-wire and catheter techniques, the catheter is advanced beyond the first-branch point into the second-order portion of the vessel (eg, splenic, common hepatic, left gastric). Flush and test injection are repeated throughout the procedure to ensure safe position and patency of catheter system. The catheter may be repositioned or exchanged over appropriate guidewire to be seated safely in the vessel. Following the imaging portion of the procedure (performed and reported separately), manual compression or closure device are utilized for closure of the arteriotomy to achieve hemostasis.

Description of Service for Code ⊙▲36247

Administer or supervise administration of conscious sedation. The access vessel is palpated and local anesthesia is administered. Using Seldinger technique, the vessel is punctured, a guidewire is passed, and a catheter and guidewire are manipulated into the aorta. After the nonselective imaging portion of the proce-dure is performed (separately reported), the catheter is exchanged over guidewire for appropriate selective catheter, which is manipulated under fluoroscopic guidance into the origin of the chosen branch vessel. Sterile saline flush and test injection of contrast are performed to ensure intraluminal and safe position of catheter. Using guidewire and catheter techniques, the catheter is advanced beyond the first-branch point into the second-order portion of the vessel (eg, splenic, common hepatic, left gastric). Flush and test injection are repeated throughout the procedure to ensure safe position and patency of catheter systems. Through the base catheter (typically 4-5 French), a second microcatheter (typically 3 French) is prepared on the back sterile table with assistant. This microcatheter and wire are introduced into the base catheter with sterile pressurized heparin flush connected and infused. Microcatheter is advanced under guidance into the third-order branch vessel (GDA, proper hepatic). Following the imaging portion of the procedure (per-formed and reported separately), manual compression or closure device are utilized for closure of the arteri-otomy to achieve hemostasis.

CODING TIP RS&I is inclusive of open or percutane-ous peripheral vessel angioplasty of the iliac, femoral/popliteal, or tibial/peroneal arteries, respectively (**37220-37235**), when performed. RS&I is also inclusive of percutaneous (**37205**, **37206**) transcatheter place-ment of intravascular stent(s) (except coronary, carotid, vertebral, iliac, and lower extremity arteries) and open stent placement (**37207**, **37208**). RS&I is also inclusive of open or percutaneous stent placement in the iliac, femo-ral, popliteal, or tibial/peroneal arteries (**37221**, **37223**, **37226**, **37227**, **37230**, **37231**, **37234**, **37235**). RS&I is inclusive of open or percutaneous peripheral vessel atherectomy of the femoral/popliteal artery(s) (**37225**, **37227**) or a tibial/peroneal artery (**37229**, **37231**, **37233**, **37235**). RS&I is inclusive of Category III codes **0234T-0238T** used for open or percutaneous peripheral vessel atherectomy of a renal artery, a visceral artery, abdominal aorta, a brachiocephalic artery, and an iliac artery, respectively.

Reporting Additional Services

While codes 36200, 36245, 36246, 36247, 36248, 36140 would not be reported separately for lower extremity transluminal angioplasty, atherectomy, and/or stent procedures, these procedures could be separately reported appropriately with the new codes in several instances, including:

1. Diagnostic angiography performed at the same time as the intervention(s) from a separate access;

2. Diagnostic angiography performed at the same time as the intervention(s), which requires a higher degree of selectivity than does the intervention;

3. Another intervention of a non-lower extrem-ity artery performed at the same time as the intervention(s) of a lower extremity that requires a separate access or a higher degree of selectivity than the lower extremity access; and

4. Another intervention of the lower extremity is performed initially (eg, thrombolysis), followed by a lower extremity transluminal angioplasty, atherec-tomy, and/or stent on a subsequent day, or a separate diagnostic study and/or intervention done through the same access (eg, renal angiogram/intervention).

In these cases, only the catheterization work related to the lower extremity transluminal angioplasty/atherec-tomy/stent is included with the codes 37220-37235. The additional catheterization(s) are also reported.

To further clarify, radiological supervision and interpretation codes **75962**, **75964**, **75960** may be reported should other interventions on non-lower extremity vessels be performed at the same setting. Codes **75962** and **75964** may be reported when angioplasty is performed in an upper extremity artery(s). Code **75960** may be reported when vascular stent placement is performed in non-coronary, non-lower extremity, and non-extracranial carotid vessels. To illustrate, an iliac stent and a renal stent could be performed during the same patient encounter. While code **75960** would be considered inherent in the iliac stent placement (**37221**), the renal stent placement may be reported using code **75960**. It is suggested that **modifier 59**, *Distinct procedural service*, be appended to reflect this circumstance.

EXAMPLE 1: An aortogram with ilio-femoral arteriography is performed on a patient with a history of 1-block calf claudication bilaterally. The femoral pulses are decreased on each side, and no prior imaging of the vessels has been performed. A right femoral approach is used for the arteriogram, which identifies 80% iliac artery stenoses bilaterally. The diagnostic catheter on the right is exchanged for a sheath. The left femoral artery is then also punctured and a sheath placed into the left common iliac artery. The left iliac stenosis is treated with angioplasty with good result. The right iliac lesion is also treated with angioplasty but results in a flow-limiting dissection, so a stent is placed to completely open the right iliac artery. Is it correct to code **36200** and **75625** along with the iliac angioplasties?

Coding Solution: The codes for intervention are **37221** for the right and **37220** for the left. A primary code is used for the first vessel treated in each vascular territory in each leg. The add-on codes **37222** and **37223** are not used in this case because the additional iliac treated is on the opposite side of the body.

Code **36200**, *Introduction of catheter, aorta*, might be reported for the right side because the catheter was advanced farther than was needed for the intervention alone. Code **36140**, *Introduction of needle or intracathete; extremity artery*, would be included in the interventional codes. On the left, the catheter/sheath was not advanced into the aorta, so no additional selectivity would be reported for the left. Sometimes the catheter must be advanced into the aorta to be able to treat an external iliac lesion, and if the placement of the catheter is done for the purpose of treating the iliac lesion, it is included in the interventional code and not separately reported. In this case, the catheter was additionally advanced into the aorta for diagnostic purposes, so it might be considered additional work beyond the catheter placement used for the intervention. The aortogram is reportable using code **75625**, *Aortography, abdominal, by serialography, radiological supervision and interpretation*, with **modifier 59**, *Distinct procedural service*, appended, or code **75630**, *Aortography, abdominal plus bilateral iliofemoral lower extremity, catheter, by serialography, radiological supervision and interpretation*, again with **modifier 59** appended, depending on the exact imaging performed. **Modifier 59** is appended to indicate that this was diagnostic work and that there was no prior angiography. Had an arterial puncture site been performed in which that specific catheter was never used for intervention, it would be separately reportable using code **36200**.

EXAMPLE 2: A peripheral arterial rotational atherectomy is performed with a device that also employs suction to remove debris and thrombi, if present. Is it appropriate to report both atherectomy (eg, **37225**, **37229**) and secondary thrombectomy (**37186**) when this device is used, or should it be reported as a single atherectomy procedure? Under what circumstances may thrombectomy be reported in addition to atherectomy when this device is used?

Coding Solution: CPT add-on code **37186**, *Secondary percutaneous transluminal thrombectomy (eg, nonprimary mechanical, snare basket, suction technique), noncoronary, arterial or arterial bypass graft, including fluoroscopic guidance and intraprocedural pharmacological thrombolytic injections, provided in conjunction with another percutaneous intervention other than primary mechanical thrombectomy (List separately in addition to code for primary procedure)*, is never used to report removal of debris at the atherectomy site itself.

It should be noted that CPT add-on code **37186** is a secondary arterial mechanical thrombectomy. This code is used to describe "rescue" thrombectomy for distal embolization that occurs at the time of a procedure or intervention that threatens flow to another vascular territory. For example, completion angiography following femoral artery angioplasty identifies an acute distal thromboembolic arterial occlusion of the common peroneal trunk that occurs after an endovascular treatment. In essence, a complication is identified where the outflow tract that was patent on pre-procedure imaging is now occluded after the endovascular therapy. Therefore, suction/mechanical removal of such debris (distal to the zone of endovascular intervention or distal to the embolic protection device when employed) is appropriately reported using code **37186**.

This code may also be used for removal of thrombus prior to intervention. In cases where prior diagnostic study has identified a stenosis and an intervention is planned, but roadmapping studies at the time of intervention show that thrombus is present at the lesion, thrombectomy may be performed prior to the primary intervention to remove the thrombus before it is embolized distally by the intervention.

These two scenarios are very different than intentional removal of plaque at the site of treatment that is inherent to an atherectomy procedure.

Codes 37225, *Revascularization, endovascular, open or percutaneous, femoral/popliteal artery(s), unilateral; with atherectomy, includes angioplasty within the same vessel, when performed*, and 37229, *Revascularization, endovascular, open or percutaneous, tibial/peroneal artery(s), unilateral initial vessel; with atherectomy, includes angioplasty within the same vessel, when performed*, describe atherectomy that may be performed primarily or secondarily and include either the manual or suction of plaque material from the vessel. An appropriate atherectomy device is chosen, advanced into the diseased segment, and positioned using fluoroscopic guidance and contrast injection. Multiple passes are made with the atherectomy device, physically removing plaque from the vessel. The atherectomy catheter may require periodic removal from the vessel to empty the collection chamber for plaque. It is then reintroduced into the vessel again over the wire, and the process is repeated until the desired amount of plaque is removed. This does not constitute an additional atherectomy procedure and does not warrant the additional reporting of either code 37225 or 37229.

Regarding thrombectomy, codes 37225 and 37229 also include the insertion of a distal embolic protection device. Predilatation may be required if tight stenosis or an area of occlusion exists. At the end of the procedure, the embolic protection device is retrieved (if used). Should a thrombus or plaque fragment be removed in the embolic protection device, this does not constitute a separate thrombectomy procedure and does not warrant additional reporting of code 37186.

ENDOVASCULAR REPAIR OF ABDOMINAL AORTIC ANEURYSM (34803)

34803   Endovascular repair of infrarenal abdominal aortic aneurysm or dissection; using modular bifurcated prosthesis (2 docking limbs)
CPT Changes: An Insider's View 2005

Intent and Use of Code 34803

Code 34803 describes endovascular repair of infrarenal abdominal aortic aneurysm (AAA) or dissection using a modular bifurcated prosthesis (with two docking limbs).

Description of Service for Code 34803

The modular bifurcated endovascular repair device is an inverted Y-shaped, three-piece modular prosthesis that is designed to cover the infrarenal abdominal aorta. The limbs extend into each iliac artery and are attached in a modular fashion after deployment of the main body. The main difference between the codes used for the modular bifurcated device and those for other AAA endovascular devices is the number of components. An open femoral or iliac artery exposure should be reported separately using code 34812 or code 34820, as appropriate. Placement of a proximal or distal extension prosthesis should also be separately reported using code 34825 for the initial vessel and code 34826 for each additional vessel. Radiological code 75952 should be used to report supervision and interpretation (S&I) work for code 34803. Code 75953 should be reported only when an extension prosthesis is required in addition to the three main components of code 34803. In addition, the arterial catheterization(s) should be separately reported. The procedure includes angioplasty and/or stent placement when performed in the target zone of the endoprosthesis.

> **CODING TIP** For endovascular repair of abdominal aortic aneurysm or dissection involving visceral vessels using a fenestrated modular bifurcated prosthesis (with two docking limbs), use Category III codes **0078T** and **0079T**.

TRANSCATHETER PLACEMENT OF EXTRACRANIAL CERVICAL CAROTID ARTERY STENTS (37215, 32716)

⊙37215   Transcatheter placement of intravascular stent(s), cervical carotid artery, percutaneous; with distal embolic protection
CPT Assistant May 05:7; CPT Changes: An Insider's View 2005

⊙37216   without distal embolic protection
CPT Assistant May 05:7; CPT Changes: An Insider's View 2005

Intent and Use of Codes ⊙37215 and ⊙37216

Extracranial cervical carotid artery angioplasty and stenting are reported with code **37215**, when performed with distal embolic protection, and with code **37216**, when performed without distal embolic protection. Both codes include all ipsilateral cervical and cerebral angiography (performed on the same day of the procedure), as well as carotid angioplasty, stent placement, deployment and removal of distal embolic protection systems, and all associated S&I services. Both codes also include a 90-day global service period. Category III codes **0075T** and **0076T** describe stenting of the extracranial vertebral or intrathoracic carotid arteries.

Code **37215** is used to report transcatheter stenting of the cervical carotid artery with use of an embolic protection system. Code **37216** is used to report transcatheter stenting of the cervical carotid artery without use of an embolic protection system.

If bilateral carotid angiography is performed on the same day as the cervical carotid stent procedure, the ipsilateral carotid angiogram (cervical and cerebral), catheter placement, and appropriate S&I services are included in codes **37215** and **37216**, and the contralateral cervical and cerebral carotid angiogram is coded separately.

Description of Service for Code ⊙37215

The electrocardiogram and hemodynamic monitors are in place and functioning. Perform all following steps under fluoroscopic guidance. Puncture the common femoral artery for the insertion of the 6F sheath. (All radiological supervision and imaging work are included.) Direct technical personnel throughout the procedure. Interpret the imaging of the vessel being treated, including complete intracranial and extracranial views of the target vessel in all views necessary. Ensure accurate radiological views, exposures, shielding, image size, injection sequences, radiation protection, and management of the patient and staff. Analyze all imaging in real time during the procedure, including pretreatment imaging, fluoroscopic and angiographic imaging throughout the procedure as required, and postprocedure fluoroscopic and angiographic imaging. This includes all imaging done to manipulate the wires, catheters, and devices into position. Ensure the embolic protection system (EPS) is positioned and deployed correctly and that the positioning of the EPS is stable throughout the procedure. Ensure that the stent and opening balloon are positioned and deployed correctly. Assess the postoperative success and complications of the procedure. Complete

the intra- and extracranial study poststent, recapture the protection device, and remove the catheters. Take a quantitative measurement of the lesion, target vessel, and the distal EPS landing zone to determine the appropriate size of the balloon, stent, and the EPS. Take continuous fluoroscopic imaging during all catheter and stent manipulations to assess the proper position of the EPS and adequate EPS performance throughout the procedure.

Baseline Cervical Cerebral Angiography and Quantitative Measurements: Advance a standard .035 guidewire into the aortic arch at the base of the great vessels. Advance a carotid configuration catheter to the aortic arch. Roadmap the common carotid artery origin and proximal segment. Remove a standard .035 wire and replace it with a .035 hydrophilic wire. Insert a carotid-selective reverse curve catheter into the sheath over the hydrophilic wire. Administer heparin intravenously. Reform the shape of the carotid-selective catheter in the aortic arch. Use the carotid catheter to selectively catheterize the origin of the common carotid artery. Inject contrast to perform an initial roadmap arteriogram of the common carotid and bifurcation. Perform a cervical carotid angiography in the anteroposterior (AP) and lateral views. Take quantitative measurements of the vessels including the area of stenosis and the area of the EPS landing zone. Perform a cerebral angiography including at minimum, lateral and AP Towne views. Place a catheter to ensure a continuous heparin flush.

Selection of Appropriate Stent and EPS: Choose equipment based on results of the quantitative measurements. Connect the side-arm of a long guiding sheath to the arterial pressure transducer. Perform a focused arteriogram of bifurcation and distal internal carotid through the guiding sheath.

Prep Distal EPS: Prep a .014 wire and ensure the filter is completely air free. Assemble the delivery system and ensure it is air free. Assemble the retrieval system and ensure it is air free.

Exchange for Guiding the Catheter/Sheath: Advance a .035 hydrophilic wire under the roadmap into the external carotid. Advance the catheter into the external carotid. Remove the hydrophilic wire and insert a stiff .035 exchange-length wire. Exchange the long guiding sheath/catheter into the common carotid. Remove the wire and carotid-selective catheter. Check ACT to ensure adequate anticoagulation.

Placement of Distal EPS: Load a .014 wire/EPS/delivery system and advance into the common carotid. Perform high magnification predeployment arteriogram of carotid bifurcation. Check the patient's neurological status and throughout the case at intervals. Advance and maneuver the .014 wire/EPS across the lesion into the distal extracranial internal carotid. Carefully position it using confirmatory angiography and roadmapping. Activate the EPS by opening the filter umbrella in the distal internal carotid. Remove the EPS deployment catheter. Assess the position of the deployed EPS with an angiogram to confirm good flow and filter/wall apposition. Reposition and repeat as necessary until the proper position is attained.

Pre-Stent Carotid Angioplasty: Prepare the angioplasty balloon and ensure it is air free. Advance a 3- to 4-mm, low-profile balloon across the lesion and check the position. Insufflate the balloon to pre-dilate the lesion. Remove the balloon.

Carotid Stent Placement: Prepare the stent delivery system and ensure it is air free. Load the appropriately sized self-expanding stent into the guiding catheter. Advance the stent delivery catheter carefully across the lesion. Perform a final angiographic check to ensure exact positioning. Deploy the stent. Remove the stent delivery device. Load and advance a 5- to 6-mm balloon. Position the balloon within the stent and inflate the balloon for post dilatation. Check the electrocardiogram for bradycardia or other arrhythmia and treat as needed with intravenous medications.

EPS Removal: Advance the EPS retrieval system through the stent to the distal EPS position. Deactivate the EPS. Remove the .014 wire and EPS.

Final Carotid and Cerebral Angiography: Perform the completion bifurcation arteriogram. Check carefully for residual stenosis, dissection, and vasospasm and treat if present (eg, use nitroglycerin for vasospasm). Perform completion intra-cerebral arteriogram in anteroposterior and lateral Towne views. Review the cerebral images in detail for emboli, vaso-spasm, and cross-filling. Insert a soft-tip .035 guidewire into a long guiding sheath/catheter. Remove the guiding sheath/catheter from the common carotid. Remove the guiding sheath and guidewire from the puncture site and attain hemostasis. Conduct a final neurological check prior to transferring the patient to the recovery area.

Description of Service for Code 37216

All radiologic imaging and supervision work is included. Technical personnel are directed throughout the procedure. Interpretation of imaging of the vessel being treated, including complete intracranial and extracranial views of the target vessel in all views necessary, is done. It is ensured that accurate radiologic views, exposures, shielding, image size, injection sequences, radiation protection, and management for patient and staff are done. Real-time analysis of all imaging during procedure, including pre-treatment imaging, fluoroscopic, and angiographic imaging are done throughout the procedure as required to perform the procedure, and postprocedure fluoroscopic and angiographic imaging are reviewed. This includes all imaging to manipulate the wires, catheters, and devices into position, plus correct positioning and deployment of the stent, opening the balloon, assessing postoperative success and complications, complete intra- and extracranial study after stenting, and removing catheters. Quantitative measurement is done of the lesion and target vessel to determine the appropriate balloon and stent sizes.

Initial Arterial Access and Monitoring: It is ensured that electrocardiographic and hemodynamic monitors are in place and functioning. All the following steps are performed under fluoroscopic guidance. The common femoral artery is punctured for insertion of a 6F sheath.

Baseline Cervical and Cerebral Angiography and Quantitative Measurement: A standard .035 guidewire is advanced into the aortic arch at the base of the great vessels. The carotid configuration catheter is advanced to the aortic arch. The common carotid artery origin and proximal segment are roadmapped. The standard .035 guidewire is removed and replaced with a .035 hydrophilic wire. A carotid-selective reverse curve catheter is inserted into the guiding sheath over the hydrophilic wire. Intravenous heparin is administered. The shape of the carotid-selective catheter is reformed in the aortic arch. This carotid catheter is used to selectively catheterize the origin of the common carotid artery. Contrast is injected to perform initial roadmap arteriogram of the common carotid and bifurcation. Cervical carotid angiography is performed in the anteroposterior (AP) and lateral views. Quantitative measurements of the vessels, including the area of stenosis, are performed. Cerebral angiography, including lateral and AP Towne views, is performed. The catheter is placed to continuous heparin flush.

Selection of Appropriate Stent: Equipment is chosen based on the results of quantitative measurements. The side arm of the long guiding sheath is connected to the arterial pressure transducer. Focused arteriogram of the bifurcation and distal internal carotid is performed through the guiding sheath.

Exchange for Guiding Catheter or Sheath: A .035 hydrophilic wire is advanced under roadmap into the external carotid. The catheter is advanced into the external carotid. The hydrophilic wire is removed, and a stiff .035 wire is inserted. A long guiding sheath is exchanged into the common carotid over the carotid-selective catheter. The wire and carotid-selective catheter are removed. The activated clotting time (ACT) is checked to ensure adequate anticoagulation.

Placement of a Small-Diameter Wire Across Lesion: A 0.014 wire is loaded and advanced into the common carotid. High-magnification predeployment arteriogram of carotid the bifurcation is performed. The patient's neurologic status is checked now and throughout the procedure at intervals. The 0.014 wire is advanced and maneuvered across the lesion into the distal extracranial internal carotid with careful positioning using confirming angiography and roadmapping.

Prestent Carotid Angioplasty: The angioplasty balloon is prepared to be air free. A 3- to 4-mm, low-profile balloon is advanced across the lesion, and its position is checked. Atropine is administered. The balloon is insufflated to predilate the lesion. The balloon is removed.

Carotid Stent Placement: The stent delivery system is prepared to be air free. An appropriately sized self-expanding stent is loaded into the guiding catheter. The stent delivery catheter is advanced very carefully across the lesion. A final angiographic check is performed to ensure exact positioning. The stent is deployed. The stent delivery device is removed. A 5- to 6-mm balloon is loaded and advanced. The balloon is positioned within the stent and inflated for postdilatation. The electrocardiography is checked for bradycardia or other arrhythmia and treated as needed with intravenous medications.

Final Carotid and Cerebral Angiography: Completion bifurcation arteriogram is performed. A careful check is done for residual stenosis, dissection, and vasospasm, and they are treated if present (eg, nitroglycerin for vasospasm). Completion intracerebral arteriogram is performed in the lateral and Towne views. The cerebral images are reviewed in detail for emboli, vasospasm, cross-filling, and so on. The .014 wire is exchanged for a .035 guidewire through the guiding sheath. The guiding sheath or catheter is removed from the common carotid, and the guiding sheath and guidewire are removed from the puncture site.

Groin Management: The sheath is removed, and hemostasis is achieved.

Neurologic Assessment: A final neurologic check is done.

> **PAYMENT POLICY ALERT** At this time, Medicare will cover carotid stent placement only when the procedure is performed as part of a clinical trial that has received Category B investigational device exemption (IDE) designation from the Food and Drug Administration (FDA) or as part of a postmarket study (PMS) for an FDA-approved carotid stent system. Carotid stenting that does not meet those criteria is currently a noncovered service.

TRANSCATHETER PLACEMENT OF EXTRACRANIAL NONCERVICAL CAROTID CEREBROVASCULAR ARTERY STENTS (0075T, +0076T)

0075T Transcatheter placement of extracranial vertebral or intrathoracic carotid artery stent(s), including radiologic supervision and interpretation, percutaneous; initial vessel
CPT Assistant May 05:7; CPT Changes: An Insider's View 2005

+0076T   each additional vessel (List separately in addition to code for primary procedure)
CPT Assistant May 05:7; CPT Changes: An Insider's View 2005

Intent and Use of Code 0075T

Category III code **0075T** describes transcatheter placement of an extracranial vertebral or intrathoracic carotid artery stent in the initial vessel. As with codes **37215** and **37216**, this code includes all associated radiological supervision and interpretation (RSI).

Intent and Use of Code +0076T

Category III add-on code **0076T** describes transcatheter placement of an extracranial vertebral or intrathoracic carotid artery stent for each additional vessel. It also includes all associated RSI.

INTRAVASCULAR ULTRASOUND (**+37250**, **+37251**)

+37250 Intravascular ultrasound (non-coronary vessel) during diagnostic evaluation and/or therapeutic intervention; initial vessel (List separately in addition to code for primary procedure)
CPT Assistant Nov 96:7, Nov 97:17, Nov 99:20; *CPT Changes: An Insider's View* 2000

+37251 each additional vessel (List separately in addition to code for primary procedure)
CPT Assistant Nov 96:7, Nov 97:17, Nov 99:20; *CPT Changes: An Insider's View* 2000

Intent and Use of Codes +37250 and +37251

According to CPT guidelines, intravascular ultrasound services include all transducer manipulations and repositioning within the specific vessel being examined, both before and after therapeutic intervention (eg, stent placement). Vascular access for intravascular ultrasound performed during a therapeutic intervention is not reported separately. Add-on code 37250 describes intravascular noncoronary ultrasound image acquisition (initial vessel). Add-on code 37251 describes image acquisition for each additional vessel.

Add-on codes 37250 and 37251 are constructed differently from the coronary ultrasound codes. Like other imaging codes, the service is broken down into the procedural component and the RSI component. As with coronary ultrasound, the CPT coding system allows peripheral ultrasound to be coded when it is performed in conjunction with a diagnostic procedure as well as a therapeutic procedure. Code 75945 describes the corresponding supervision and interpretation of those images (initial vessel). Code 75946 describes the imaging supervision and interpretation for each additional vessel. Use code 75946 in conjunction with code 75945.

Diagnostic Radiological Services

Technical Versus Professional Services

Diagnostic services are performed for inpatients and outpatients. Outpatient services are provided in various locations, such as physicians' offices, hospital outpatient departments, diagnostic centers, mobile facilities, and other locations.

Third-party payers require that submitted claims clearly define whether a complete technical or professional service was provided in order for physicians to receive appropriate reimbursement. Thus, an understanding of a complete service and its technical and professional components is critical to making an appropriate claim for reimbursement.

A *complete service,* as defined by the Centers for Medicare & Medicaid Services (CMS), is one in which the physician provides everything needed for the entire service, including equipment, supplies, technical personnel, and the physician's personal professional services. The complete service can then be divided into a technical component and a professional component.

The technical component includes equipment, supplies, technical personnel, and the costs attendant to the performance of the procedure other than professional services.

The professional component encompasses all of the physician's work in providing the service, including a complete interpretation and report by the physician performing the service. In some instances, a separate CPT code has been developed to describe the professional component. In others, **modifier 26** is required to identify the professional component of a service. For some services, the interpretation and report make up the entire professional component. Generally, the physician reports only the professional component of a service when that service is provided in a setting where the physician does not own the equipment (such as a hospital). (Refer to Appendix B for the list of CPT codes having technical and professional components.)

SUPERVISION

The three levels of supervision (general, direct, and personal) apply to diagnostic tests performed in a nonhospital setting. *General supervision* means the procedure is performed under the physician's overall direction and control, but the physician's presence is not required during the test. The physician remains responsible for the nonphysician personnel performing the procedure. *Direct supervision* in the office setting means the physician must be present in the office suite and immediately available to furnish assistance and direction but does not need to be physically present during the test. *Personal supervision* means a physician must be in attendance in the room during the procedure.

Different supervision requirements apply in the hospital setting. For hospitals, there are few Medicare requirements on physician supervision unless a resident is performing a procedure, in which case teaching physician rules apply. Supervision levels are reflected in the CMS public use files. The levels are described in section 2070 of the *Medicare Carriers Manual.*

Cardiac Diagnostic Imaging

The fluoroscopic guidance for pacemaker insertion (**71090**) was deleted for *CPT 2012*. Pacemaker or pacing cardioverter-defibrillator lead insertion, replacement, or revision procedures with fluoroscopic guidance are reported using codes **33206-33249**. To report fluoroscopic guidance for diagnostic lead evaluation without lead insertion, replacement, or revision procedures, use code **76000**, *Fluoroscopy (separate procedure), up to 1 hour physician time, other than 71023 or 71034 (eg, cardiac fluoroscopy)*. Because code **76000** is designated as a CPT "separate procedure," it will be necessary to append **modifier 59**, *Distinct Procedural Service*.

CARDIAC MAGNETIC RESONANCE IMAGING (**75557-+75565**)

75557   Cardiac magnetic resonance imaging for morphology and function without contrast material;

   CPT Changes: An Insider's View 2008; Clinical Examples in Radiology Spring 09:2

75559   with stress imaging

   CPT Changes: An Insider's View 2008; Clinical Examples in Radiology Spring 09:2

75561   Cardiac magnetic resonance imaging for morphology and function without contrast material(s), followed by contrast material(s) and further sequences;

   CPT Changes: An Insider's View 2008; Clinical Examples in Radiology Spring 09:2

75563   with stress imaging

   CPT Changes: An Insider's View 2008; Clinical Examples in Radiology Spring 09:2

+75565   Cardiac magnetic resonance imaging for velocity flow mapping (List separately in addition to code for primary procedure)

   CPT Assistant Jul: 10:7; CPT Changes: An Insider's View 2010

Intent and Use of Codes 75557-75565

Codes **75557-75565** are used to report the various combinations and permutations of imaging protocols with sufficient granularity for cardiac magnetic resonance (MR) of the heart patterns and to more accurately describe cardiac magnetic resonance imaging (MRI) services as they are currently performed.

As indicated in the CPT guidelines, cardiac magnetic imaging differs from traditional MRI in its ability to provide a physiologic evaluation of cardiac function. Traditional MRI relies on static images to obtain clinical diagnoses based on anatomic information. Improvement in spatial and temporal resolution has expanded the application from an anatomic test and includes physiologic evaluation of cardiac function. Flow and velocity assessment for valves and intracardiac shunts is performed in addition to a function and morphologic evaluation. Use code **75559** with code **75565** to report flow with pharmacologic wall motion stress evaluation without contrast. Use code **75563** with code **75565** to report flow with pharmacologic perfusion stress with contrast.

Cardiac MRI for velocity flow mapping can be reported in conjunction with code **75557, 75559, 75561,** or **75563**.

Listed procedures may be performed independently or in the course of overall medical care. If the physician providing these services is also responsible for diagnostic workup and/or follow-up care of the patient, see appropriate sections also. Only one procedure in the code series **75557-75563** is appropriately reported per session. Only one add-on code for flow velocity can be reported per session.

Cardiac MRI studies may be performed at rest and/or during pharmacologic stress. Therefore, the appropriate stress testing code from the **93015-93018** series should be reported in addition to code **75559** or **75563**.

> **CODING TIP** Cardiac MR can be used in a patient to evaluate myocardial ischemia and to identify myocardial scar and viability before revascularization. Pharmacologic stress testing to identify myocardial ischemic risk can be done using wall motion techniques (similar to stress echocardiography) or perfusion techniques (similar to radionuclide techniques).

Intent and Use of Code 75557

Code **75557** describes the cardiac MRI for morphology and function without the use of contrast material.

Clinical Example for Code 75557

A 36-year-old male has syncope and nonsustained ventricular tachycardia suggesting an origin in the right ventricle and a family history of sudden cardiac death. Cardiac MRI is ordered to assess the right ventricular structure and function.

Description of Service for Code 75557

The setup is supervised for different anatomic imaging planes. The study images are reviewed, and input is provided on whether to obtain additional imaging planes or sequences. Reconstructions of the heart and mediastinum are supervised and/or created using an independent workstation. The projection of the reconstructions is adjusted to optimize visualization of anatomy and diseased areas. The source and reformatted images resulting from the study are interpreted, typically including cine review with the following specific activities: evaluation of the morphologic findings in multiple planes; assessment of biventricular function with ejection fraction and characterization of wall motion abnormalities; and comparison with all pertinent available prior studies. The report is dictated for the medical record.

Intent and Use of Code 75559

Code **75559** describes the cardiac MRI for morphology and function with the use of stress imaging.

Clinical Example for Code 75559

A 65-year-old hypertensive female with chronic obstructive pulmonary disease and worsening shortness of breath is scheduled for abdominal aortic aneurysm resection. Preoperative assessment for myocardial ischemia with cardiac MRI is requested.

Description of Service for Code 75559

The setup is supervised for different anatomic imaging planes. The study images are reviewed, and input is provided on whether to obtain additional imaging planes or sequences. Reconstructions of the heart and mediastinum are supervised and/or created using an independent workstation. The projection of the reconstructions is adjusted to optimize visualization of anatomy and diseased areas. The source and reformatted images resulting from the study are interpreted, typically including cine review with the following specific activities: evaluation of the morphologic findings in multiple planes; assessment of biventricular function with ejection fraction and characterization of wall motion abnormalities; evaluation of multiple cardiac segments at incremental levels of stress for abnormal wall motion; and comparison with all pertinent available prior studies.

Intent and Use of Code 75561

Code **75561** describes a cardiac MRI study without contrast material, followed by contrast material to assess cardiac myocardial viability.

Clinical Example for Code 75561

A 55-year-old male with multivessel coronary artery disease and severe reduced left ventricular systolic function is scheduled for bypass surgery. A cardiac MRI with contrast material is scheduled to assess cardiac myocardial viability before surgery.

Description of Service for Code 75561

The setup is supervised for different anatomic imaging planes. The study images are reviewed, and input is provided on whether to obtain additional imaging planes or sequences. Reconstructions of the heart and mediastinum are supervised and/or created using an independent workstation. The projection of the reconstructions is adjusted to optimize visualization of anatomy and diseased areas. The source and reformatted images resulting from the study are interpreted, typically including cine review with the following specific activities: evaluation of the morphologic findings in multiple planes; assessment of biventricular function with ejection fraction and characterization of wall motion abnormalities; interpretation of precontrast and postcontrast images to assess myocardial viability; and comparison with all pertinent available prior studies. The report is dictated for the medical record.

Intent and Use of Code 75563

Code **75563** describes a cardiac MRI study without contrast material, followed by contrast material, and includes stress imaging.

Clinical Example for Code 75563

A 75-year-old diabetic male with new-onset chest pain has known severe, diffuse, three-vessel coronary artery disease; has undergone coronary artery bypass surgery; and has known saphenous vein graft disease. He is referred for adenosine stress testing to determine the culprit lesion for possible cardiac intervention, depending on the remaining viable myocardium at risk.

Description of Service for Code 75563

The setup is supervised for different anatomic imaging planes. The study images are reviewed, and input is provided on whether to obtain additional imaging planes or sequences. Reconstructions of the heart and mediastinum are supervised and/or created using an independent workstation. The projection of the reconstructions is adjusted to optimize visualization of anatomy and diseased areas. The source and reformatted images resulting from the study are interpreted, typically including cine review with the following specific activities: evaluation of the morphologic findings in multiple planes; assessment of biventricular function with ejection fraction and characterization of wall motion abnormalities; evaluation of multiple cardiac segments at incremental levels of stress for abnormal wall motion and viability; interpretation of precontrast and postcontrast images to assess myocardial ischemia and viability; and comparison with all pertinent available prior studies. The report is dictated for the medical record.

Intent and Use of Code +75565

Traditional MRI uses static images to obtain clinical diagnoses based upon anatomic information, whereas cardiac MRI also provides a physiologic evaluation of cardiac function. Cardiac MRI may be indicated in selected patients with diagnosis and treatment planning in several conditions including coronary artery disease, cardiac valvular disease, and congenital heart disease. It may also be indicated for imaging of cardiac anatomy for treatment planning. Add-on code **75565** describes cardiac MRI for velocity flow mapping. This code is reported only once per session. Add-on code **75565** is reported in conjunction with cardiac MRI codes **75557, 75559, 75561,** and **75563.** It is not appropriate to report the three-dimensional rendering codes **76376** and **76377** separately with code **75565.**

CODING TIP When flow velocity quantification is the only examination performed, it should be reported using code **76498,** *Unlisted magnetic resonance procedure (eg, diagnostic, interventional).*

Clinical Example for Code +75565

A 55-year-old male presents with heart failure, an enlarged cardiac silhouette on chest x-ray, and an eccentric jet of aortic regurgitation echocardiography. He is undergoing cardiac MRI to evaluate ventricular size and function. Flow velocity quantification is also requested.

Description of Service for Code +75565

Supervise the setup of flow quantification scan planes. Scan using flow protocols to obtain data to quantify valve function. Adjust the parameters to optimize

data accuracy. Analyze the velocity/flow data on an independent workstation. Calculate the regurgitation fraction, gradients, or shunt ratio using the velocity/flow data obtained.

NON-INVASIVE COMPUTED TOMOGRAPHIC ANGIOGRAPHY (CTA) (**75571-75574, 75635**)

75571   Computed tomography, heart, without contrast material, with quantitative evaluation of coronary calcium
CPT Assistant: Jul: 10:7; *CPT Changes: An Insider's View* 2010

75572   Computed tomography, heart, with contrast material, for evaluation of cardiac structure and morphology (including three-dimensional image postprocessing, assessment of cardiac function, and evaluation of venous structures, if performed)
CPT Assistant: Jul: 10:7; *CPT Changes: An Insider's View* 2010

75573   Computed tomography, heart, with contrast material, for evaluation of cardiac structure and morphology in the setting of congenital heart disease (including three-dimensional image postprocessing, assessment of LV cardiac function, RV structure and function and evaluation of venous structures, if performed)
CPT Assistant: Jul: 10:7; *CPT Changes: An Insider's View* 2010

75574   Computed tomographic angiography, heart, coronary arteries and bypass grafts (when present), with contrast material, including three-dimensional image postprocessing (including evaluation of cardiac structure and morphology, assessment of cardiac function, and evaluation of venous structures, if performed)
CPT Assistant: Jul: 10:7; *CPT Changes: An Insider's View* 2010

75635   Computed tomographic angiography, abdominal aorta and bilateral iliofemoral lower extremity runoff, with contrast material(s), including noncontrast images, if performed, and image postprocessing
CPT Assistant Jul 01:4-5, Dec 05:7, Jan 07:31; *CPT Changes: An Insider's View* 2001, 2008; *Clinical Examples in Radiology* Spring 06:1-3, Summer 08:7

Computed tomographic angiography (CTA) is a *non-invasive* (ie, non-catheter-based) technique for imaging vessels. The information obtained from the CTA is used in the evaluation of vascular anatomy (eg, renal or liver transplant donors, congenital anomalies); vascular disorders (eg, aortic or intracranial aneurysms, renal artery or carotid stenosis); vascular trauma (eg, aortic laceration); and in the follow-up of organ transplantation. The key distinction between CTA and computed tomography (CT) is that CTA includes reconstruction postprocessing of angiographic images and interpretation. If reconstruction postprocessing is not done, it is not a CTA study. Injection of contrast material is part of the "with contrast" CTA procedure; therefore, it is not appropriate to report separately the code for the administration of contrast.

Intent and Use of Codes 75571-75574

Cardiac CT and CTA provide imaging of the heart. These studies include the axial source images of the precontrast, arterial phase sequence and venous phase sequence (if performed), as well as the two-dimensional and three-dimensional reformatted images resulting from the study, including cine review. Contrast enhanced cardiac CT and coronary CTA codes 75571-75574 include any quantitative assessment when performed as part of the same encounter. Only one computed tomography heart service should be reported per encounter. The three-dimensional rendering codes 76376 and 76377 are considered an integral part of codes 75571-75574 and thus are not reported separately.

(Refer to Chapter 5 for further information pertaining to cardiac catheterization procedures.)

Intent and Use of Code 75571

Code 75571 describes CT study of the heart without the use of contrast material for quantitative evaluation of coronary calcium.

Clinical Example for Code 75571

A 45-year-old male presents for evaluation. Although he is asymptomatic, his family history is significant for coronary disease, with his father having suffered a myocardial infarction at the age of 58. A lipid profile is as follows: total cholesterol, 245 mg/dL; LDL low-density lipoprotein cholesterol, 156 mg/dL; HDL high-density lipoprotein cholesterol, 34 mg/dL; and triglycerides, 190 mg/dL. A risk assessment calculates a 10% risk of coronary disease over the next 10 years. A calcium score is ordered to help support the initiation of therapy with lipid-lowering agents.

Intent and Use of Code 75572

Code 75572 describes CT of the heart with the use of contrast material and includes three-dimensional imaging with postprocessing, assessment of cardiac function, and evaluation of venous structures, when performed.

Clinical Example for Code 75572

A 66-year-old female is seen for treatment of atrial fibrillation. A 48-hour monitor now shows her to be in atrial fibrillation approximately 12% of the time. Radiofrequency ablation is planned to isolate the pulmonary veins and eliminate the focus of atrial fibrillation. A cardiac CT scan is ordered by the electrophysiologist to identify the number, location, and morphology of the pulmonary veins as they enter the left atrium, the contours of the endoluminal surface of the left atrium, and the location of the esophagus in relation to the pulmonary veins.

Intent and Use of Code 75573

Code 75573 describes CT of the heart for evaluation of cardiac structure and morphology for congenital heart disease. This code also includes three-dimensional image postprocessing, assessment of LV cardiac function, RV structure and function, and evaluation of venous structures, when performed.

Clinical Example for Code 75573

A 12-year-old male presents for evaluation. As an infant, he underwent bilateral modified Blalock-Taussig shunts for tetralogy of Fallot with pulmonary atresia. Subsequent to that, he underwent total repair that included an aortic homograft Rastelli conduit from the right ventricle to the pulmonary arteries. Echocardiography reveals pulmonary pressures that are 65% of systemic pressures. There is minimal Rastelli valve stenosis but marked insufficiency and right ventricular enlargement. Bilateral peripheral pulmonary arterial stenosis is suspected, but branch pulmonary arteries are not visualized on echocardiography. The patient is referred for cardiac CT to measure right ventricular volume to determine whether he is a candidate for pulmonic valve replacement and to define branch pulmonary arteries to rule out significant peripheral pulmonary stenosis.

Intent and Use of Code 75574

Code 75574 describes computed tomographic angiography of the heart and coronary arteries, as well as any present bypass grafts with the use of contrast material. This code also includes three-dimensional image postprocessing with evaluation of cardiac structure and morphology and assessment of cardiac function, and evaluation of venous structures when performed.

CHAPTER 4

Clinical Example for Code 75574

A 52-year-old female presents for evaluation and possible treatment for retrosternal chest pain radiating to her left shoulder. Her physician determines that she is at intermediate risk for coronary artery disease. Her previous stress evaluations have been nondiagnostic. She is referred for cardiac CTA for evaluation of her coronary anatomy and left ventricular function.

Intent and Use of Code 75635

Computed tomographic angiography uses images obtained with a large volume of rapidly injected intravenous contrast, acquired with narrow collimation and reconstructed at narrower intervals than standard CT images. The scans are optimized specifically for visualization of the arterial and venous anatomy and any associated vascular anomalies *and* with CTA, additional information is provided, including vessel wall thickness, relationship to adjacent structures, enhanced depiction of the venous anatomy and parenchymal information of the target organ, and other structures within the scan range and field of view.

Code **75635** is the appropriate code to report CTA of the abdomen, pelvis, and bilateral lower extremities and reported for CTA of aorto-iliofemoral runoff. Code **75635** is an all-inclusive code that was designed and valued to reflect a complete evaluation of all three contiguous body parts (abdomen, pelvis, lower extremities). Coding this procedure as three separate studies (**72191**, **73706**, **74175**) would be considered unbundling and would not meet the CPT guidelines that one must select the code that accurately identifies the services performed.

Computed tomographic angiography uses images obtained with a large volume of rapidly injected intravenous contrast, acquired with narrow collimation and reconstructed at narrower intervals than standard CT images. The scans are optimized specifically for visualization of the arterial and venous anatomy and any associated vascular anomalies. The acquired data set is then evaluated with the aid of computer reconstruction. Cine display (mouse-driven sequential viewing of the images) greatly facilitates the examination of large stacks of slices. Two-dimensional reformatted images can be created in multiple planes, then interpreted, annotated, and archived as hard copy, electronically, or both. Three-dimensional or volume-rendered reconstructions are typically performed and evaluated in multiple projections. The phrase "image postprocessing" in the CTA descriptors refers to the two- and three-dimensional reconstructions. CPT codes **76376** and **76377** should not be coded separately for CTA studies.

With CTA, additional information is provided, including vessel wall thickness, relationship to adjacent structures, and enhanced depiction of the venous anatomy and parenchymal information of the target organ and other structures within the scan range and field of view.

Injection of contrast material is part of the "with contrast" CTA procedure; therefore, it is not appropriate to separately report the code for the administration of contrast. Sometimes a noncontrast sequence(s) is performed for localization of the anatomic region to be evaluated during the contrast scan. This is not separately reportable as, with all CTA codes, noncontrast images are included, if performed.

> **CODING TIP** Code **73706** is an inclusive component of code **75635**. Do not report **75635** in conjunction with codes **72191**, **73706**, **74175**, or **74174**.

Description of Service for Code 75635

Obtain and interpret scout views of area to be imaged. Obtain and review noncontrast CT images to localize the vascular phase sequence and to screen the patients who are not candidates for the arterial phase component of the study. Supervise low- or iso-osmolar contrast injection. Obtain the arterial phase CT images and review to ensure adequate anatomic coverage. Obtain and review delayed parenchymal phase CT images. Create and/or supervise two-dimensional reconstructions of the vasculature and associated organs, interpret, and annotate. Supervise and/or create three-dimensional reconstructions of the vasculature and associated organs. Adjust the projection of the three-dimensional reconstructions to optimize visualization of anatomy or pathology. Interpret the axial source images of the precontrast sequence, arterial phase sequence, and parenchymal phase sequence, as well as the two-dimensional and three-dimensional reformatted images resulting from the study, often including cine review. Compare with all pertinent available prior studies.

CATHETER-BASED PERIPHERAL ANGIOGRAPHY

Angiographic procedures done in conjunction with cardiac catheterization are significantly different from coding conventions for cardiac catheterization services. Cardiac catheterization is an invasive diagnostic medical procedure that includes several components. The procedure begins when the physician introduces one or more catheters into peripheral arteries and/or veins. The most common access point for cardiac catheterization is the femoral artery (used for left heart catheterization, aortography, coronary angiography, internal mammary artery injection, vein bypass graft injection, and for other left heart procedures and coronary artery interventions). Right heart catheterization (as well as pulmonary arteriography) is most often accomplished by initial entry in the right femoral vein. Each catheter is then positioned in a branch vessel or a cardiac chamber. During the catheterization procedure, recordings are made of intracardiac and intravascular pressure, blood samples are obtained for measurement of oxygen saturation or blood gases and cardiac output measurements are made.

Diagnostic angiography (radiological supervision and interpretation) codes should *not* be used with interventional procedures for:

1. Contrast injections, angiography, road mapping, and/or fluoroscopic guidance for the intervention;

2. Vessel measurement; and

3. Postangioplasty, stent, or atherectomy angiography because this work is captured in the radiological supervision and interpretation code(s). In the therapeutic codes that include radiological supervision and interpretation, this work is captured in the therapeutic code.

Diagnostic angiography performed at the time of an interventional procedure is separately reportable if:

1. No prior catheter-based angiographic study is available and a full diagnostic study is performed, and the decision to intervene is based on the diagnostic study, *or*

2. A prior study is available, but as documented in the medical record:

   a. The patient's condition with respect to the clinical indication has changed since the prior study, *or*

   b. There is inadequate visualization of the anatomy and/or pathology, *or*

   c. There is a clinical change during the procedure that requires new evaluation outside the target area of intervention.

Diagnostic angiography performed at a separate session from an interventional procedure is separately reported. If diagnostic angiography is necessary, is performed at same session as the interventional procedure, and meets the aforementioned criteria, **modifier 59** must be appended to the diagnostic radiological supervision and interpretation code(s) to denote that diagnostic work has been done following these guidelines. (Refer

to Chapter 6 for further discussion regarding use of **modifier 59**.)

Diagnostic angiography performed at the time of an interventional procedure is *not* separately reportable if it is specifically included in the interventional code descriptor.

In recognition of the complexity of interventional radiology services and their proper description, complete procedure codes were deleted from the CPT nomenclature in 1992 and "component" coding was introduced. Component coding facilitates more accurate coding by helping to completely describe the various procedures performed.

It allows for the following:

- Accurate tracking of professional services for outcome analysis, utilization review, and billing purposes

- Accurate service reporting whether one provider performs all services or multiple providers work in concert to perform the services (eg, one physician performs the procedure and another physician provides imaging supervision and interpretation)

- Tracking and reporting of interventional radiological hospital services in a manner exactly the same as other surgical and radiological services

- Fair relative valuation of similar types of services without regard to the specialty of the provider

AORTOGRAPHY (**75600-75630**)

75600	Aortography, thoracic, without serialography, radiological supervision and interpretation
75605	Aortography, thoracic, by serialography, radiological supervision and interpretation *CPT Assistant* Spring 1994:29, Dec 1998:9
75625	Aortography, abdominal, by serialography, radiological supervision and interpretation *CPT Assistant* Fall 1993:16, Jan 2001:14, Dec 2007:14, Apr 2008:11, Dec 2009:13; *Clinical Examples in Radiology* Winter 2008:1,2,4,5,9
75630	Aortography, abdominal plus bilateral iliofemoral lower extremity, catheter, by serialography, radiological supervision and interpretation *CPT Assistant* Fall 93:16, Jan 01:14, Apr 08:11, Dec 09:13

Imaging of the aorta may be performed independent of cardiac catheterization. In this circumstance,

FIGURE 4-1. Aortography **75600-75630**

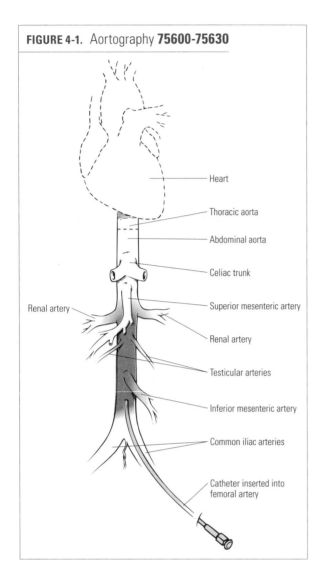

- Heart
- Thoracic aorta
- Abdominal aorta
- Celiac trunk
- Superior mesenteric artery
- Renal artery
- Renal artery
- Testicular arteries
- Inferior mesenteric artery
- Common iliac arteries
- Catheter inserted into femoral artery

introduction of a catheter into the aorta with injection procedures for an arch aortography, thoracic aortography, and abdominal aortography would be reported with the following codes:

⊙▲**36200**   Introduction of catheter, aorta

> *CPT Assistant* Fall 93:16, Aug 96:3, Jul 06:7, Dec 07:10, 14, Apr 08:11, Dec 09: 13; *CPT Changes: An Insider's View* 2012

75605   Aortography, thoracic, by serialography, radiological supervision and interpretation

75625   Aortography, abdominal, by serialography, radiological supervision and interpretation

75650   Angiography, cervicocerebral, catheter, including vessel origin, radiological supervision and interpretation

In this example, only one code is reported for the catheter placement in the aorta. However, three separate codes are necessary to completely report the radiological supervision and interpretation portion of the service. Code **75650** is reported for the arch aortography, code **75605** for the thoracic aortography, and code **75625** for the abdominal aortography.

However, if performing and imaging of the aortic root or ascending aorta at the time of a cardiac catheterization, this procedure is reported using add-on code **93567**, *Injection procedure during cardiac catheterization including imaging supervision, interpretation, and report; for supravalvular aortography (List separately in addition to code for primary procedure)*. Anatomically, the ascending aorta is the section between the heart and the arch of aorta. Add-on code **93567** represents supravalvular aortography that involves injection of contrast into the aorta, just above the aortic valve, to image the ascending aorta; for example when evaluating aortic insufficiency, ascending aortic dissection or ascending aortic aneurysm. Also, add-on code **93567** does not include any of the work that is reported with the base cardiac catheterization codes.

However, arch aortogram, descending thoracic aortogram, and abdominal aortogram are not routinely, but sometimes, performed during the same cardiac catheterization session. It is appropriate to additionally report a diagnostic abdominal (**75625**) or thoracic (**75605**) aortogram if performed at the same time as a diagnostic cardiac catheterization study and when performed in addition to supravalvular aortography (**93567**).

There are instances wherein "angiography of the peripheral vessel(s)" may be required. The imaging described by code **75630** is **not** inclusive of any of the cardiac catheterization procedures described by codes **93451-93462**. Therefore, when performed at the time of cardiac catheterization, it is appropriate to additionally report code **75630**, in addition to any of the cardiac catheterization codes **93451-93462**.

EXAMPLE: The right brachial artery is entered and a coronary catheter is advanced to the aortic root. Selective angiograms are made of the right coronary artery and the left coronary arteries. The coronary catheter is withdrawn and exchanged for a catheter that is then positioned in the infrarenal aorta for injection of contrast for aortography and bilateral iliofemoral angiograms with runoff films. The catheter is removed and hemostasis is achieved.

Coding Solution: In the above scenario, codes **93454**, *Catheter placement in coronary artery(s)*

for coronary angiography, including intraprocedural injection(s) for coronary angiography, imaging supervision and interpretation, and **75630** should be reported.

ABDOMINAL AORTOGRAPHY AND ILIOFEMORAL LOWER EXTREMITY RUNOFF (**75625**, **75630**, **75710**, **75716**, **+75774**)

75625 Aortography, abdominal, by serialography, radiological supervision and interpretation
CPT Assistant Fall 1993:16, Jan 2001:14, Dec 2007:14, Apr 2008:11, Dec 2009:13; *Clinical Examples in Radiology* Winter 2008:1, 2, 4, 5, 9

75630 Aortography, abdominal plus bilateral iliofemoral lower extremity, catheter, by serialography, radiological supervision and interpretation
CPT Assistant Fall 93:16, Jan 01:14, Apr 08:11, Dec 09:13

75710 Angiography, extremity, unilateral, radiological supervision and interpretation
CPT Assistant Apr 99:11, Jan 01:14

75716 Angiography, extremity, bilateral, radiological supervision and interpretation
CPT Assistant Fall 93:16, Jan 01:14, Dec 07:14, Apr 08:11, Dec 09:13; *Clinical Examples in Radiology* Winter 08:1, 2, 4, 5, 9

+75774 Angiography, selective, each additional vessel studied after basic examination, radiological supervision and interpretation (List separately in addition to code for primary procedure)
CPT Assistant Fall 1993:17, Spring 1994:29;*Clinical Examples in Radiology* Winter 2008:1, 2,4, 5, Summer 2008:1, 2, 3

When an abdominal aorta and bilateral iliofemoral lower extremity runoff study is performed, the evaluation also should include both the iliac and femoral arteries in the lower extremities at least to the level of the knees and usually to the level of the ankles.

For a procedure described as a full and complete arteriogram study of the abdominal aorta and a full and complete arteriogram evaluation of the lower extremities, code **36200**, *Introduction of catheter, aorta,* should be reported for placement of the catheter.

For a full and complete arteriogram of the abdominal aorta, one should report code **75625**, *Aortography, abdominal, by serialography radiological supervision and interpretation.*

For a full and complete arteriogram of the bilateral lower extremities, code **75716**, *Angiography, extremity,*

bilateral, radiological supervision and interpretation, is reported. Both codes **75625** and **75716** are reported when the catheter is placed at the level of the renal arteries for imaging of the entire abdominal aorta and then repositioned just above the aortic bifurcation for imaging of the distal aorta, the iliac arteries, and both lower extremities. Code **75630** is not reported as both studies are described as "full and complete" and when the catheter is repositioned for lower extremity imaging. To further clarify, code **75630**, *Aortography, abdominal plus bilateral iliofemoral lower extremity, catheter, by serialography, radiological supervision and interpretation,* is only reported when the abdominal aorta and runoff vessels in the lower extremities are studied with a single catheter position. Codes **75625**, *Aortography, abdominal, by serialography, radiological supervision and interpretation,* and **75716**, *Angiography, extremity, bilateral, radiological supervision and interpretation,* are for imaging of the aorta and [bilateral] runoff vessels when the physician images the aorta at one catheter position and performs the extremity vessel runoff after moving the catheter to another location.

To report an abdominal aortogram, code **75625** may be reported. If the physician performs an abdominal aortogram and repositions the catheter to image a unilateral lower extremity, codes **75625** and **75710** may be reported. If the physician performs both an abdominal aortogram and bilateral lower-extremity angiograms, codes **75625** and **75716** may be reported. Therefore, the physician's catheter movement is critical to support reporting of either of the extremity angiography codes (**75716** or **75710**). Even so, catheter movement will not always qualify reporting of a separate study, because some "abdominal only" studies (such as abdominal aortic aneurysm evaluation) may include more than one catheter position.

> **CODING TIP** Interventional radiology procedures are reported according to the documentation provided on a case-by-case basis. The operative note should reflect catheter movement and abdominal and extremity study findings before one reports the extremity study in addition to the abdominal study.

When the catheter is advanced to the aorta, then retracted back into the right common iliac artery ipsilaterally for additional study, no additional catheterization code (eg, **36140**) should be reported because the catheter was merely "pulled back" through the vessel. However, is performed contralaterally, code **36246**, *Selective catheter placement, arterial system; initial second order abdominal, pelvic, or lower extremity artery branch,* *within a vascular family*, should be reported for the second order contralateral selection.

Any additional selective imaging of the leg performed after the basic examination is reported with add-on code **+75774**, *Angiography, selective, each additional vessel studied after basic examination, radiological supervision and interpretation (List separately in addition to code for primary procedure).* The rationale for **not** coding **36140** with **36246** is the same as for doing a thoracic aortogram and then pulling the catheter back to do an abdominal aortogram. The work of placing the catheter in the second non-selective position is included in the work of the first non-selective position, or in the work of the higher-order selective placement.

> **CODING TIP** Code **75722** has been deleted. To report, see **36251**, **36253**, as appropriate. Code **75724** has also been deleted. To report, see **36252**, **36254**, as appropriate.

PERIPHERAL ANGIOGRAPHY DURING CARDIAC CATHETERIZATION (**75650-+75774**)

75650   Angiography, cervicocerebral, catheter, including vessel origin, radiological supervision and interpretation
CPT Assistant Spring 94:29, Apr 98:9, Oct 00:6

75658   Angiography, brachial, retrograde, radiological supervision and interpretation

75660   Angiography, external carotid, unilateral, selective, radiological supervision and interpretation
CPT Assistant Apr 11:12; *Clinical Examples in Radiology* Winter 09:2

75662   Angiography, external carotid, bilateral, selective, radiological supervision and interpretation
Clinical Examples in Radiology Spring 09:2, Winter 09:2

75665   Angiography, carotid, cerebral, unilateral, radiological supervision and interpretation
Clinical Examples in Radiology Winter 09:2

75671   Angiography, carotid, cerebral, bilateral, radiological supervision and interpretation
CPT Assistant Oct 00:6; *Clinical Examples in Radiology* Summer 07:1, 2, Winter 09:2

75676   Angiography, carotid, cervical, unilateral, radiological supervision and interpretation
Clinical Examples in Radiology Winter 09:2

75680   Angiography, carotid, cervical, bilateral, radiological supervision and interpretation
CPT Assistant Oct 00:6; *Clinical Examples in Radiology* Summer 07:1,2, Winter 09:2

75685   Angiography, vertebral, cervical, and/or intracranial, radiological supervision and interpretation
CPT Assistant Oct 00:6

75705   Angiography, spinal, selective, radiological supervision and interpretation

75726   Angiography, visceral, selective or supraselective (with or without flush aortogram), radiological supervision and interpretation
Clinical Examples in Radiology Summer 08:1, 2, 3

75731   Angiography, adrenal, unilateral, selective, radiological supervision and interpretation

75733   Angiography, adrenal, bilateral, selective, radiological supervision and interpretation

75736   Angiography, pelvic, selective or supraselective, radiological supervision and interpretation
Clinical Examples in Radiology Spring 05:14, Winter 08:4, 5

+75774   Angiography, selective, each additional vessel studied after basic examination, radiological supervision and interpretation (List separately in addition to code for primary procedure)
CPT Assistant Fall 1993:17, Spring 1994:29; *Clinical Examples in Radiology* Winter 2008:1, 2, 4, 5, Summer 2008:1, 2, 3

Often, diagnostic and therapeutic services are provided in a variety of combinations and permutations determined by the underlying disease process, the clinical evaluation of the patient, and the intraprocedural interpretation of the diagnostic portion of the service (including physiologic data and images obtained). These contingencies may result in several coding possibilities.

All noncoronary vascular procedures, whether diagnostic or therapeutic, begin with establishment of vascular access (vascular catheterization). The codes available for reporting the catheterization portion of the procedure are found in the vascular injection procedures series of codes (**36000-36299**).

Often, there is not a one-to-one relationship between the number of codes reported for the catheterization and the number of codes reported from the **70000** series for the radiological supervision and interpretation portion of the service.

When multiple selections are performed in different vascular families, then the highest level of selectivity is reported for each vascular family. However, this catheterization was performed within the same family. Therefore, it would be appropriate to report only one code for the selective catheterization. The final destination of the catheter on the left side is not clear. If the final destination of the catheter involved selective positioning of the catheter into the right common iliac from the left common femoral access, it would be appropriate to report only code **36245** because this would be a first-order selection from the left common femoral artery. If a more selective catheterization than a first order were performed in the left femoral system, it would be appropriate to report a single code only for the highest order of selection in the catheterization of the left and right arteries. (Refer to Chapter 3 for further information regarding lower extremity revascularization [37222-37235].)

Interventional radiology procedures are reported according to the documentation provided on a case-by-case basis. The operative note should reflect catheter movement and abdominal and extremity study findings before one reports the extremity study in addition to the abdominal study. (Refer to Chapter 3 for further information and examples regarding the renal angiography performed independent of cardiac catheterization. Refer to Chapter 5 for further information regarding the reporting of cardiac catheterization and iliac and renal angiography [G0275 and G0278].)

RIGHT/LEFT INTERNAL MAMMARY ANGIOGRAPHY DURING CARDIAC CATHETERIZATION (**75756**)

75756 Angiography, internal mammary, radiological supervision and interpretation

Although not typically studied "in preparation" for bypass surgery, should angiography be performed to evaluate the left or right internal mammary artery (LIMA, RIMA), for example, due to prior thoracic surgery or radiation, the appropriate diagnostic cardiac catheterization with angiography code (**93455, 93457, 93459,** or **93461**) should be reported, based on the catheterization approach performed.

However, in the absence of another diagnostic cardiac catheterization procedure, selective catheterization of the left internal mammary artery is reported using code **36216**. The selective catheter placement of the right internal mammary artery is reported using code **36217** because for the RIMA one has to traverse the

innominate and then the subclavian. The radiological supervision and interpretation for right and left internal mammary artery angiography is reported using code **75756**, which may be reported twice, either by appending **modifier 50**, *Bilateral Procedure,* or **modifier 59**, *Distinct Procedural Service.*

CODING TIP The noncongenital cardiac catheterization codes include the phrase "free arterial." A free arterial graft means that it is completely disconnected from its source and then sewn distally to a coronary artery and proximally to the aorta or to another graft. It can be a segment of internal mammary artery (IMA), radial artery, or any other arterial conduit. A regular IMA graft is still left in situ proximally, so there is only a distal anastomosis. If the IMA is disconnected proximally, as is sometimes necessary for a right IMA, then it is a free graft. A radial graft is always a free graft.

PULMONARY VEIN ANGIOGRAPHY DURING CARDIAC CATHETERIZATION (**75741-75746**)

75741 Angiography, pulmonary, unilateral, selective, radiological supervision and interpretation

75743 Angiography, pulmonary, bilateral, selective, radiological supervision and interpretation
CPT Assistant Spring 94:29, Apr 98:7

75746 Angiography, pulmonary, by nonselective catheter or venous injection, radiological supervision and interpretation

Selective injection and diagnostic imaging of the pulmonary *veins* during cardiac catheterization is additionally reported using code **93541**, *Injection procedure during cardiac catheterization; for pulmonary angiography,* and either code **75743**, *Angiography, pulmonary, bilateral, selective, radiological supervision and interpretation,* or code **75741**, *Angiography, pulmonary, unilateral, selective, radiological supervision and interpretation.*

However, because the cardiac catheterization codes for congenital anomalies may require additional access to other vessels not normally required in normal cardiac anatomy (eg, pulmonary vein, azygous vein), it is appropriate to additionally report selective catheterization codes from the 36200-36248 series and/or their respective radiologic supervision and interpretation codes. Therefore, if evaluating each of the four pulmonary veins, the codes would be reported four times. (Refer to Chapter 5 for further information and reporting example of pulmonary vein angiography at the time of cardiac catheterization.) The examples reflect reporting during a congenital cardiac catheterization; however, this reporting usage is appropriate for noncongenital cardiac catheterization as well.

Furthermore, when reporting only the professional component of the service, **modifier 26** should be appended to the radiological supervision and interpretation code reported (eg, if the procedure is performed on hospital or facility-owned equipment). (Refer to Chapter 6 for further discussion regarding the use of **modifier 26**.)

(Refer to Chapter 5 for further information pertaining to reporting diagnostic angiography **70000** codes in addition to cardiac catheterization.)

ANGIOGRAPHY OF ARTERIOVENOUS SHUNT (EG, DIALYSIS) (**75791**)

75791   Angiography, arteriovenous shunt (eg, dialysis patient fistula/graft), complete evaluation of dialysis access, including fluoroscopy, image documentation and report (includes injections of contrast and all necessary imaging from the arterial anastomosis and adjacent artery through entire venous outflow including the inferior or superior vena cava), radiological supervision and interpretation
CPT Changes: An Insider's View 2010

Intent and Use of Code 75791

Code **75791** describes the performance of a radiological evaluation through an already existing access site into the shunt or from an access site that is not a direct puncture of the shunt. Code **75791** is not reported in conjunction with codes **36147** and **36148**. Codes **36140**, **36215-36217**, and **36245-36247**, as appropriate, should also be reported in addition to code **75791** for introduction of a catheter. Code **36147** differs in that it represents a complete radiological evaluation with needle/catheter introduction of an AV dialysis shunt.

Clinical Example for Code 75791

A patient with end-stage renal disease (ESRD) is found to have poor flows during dialysis with clotting of the needle such that dialysis cannot be completed. The patient is sent to the angiographic suite with needles in place for a diagnostic study to evaluate the arteriovenous shunt.

Description of Service for Code 75791

Angiography is performed to include the entire length of the graft and all outflow veins to the level of the superior vena cava. Compression may be applied to allow visualization of the arterial anastomosis. Technical personnel are directed throughout. Interpretation of the imaging of all views is obtained.

THREE-DIMENSIONAL RENDERING (**76376**, **76377**)

76376   three-dimensional rendering with interpretation and reporting of computed tomography, magnetic resonance imaging, ultrasound, or other tomographic modality; not requiring image postprocessing on an independent workstation
CPT Assistant Dec 05:1,7, Jan 07:31, Jul 08:3, May 09:9, Jun 09:9, Jul 09:10, Apr 10:5,9, Jul 10:7; CPT Changes: An Insider's View 2006; Clinical Examples in Radiology Winter 06:17, Spring 06:8-9, Fall 06:9-10, Winter 07:4-5, Summer 08:8, Fall 08:12, Spring 09:4

76377   requiring image postprocessing on an independent workstation
CPT Assistant Dec 05:1, Jan 07:31, Jul 08:3, May 09:9, Jun 09:9, Jul 09:10, Dec 09:13, Feb 10:6, Apr 10:5,9, Jul 10:7; CPT Changes: An Insider's View 2006; Clinical Examples in Radiology Winter 06:17, Spring 06:8-9, Fall 06:9-10, Winter 07:4-5, Summer 07:1,2, Summer 08:8, Fall 08:12, Spring 09:5

Intent and Use of Codes 76376-76377

Code **76376** is used to report three-dimensional rendering with interpretation and reporting of CT, MRI, ultrasound, or other tomographic modality not requiring postprocessing on an independent workstation.

Code **76377** is used to report three-dimensional rendering with interpretation and reporting of CT, MRI, ultrasound, or other tomographic modality requiring image postprocessing on an independent workstation.

The three-dimensional image rendering codes **76376** and **76377** reflect the levels of complexity of image postprocessing and rendering currently being performed. Advances in technology have, in many situations, expedited two-dimensional image reformatting so that it can now be performed rapidly by a technologist without a separate workstation or the need to take a scanner off-line for image processing. On the other hand, complex three-dimensional image rendering often requires extensive independent workstation processing by a supervising physician and specially trained technologist. A few applications can be performed on the scanner using optional and expensive hardware and software. In addition, with the evolution of scanner capabilities to produce two-dimensional reformatting virtually in real time, it is thought that the two-dimensional reformats should be included in the base procedure code and not separately reported. The new three-dimensional rendering codes address complex renderings such as shaded surface rendering, volumetric rendering, maximum intensity projections, fusion imaging, and quantitative analysis (segmental volumes and surgical planning).

According to the American College of Radiology, the three-dimensional rendering codes address complex renderings such as shaded surface rendering, volumetric rendering, quantitative analysis (segmental volumes and surgical planning), and maximum intensity projections when such renderings can be performed on the scanner or when it requires the use of an independent workstation.

While it is generally understood in an individual practice that three-dimensional renderings are performed on the scanner (as with ultrasound) or on an independent workstation, making an explicit statement in the report will avoid ambiguity and aid the coder in accurately coding the procedure. Some practices may document this separately (eg, as part of an electronic medical record) but not actually in the report.

Whether three-dimensional rendering should be performed is determined by the referring physician, sometimes with consultation from, or at the recommendation of, the radiologist. Theoretically, within a Medicare facility, a radiologist can order three-dimensional rendering on Medicare beneficiaries independent of the treating physician. This is not the case in an independent diagnostic testing facility or other nonhospital setting. It is a stretch to invoke the radiology exemption to the Ordering of Diagnostic Tests Rule as justification for a radiologist to perform three-dimensional rendering without an order from the treating physician in the nonfacility setting. Because of the potential for abuse and the risk of an Office of the Inspector General inspection, it is generally thought to be prudent that medical necessity for three-dimensional rendering be based on the referring physician's request, regardless of the clinical setting. Payers want to be assured that the three-dimensional studies are adding valuable clinical information; therefore, they want a request to perform three-dimensional to come from the treating physician on a case-by-case basis.

The three-dimensional rendering codes are not to be used in conjunction with CTA, magnetic resonance angiography, nuclear medicine studies (including codes

74261, 74262 CT colonography), or cardiac CT and CTA procedures because all of these procedures have three-dimensional rendering valued into the codes.

However, codes **76376** and **76377** are used in conjunction with a primary base procedure code, such as CT, MR, ultrasound, or other tomographic modality. For example, if a physician reports that three-dimensional rendering is performed on an independent workstation, CPT code **76377** should be reported.

Code **76376** is reported in conjunction with code(s) for base imaging procedure(s). Because echocardiography is defined in the CPT codebook as an ultrasound examination of the cardiac chambers and valves, the adjacent great vessels, and the pericardium, CPT coding rules do not prohibit the use of CPT codes **93307** and **93350** (both listed in the echocardiography section of the CPT codebook), provided three-dimensional images are obtained as outlined in the following intraservice descriptions.

CODING TIP Do not report code **76376** in conjunction with codes **31627, 70496, 70498, 70544-70549, 71275, 71555, 72159, 72191, 72198, 73206, 73225, 73706, 73725, 74174, 74175, 74185, 74261-74263, 75557, 75559, 75561, 75563, 75565, 75571-75574, 75635, 76377, 78000-78999**, or **0159T**.

CODING TIP Do not report code **76377** in conjunction with codes **70496, 70498, 70544-70549, 71275, 71555, 72159, 72191, 72198, 73206, 73225, 73706, 73725, 74174, 74175, 74185, 74261-74263, 75557, 75559, 75561, 75563, 75565, 75571-75574, 75635, 76376, 78000-78999**, or **0159T**.

Description of Service for Code 76376

The physician supervises the technologist in creating the three-dimensional images, interprets the images, and dictates a report for the medical record.

Description of Service for Code 76377

The physician supervises and/or creates three-dimensional reconstructions of the organs of interest using an independent workstation. He or she adjusts the projection of the three-dimensional reconstructions to optimize visualization of the anatomy or pathology. The physician interprets the three-dimensional reformatted images resulting from the study, typically including cine review. The images are compared with all pertinent available prior studies, and a report is dictated for the medical record.

MYOCARDIALPERFUSION IMAGING (78451-78454)

78451   Myocardial perfusion imaging, tomographic (SPECT) (including attenuation correction, qualitative or quantitative wall motion, ejection fraction by first pass or gated technique, additional quantification, when performed); single study, at rest or stress (exercise or pharmacologic)
CPT Assistant May 10:5, 11; CPT Changes: An Insider's View 2010

78452   multiple studies, at rest and/or stress (exercise or pharmacologic) and/or redistribution and/or rest reinjection
CPT Assistant May 10:5, 11; CPT Changes: An Insider's View 2010

78453   Myocardial perfusion imaging, planar (including qualitative or quantitative wall motion, ejection fraction by first pass or gated technique, additional quantification, when performed); single study, at rest or stress (exercise or pharmacologic)
CPT Assistant May 10:5, 11; CPT Changes: An Insider's View 2010

78454   multiple studies, at rest and/or stress (exercise or pharmacologic) and/or redistribution and/or rest reinjection
CPT Assistant May 10:5, 11; CPT Changes: An Insider's View 2010

Intent and Use of Codes 78451-78454

Myocardial perfusion is performed to diagnose or manage conditions such as myocardial ischemia, coronary artery disease, and myocardial infarction. Single photon emission-computed tomography (SPECT) myocardial perfusion imaging (MPI) was one of the earliest cardiovascular diagnostic tests developed. As more clinical evidence-based studies were subsequently performed, the changing technology has enabled SPECT to be performed in a physician's office or hospital outpatient setting.

The common indications for the performance of the MPI tests include the following:

- assessment of the presence, location, and severity of myocardial perfusion abnormalities;

- identification and confirmation of possible ischemic myocardium; and

- determination of the significance of anatomic lesions detected by angiography.

The two forms of MPI stress include exercise induced and pharmacologically induced. All stress procedures must be supervised by a health care professional and must be continually monitored.

Exercise Stress

Exercise stress is typically performed with a treadmill or bicycle, with the patient fasting at least four hours before the test. Exercise stress is the preferred method because of its ability to collect additional prognostic information and evaluate exercise-related symptoms. However, patients with medical conditions that would result in the inability to perform adequate exercise stress may need to undergo pharmacologic stress. Similarly, patients unable to stop medications that modulate heart rate and blood pressure response, such as beta-blocking and calcium channel–blocking drugs, may also need to undergo pharmacologic stress.

Pharmacologic Stress

Two types of pharmacologic stress are used to evaluate myocardial perfusion:

Vasodilator stress agents, such asdipyridamole, adenosine, and regadenoson, are administered to create coronary hyperemia. Caffeinated beverages and methylxanthine-containing medications, which interfere with coronary hyperemia, should be discontinued for at least 12 hours before pharmacologic-induced stress imaging. If not medically contraindicated, patients may also perform low-level exercise to minimize symptoms associated with vasodilators and to minimize subdiaphragmatic tracer absorption.

Inotropic or chronotropic adrenergic agents, such as dobutamine, are administered to increase myocardial oxygen demand. If not medically contraindicated, certain medications such as beta-adrenergic blocking agents, which modulate the chronotropic response to the adrenergic stimulation with dobutamine, should be discontinued before the procedure. (Warning: Abrupt withdrawal of beta blockade can result in myocardial infarction or acute coronary syndromes.) Some patients may require atropine to increase the heart rate response. However, increasing heart rate by administrating atropine does not give the same result of an increase in coronary blood flow induced by exercise.

Image Acquisition

SPECT imaging *slices* the area of the body into three planes: front-to-back, side-to-side, or head-to-toe (X, Y, and Z axes). The gamma camera acquires the imaging data, and the computers process the data to enable the physician to meticulously examine a specific area in multiple planes and to determine the precise location of any abnormal areas.

Data from perfusion images are acquired and recorded using planar and/or SPECT techniques. To illustrate the distribution of blood perfusion within the myocardium, intravenous radiopharmaceuticals are administered (such as 201Tl and 99mTc sestamibi, and 99mTc tetrofosmin), extracted, and retained for a time by the myocardium. This allows the identification of areas with reduced myocardial blood flow associated with ischemia or scar. The data are analyzed by visual inspection and/or by quantitative or qualitative techniques. Patients with significant coronary artery narrowing will have an area of reduced concentration of the radiopharmaceutical, confirming the location of decreased perfusion. If the location or severity of decreased radiopharmaceutical concentration is worse with administration during stress, the area of decreased concentration presumably signifies ischemia. Conversely, if the location or severity of diminished radiopharmaceutical concentration remains unchanged during stress, the defect generally signifies a scar. However, this may also represent severely underperfused myocardium.

CODING TIP With codes **78451-78454**, a single or dual isotope technique may be used.

Intent and Use of Code 78451

Code 78451 describes myocardial perfusion imaging specifically for single SPECT imaging studies. This code is reported when the examination is performed at rest or with stress, but not both. When both stress and rest are used, the multiple study code (**78452**) should be reported.

Description of Service for Code 78451

The study consists of an acquisition of a stress or a rest tomographic (SPECT) data set synchronized (gated) to the patient's electrocardiogram when performed. The physician verifies the completeness and adequacy of the data before completion of the study and may order additional imaging if necessary. The images are reviewed for artifacts and abnormal extracardiac

distribution. Three different tomographic data sets are reviewed and reconstructed, if necessary. The physician compares the three tomographic views for differences or similarities that would suggest ischemia or scar. Qualitative assessment of ventricular wall function and perfusion are made in a standardized manner, with each segment scored on a semiquantitative scale when performed. Wall motion is qualitatively scored for motion and thickening. This occurs in a standardized segment model for the data set with each segment scored as normal, mildly hypokinetic, moderately hypokinetic, severely hypokinetic, akinetic, or dyskinetic. Attention is given to the assessment of regional myocardial function and to the percentage of myocardium that is regionally dysfunctional in order to judge the amount of underlying myocardial scar (or stress-induced ischemia). The extent and severity of perfusion defects and their relationship to vascular geographic territories are noted.

When performed, wall motion and thickening quantitative data are generated and reviewed for the image set. The segmental wall motion data are compared with the perfusion images to generate a clinically relevant wall motion analysis for an individual patient. When performed, left ventricular ejection fraction is reported after confirming the correctness of the regions of interest that were selected for the calculation. Digital data of perfusion and ventricular function are reviewed after the qualitative assessment, in part to refine the qualitative impression. Comparison with relevant prior studies is done. A report is dictated for the medical record.

CODING TIP Wall motion, ejection fraction, and attenuation correction, when performed, are inclusive in codes **78451-78454** and may not be reported separately.

Intent and Use of Code 78452

Code 78452 describes myocardial perfusion imaging specifically for multiple SPECT imaging studies. This code is reported when the examination is performed for multiple studies of rest, stress, and/or redistribution. If the protocol is performed over several days, code 78452 would still be reported. However, it would not be appropriate to separately report a single SPECT study for each day; such a practice would be considered unbundling.

Description of Service for Code 78452

The study consists of acquisition of stress and rest (and/or redistribution) tomographic (SPECT) data sets synchronized (gated) to the patient's electrocardiogram when performed. The physician verifies the completeness and adequacy of the data sets before completion of the study and may order additional imaging if necessary. The images are reviewed for artifacts and abnormal extracardiac distribution. Three different tomographic data sets are reviewed for each acquisition and reconstructed, if necessary. The physician compares the tomographic data sets for differences or similarities that would suggest ischemia or scar. Qualitative assessment of ventricular wall function and perfusion are made in a standardized manner, with each segment scored on a semiquantitative scale when performed. Wall motion is qualitatively scored for motion and thickening. This occurs in a standardized segment model for the data set with each segment scored as normal, mildly hypokinetic, moderately hypokinetic, severely hypokinetic, akinetic, or dyskinetic. Attention is given to the assessment of regional myocardial function and to the percentage of myocardium that is regionally dysfunctional in order to judge the amount of underlying myocardial scar (or stress-induced ischemia). The extent and severity of perfusion defects and their relationship to vascular geographic territories are noted. When performed, wall motion and thickening quantitative data are generated and reviewed. The segmental wall motion data are compared with the perfusion images to generate a clinically relevant wall motion analysis for an individual patient. When performed, left ventricular ejection fraction is noted after confirming the correctness of the regions of interest that were selected for the calculation. Digital data of perfusion and ventricular function are reviewed after the qualitative assessment, in part to refine the qualitative impression. Comparison with relevant prior studies is done. A report is dictated for the medical record.

Intent and Use of Code 78453

Code 78453 describes myocardial perfusion imaging specifically for two-dimensional planar imaging studies. This code is reported when the examination is performed at rest or with stress, but not both. When both rest and stress MPI studies are performed, the multiple study code (78454) should be reported.

> **CODING TIP** It would not be appropriate to separately report codes **78481** or **78483** for the first-pass technique on a separate camera with any of the MPI codes **78451-78454**.

Description of Service for Code 78453

The study consists of a single study acquisition of a stress or rest set of planar images synchronized (gated) to the patient's electrocardiogram when performed. The physician verifies the completeness and adequacy of the data before completion of the study and may order additional imaging if necessary. The planar images are reviewed for artifacts and abnormal extracardiac distribution. The cardiac images, which are acquired in at least three different projections (eg, anterior, LAO, and lateral), are reviewed. The physician compares the acquisition data sets for differences or similarities that would suggest ischemia or scar. Qualitative assessment of myocardial perfusion is made in a standardized manner, with each segment scored on a semiquantitative scale. Qualitative assessment of left ventricular global function is made, when performed. Wall motion is qualitatively scored for motion and thickening, when performed. This occurs in a standardized segment model for each data set with each segment scored as normal, mildly hypokinetic, moderately hypokinetic, severely hypokinetic, akinetic, or dyskinetic. Attention is given to the assessment of regional myocardial function and to the percentage of myocardium that is regionally dysfunctional in order to judge the amount of underlying myocardial scar (or stress-induced ischemia). The extent and severity of perfusion defects and their relationship to vascular geographic territories are noted. When performed, wall motion and thickening quantitative data are generated and reviewed for the image set. The segmental wall motion data are compared with the perfusion images to generate a clinically relevant wall motion analysis for an individual patient. When performed, the left ventricular ejection fraction is noted after confirming the correctness of the regions of interest that were selected for the calculation. Digital data of perfusion and ventricular function are reviewed after the qualitative assessment, in part to refine the qualitative impression. Comparison with relevant prior studies is done. A report is dictated for the medical record.

Intent and Use of Code 78454

Code 78454 describes myocardial perfusion imaging specifically for two-dimensional planar imaging studies. Code 78454 is reported when the examination is performed for multiple studies of rest, stress, and/or redistribution. If the protocol is performed over several days, code 78454 would still be reported. It would not be appropriate to separately report a single two-dimensional planar imaging study for each day, which would be considered unbundling.

CHAPTER 4

CODING TIP When performing the MPI procedures described in codes **78451-78454** with stress, the physician performing the stress test will report that service with the appropriate code from the cardiovascular stress testing code series **93015-93018**. HCPCS Level II codes may be utilized for other nonradioactive drugs utilized in the study (eg, adenosine, dipyridamole, and regadenoson).

Description of Service for Code 78454

The study consists of acquisition of stress and rest (or redistribution) planar image sets synchronized (gated) to the patient's electrocardiogram when performed. The physician verifies the completeness and adequacy of the images before completion of the study and may order additional imaging if necessary. The planar images are reviewed for artifacts and abnormal extracardiac distribution. The cardiac images, which are acquired in at least three different projections (eg, anterior, LAO, and lateral) for the rest and stress sets of images are reviewed. The physician compares the acquisition datasets for differences or similarities that would suggest ischemia or scar. Qualitative assessment of myocardial perfusion is made in a standardized manner, with each segment scored on a semiquantitative scale. Qualitative assessment of left ventricular global function is made, when performed. Wall motion is qualitatively scored for motion and thickening, when performed. This occurs in a standardized segment model for each data set with each segment scored as normal, mildly hypokinetic, moderately hypokinetic, severely hypokinetic, akinetic, or dyskinetic. Attention is given to the assessment of regional myocardial function and to the percentage of myocardium that is regionally dysfunctional in order to judge the amount of underlying myocardial scar (or stress-induced ischemia). The extent and severity of perfusion defects and their relationship to vascular geographic territories are noted. When performed, wall motion and thickening quantitative data are generated and reviewed for the image set. The segmental wall motion data are compared with the perfusion images to generate a clinically relevant wall motion analysis for an individual patient. When performed, the left ventricular ejection fraction is noted after confirming the correctness of the regions of interest that were selected for the calculation. Digital data of perfusion and ventricular function are reviewed after the qualitative assessment, in part to refine the qualitative impression. Comparison with relevant prior studies is done. A report is dictated for the medical record.

MYOCARDIAL INFARCT-AVID IMAGING (78466-78469)

78466   Myocardial imaging, infarct avid, planar; qualitative or quantitative

78468   with ejection fraction by first pass technique
CPT Assistant May 10:5, 11

78469   tomographic SPECT with or without quantification
CPT Assistant May 10:5, 11

Intent and Use of Codes 78466-78469

Codes **78466-78469** apply to myocardial infarct-avid imaging, which is used as an adjunct to more common approaches for the diagnosis of myocardial infarction. Two infarct-avid agents are currently available: technetium-99m stannous pyrophosphate, the bone imaging tracer, and a specific antibody to cardiac myosin.

Code **78466** designates a planar imaging study.

Code **78469** designates a SPECT imaging study.

Code **78468** is used if first-pass imaging is performed during a bolus injection of the tracer to determine ejection fraction.

CARDIAC BLOOD POOL IMAGING (MUGA) (78472-78483) AND MYOCARDIAL IMAGING (PET) (78491-78492)

78472   Cardiac blood pool imaging, gated equilibrium; planar, single study at rest or stress (exercise and/or pharmacologic), wall motion study plus ejection fraction, with or without additional quantitative processing
CPT Assistant Nov 98:22, Jun 99:8, Nov 99:44, May 10:5, 11; *CPT Changes: An Insider's View* 2000

78473   multiple studies, wall motion study plus ejection fraction, at rest and stress (exercise and/or pharmacologic), with or without additional quantification
CPT Assistant Jun 99:11, May 10:5, 11

78481   Cardiac blood pool imaging (planar), first pass technique; single study, at rest or with stress (exercise and/or pharmacologic), wall motion study plus ejection fraction, with or without quantification multiple studies, at rest and with stress (exercise and/or pharmacologic), wall

motion study plus ejection fraction, with or without quantification
CPT Assistant May 10:5, 11

78483   multiple studies, at rest and with stress (exercise and/or pharmacologic), wall motion study plus ejection fraction, with or without quantification

78491   Myocardial imaging, positron emission tomography (PET), perfusion; single study at rest or stress
CPT Assistant Nov 97:27, May 10:5, 11

78492   multiple studies at rest and/or stress
CPT Assistant Nov 97:27, May 10:5, 11

78494   Cardiac blood pool imaging, gated equilibrium, SPECT, at rest, wall motion study plus ejection fraction, with or without quantitative processing
CPT Assistant Nov 98:22, Jun 99:3, May 10:5, 11

+78496   Cardiac blood pool imaging, gated equilibrium, single study, at rest, with right ventricular ejection fraction by first pass technique (List separately in addition to code for primary procedure)
CPT Assistant Nov 98:22, Jun 99:3,11, May 10:5, 11

78499   Unlisted cardiovascular procedure, diagnostic nuclear medicine
CPT Assistant Dec 05:7, May 10:5, 11; *Clinical Examples in Radiology* Summer 08:12

Intent and Use of Codes 78472, 78473, 78494, and +78496

Codes **78472**, **78473**, and **78494** are used to report cardiac blood pool imaging. In these studies, the tracer remains within the blood pool, generally through labeling of red blood cells with technetium-99m.

Code **78472** refers to planar electrocardiographic-gated equilibrium studies performed at rest only.

Code **78473** refers to planar electrocardiographic-gated equilibrium studies performed with supine or upright exercise or with pharmacologic stress (eg, dobutamine). Typically, these studies will include several acquisitions at one or more levels of exercise. Exercise studies are used to detect regional and global dysfunctions that are a consequence of coronary artery disease. Such data appear to be of value for the diagnosis and risk assessment. Usually rest and exercise acquisitions are made.

Code **78494** is used to report gated equilibrium studies in combination with SPECT performed at rest only.

Code **78496** is used when a first-pass study is performed in addition to a gated equilibrium study to

assess the right ventricle ejection fraction. It is considered an add-on code, to be used with code **78472**.

Codes **78481** and **78483** refer to first-pass studies in which the data are acquired rapidly after a bolus of radiotracer has been injected. Serial images are acquired as the bolus passes from the superior vena cava through the cardiac chambers and great vessels. The codes used are similar to those for the equilibrium studies described above, with code **78481** used for rest-only studies and code **78483** used for rest-plus-exercise studies. It is important to note that, while the equilibrium approach allows multiple acquisitions at rest and with various levels of stress, the first-pass approach requires another injection of tracer for each acquisition. Thus, only a limited number of physiologic states can be assessed.

> **CODING TIP** It is not appropriate to report codes **78481-78483** in conjunction with codes **78451-78454**, for first pass technique on a separate camera because the first pass study for ejection fraction, if performed, is considered inclusive.

PULMONARY PERFUSION IMAGING (●78579-78598)

●**78579**   Pulmonary ventilation imaging (eg, aerosol or gas)
CPT Changes: An Insider's View 2012

▲**78580**   Pulmonary perfusion imaging (eg, particulate)
CPT Assistant Mar 1999:4, Dec 2005:7; *CPT Changes: An Insider's View* 2012

●**78582**   Pulmonary ventilation (eg, aerosol or gas) and perfusion imaging
CPT Changes: An Insider's View 2012

●**78597**   Quantitative differential pulmonary perfusion, including imaging when performed
CPT Changes: An Insider's View 2012

●**78598**   Quantitative differential pulmonary perfusion and ventilation (eg, aerosol or gas), including imaging when performed
CPT Changes: An Insider's View 2012

Intent and Use of Codes 78579-78598

These nuclear medicine studies are diagnostic studies associated, for example, with pulmonary embolism, bronchopulmonary sequestration, or pulmonary trauma. Two isotopic methods are used to obtain ventilation data: one with gaseous radioactive xenon; the other with inhaled radioactive aerosol.

Codes **78579-78598** may be used: (1) when imaging is performed for aerosols *or* gases (because testing for aerosols or gases are performed using the same methods); and (2) eliminate confusion regarding pulmonary function quantification by differentiating between ventilation procedures and perfusion procedures. The codes distinctly identify the type of testing procedure that is done and not according to the type of product being tested (ie, ventilation testing vs perfusion imaging and not gas vs aerosol). This includes development of codes that identify multiple services (eg, ventilation *and* perfusion identified by code **78582**).

Description of Procedure for Code 78579

A 52-year-old male has recent onset of obstructive pulmonary disease. A pulmonary ventilation study is ordered to determine the extent of disease. Lung ventilation scintigraphy is a radionuclide diagnostic imaging study that records the bronchopulmonary distribution of an inhaled radioactive aerosol or gas within the lungs. Multiple images of the lungs are acquired.

Description of Procedure for Code 78580

Lung perfusion scintigraphy is a radionuclide diagnostic imaging study that records the distribution of pulmonary arterial blood flow within the lungs. Multiple images of the lungs are acquired. Under the supervision of the physician, the technologist administers the radiopharmaceutical. The study consists of multiple images, in multiple projections (eg, anterior, posterior, right and left anterior and posterior obliques, right and left laterals), and documentation regarding patient position. The physician verifies the adequacy of the imaging data before completion of the study, and directs the technologist to obtain additional views, when necessary. The data are formatted for film and/or digital display and analysis. The physician reviews the study for artifacts and abnormal distribution. The processed and raw images (eg, upright or supine, posterior, anterior, obliques and laterals, etc) are compared to a current chest X ray.

Description of Procedure for Code 78582

Lung ventilation and perfusion scintigraphy is a combination of two radionuclide diagnostic imaging procedures that record both the bronchopulmonary distribution of an inhaled radioactive aerosol or gas and the distribution of pulmonary arterial blood flow within the lungs. Multiple images of pulmonary ventilation and perfusion are acquired and compared. Under the supervision of the physician, the technologist gives specific breathing instructions to the patient while administering the radiopharmaceuticals. The

complete study consists of administration of two different radiopharmaceuticals, one by inhalation and the other by intravenous injection, acquisition of two (2) sets of multiple images in a variety of projections, (eg, anterior, posterior, right and left anterior and posterior obliques, right and left laterals) and documentation of patient position. The physician verifies the adequacy of the imaging data before completion of the study, and directs the technologist to obtain additional views, when necessary. The data are formatted for film and/or digital display and analysis. The physician reviews the study for artifacts and abnormal distribution. The processed and raw images (eg, upright or supine, posterior, anterior, obliques and laterals, etc) of both ventilation and perfusion imaging sets are compared to a current chest X ray and any additional relevant prior studies, and formally interpreted, ie, a report is dictated for the medical record.

Description of Procedure for Code 78597

Quantitative lung perfusion scintigraphy is a radionuclide diagnostic imaging study that records the relative distribution of pulmonary arterial blood flow in each lung (left, right), and within comparable areas within each lung (eg, upper, middle and lower thirds). Under the supervision of the physician, the technologist administers the radiopharmaceutical. The study consists of acquisition of timed imaging data from both the anterior and posterior projections, and may include comparable lateral projections. Measurements of relative radioactivity are made and the results expressed as percentages of the whole. The physician verifies the adequacy of the imaging data before completion of the study, and directs the technologist to obtain additional views or reprocess data, when necessary. The data are formatted for film and/or digital display and analysis. The physician reviews the study for artifacts and abnormal distribution. Quantitative evaluation of the images, including but not limited to anterior, posterior, and the geometric mean(s) for global and regional perfusion is (are) calculated and recorded. The processed and raw images when performed (eg, upright or supine, posterior, anterior, etc) are compared to a current chest X ray and any additional relevant prior studies, and formally interpreted, ie, a report is dictated for the medical record.

Description of Procedure for Code 78598

Quantitative lung ventilation and perfusion scintigraphy is a combination of two radionuclide diagnostic imaging studies that measure the bronchopulmonary distribution of an inhaled radioactive aerosol or gas and the relative distribution of pulmonary arterial blood flow in each lung (left, right) and within comparable areas within each lung (eg, upper, middle and lower thirds). Under the supervision of the physician, the technologist gives specific breathing instructions to the patient while administering the radiopharmaceuticals. The study consists of multiple acquisitions of timed imaging data from both the anterior and posterior projections, and may include comparable lateral projections. Measurements of relative radioactivity are made and the results expressed as percentages of the whole. The physician verifies the adequacy of the imaging data before completion of the study, and directs the technologist to obtain additional views or reprocess data, when necessary. The data are formatted for film and/or digital display and analysis. The physician reviews the study for artifacts and abnormal distribution. Quantitative evaluation of the images, including but not limited to anterior, posterior and the geometric mean(s) for global and regional perfusion is/are calculated and recorded. The processed and raw images when performed (eg, upright or supine, posterior, etc) are compared to a current chest X ray and any additional relevant prior studies, and formally interpreted, ie, a report is dictated for the medical record.

Cardiovascular Procedures and Services

An intricate electrical pathway throughout the heart controls the heartbeats. There is a special group of cells within the heart that have the ability to generate electrical activity on their own. These cells separate charged particles. Then they spontaneously leak certain charged particles into the cells. This produces electrical impulses in the pacemaker cells, which spread over the heart, causing it to contract. These cells do this more than once per second to produce a normal heart beat of 72 beats per minute.

Each heartbeat begins from an electrical signal initiated by the sinoatrial (SA) node—the heart's natural pacemaker—located in the right atrium. The heart also contains specialized fibers that conduct the electrical impulse from the SA node to the rest of the heart. The electrical impulse leaves the SA node and travels to the right and left atria, causing them to contract together. This takes .04 seconds. A natural delay enables the atria to contract and the ventricles to fill up with blood. When the signal arrives at the junction of the atria and ventricles, the atrioventricular (AV) node carries the signal down and through the ventricles. The AV node distributes this signal to both the left and right ventricles via special fibers called Purkinje fibers, which causes the ventricles to contract at the same time.

What Is an Electrocardiogram?

The activity that controls the heartbeat produces measurable electrical waves. An electrocardiogram (ECG, also abbreviated EKG) is the visual representation of the electrical conduction of the heart. As each signal travels from the atria to the ventricles, it can be recorded on paper. The travel of this electrical signal is what is represented as an ECG.

The following three waves are typically recorded by an ECG:

- The P wave represents the electrical signal as it travels through the atria; the atria contract, and blood is forced into the ventricles.

- The QRS waves represent the signal as it travels through the ventricles; the ventricles contract, and blood is forced into the arteries.

- The T wave represents the heart at rest prior to the next beat.

What Is an Arrhythmia?

An arrhythmia is a common condition in which the heart beats at an irregular pace. It may or may not correspond to a patient's symptoms of palpitations, as detected by monitoring tests. While an arrhythmia is generally benign (not associated with death), it may be associated with significant morbidity and require treatment. Arrhythmias often reflect coexistent heart disease. In some cases, however, an arrhythmia may be malignant (associated with an increased incidence of death) and require medical therapy and/or devices or procedures for treatment.

TYPICAL CAUSES AND SYMPTOMS

Arrhythmias may occur under the following circumstances:

- the heart's natural pacemaker develops an abnormal rate or rhythm;

- the normal conduction pathway is interrupted; or

- there is a problem with impulse conduction due to a blockage.

FIGURE 5-1. Echocardiogram (ECG)

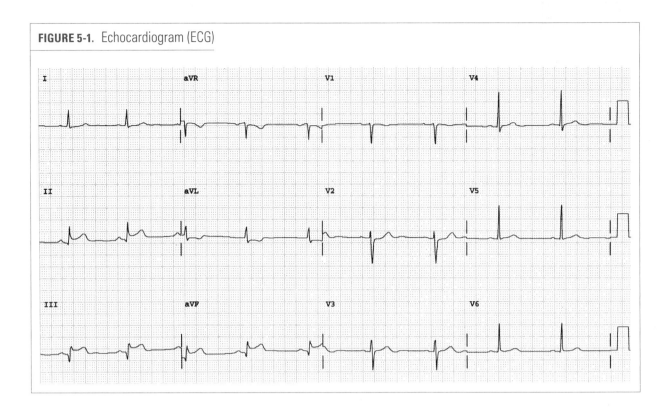

Individuals experience arrhythmias differently. The most common symptoms include:

- palpitations or fluttering,

- shortness of breath,

- fainting or dizziness, and

- chest pain.

Therapeutic services may be divided into two categories: medical and surgical. These services may be provided by cardiologists, surgeons, and/or other specialists. In some instances, surgeons and cardiologists collaborate to provide services.

CARDIOPULMONARY RESUSCITATION (**92950**)

92950   Cardiopulmonary resuscitation (eg, in cardiac arrest)
            CPT Assistant Jan 96:7, Oct 04:14, Nov 07:5

Intent and Use of Code 92950

Code **92950** describes the complete cardiopulmonary resuscitation service that may be rendered by any physician in any specialty. The physician should bill for this service if it was provided as an isolated event.

If the physician manages the cardiopulmonary resuscitation (and is present face-to-face), the physician may report code **92950**. It is not required that the physician him- or herself perform the actual chest compressions and/or mouth-to-mouth or bagging. It is appropriate for a physician to report code **92950** in addition to codes **99291**, **99292**, **99466**, **99467**, or **99468-99476** (for the critical care services) when cardiopulmonary resuscitation and critical care services are performed on the same day by the same physician. Both services should be clearly documented in the medical record.

Code **92950** is used to describe procedures in response to a failure in cardiovascular function and perfusion leading to the need for cardiac support in the form of chest compressions. This code is intended to describe cardiopulmonary resuscitation (CPR) to restore and maintain the patient's respiration and circulation after cessation of heartbeat and breathing. Code **92950** does not include endotracheal intubation, which is additionally reported with code **31500**, *Intubation, endotracheal, emergency procedure.* Basic CPR consists of assessing the victim, opening the airway, restoring breathing (eg, mouth-to-mouth, bag valve mask), then restoring circulation (eg, closed-chest cardiac massage). Advanced life support interventions such as drug therapy (eg, administration of lidocaine, atrophine, etc) should be reported with the critical care code(s) (**99291-99292**, **99466-99467**, **99468-99476**) from the Evaluation and Management (E/M) section of the *Current Procedural Terminology* (CPT®) codebook.

When advanced life support interventions and CPR are performed at the same session, code **92950** should be reported in addition to code **99291**, **99292**, **99466**, **99467**, or **99468-99476**.

Therefore, based on CPT coding guidelines, cardiopulmonary resuscitation is reported separately from critical care services, but the time spent performing CPR is not counted toward determining total critical care time. Code **92950** is reported for the 30 minutes of CPR performed. The critical care codes **99291** and **99292** or codes **99466-99467** would be reported for the remaining 90 minutes of critical care time. The time spent performing CPR is subtracted from the total critical care time as CPR was provided during the hour(s) of critical care services. Documentation in the patient's record should indicate that the critical care time does not include the time spent performing CPR (30 minutes).

TEMPORARY TRANSCUTANEOUS PACING (⊙**92953**)

⊙**92953** Temporary transcutaneous pacing
CPT Assistant Nov 99:49, Feb 07:10, Jul 07:1

Intent and Use of Code ⊙**92953**

Code **92953** is used to treat clinically significant bradycardia. It is particularly useful as a bridge to transvenous pacing or in the setting of acute hemodynamic deterioration caused by bradycardia.

Code **99288** should be reported when temporary transcutaneous pacing is initiated by personnel outside the hospital at the direction of the physician.

Description of Service for Code ⊙**92953**

Transcutaneous pacing pads are applied to the patient's anterior and posterior chest. Sedation is provided as needed, and the patient's cardiac rhythm is monitored. Pacer output and rate are increased until the pacemaker overdrives the patient's native heart rhythm. Hemodynamic stability with the paced rhythm is assessed, and additional sedation is provided as needed. Plans for temporary transvenous pacemaker insertion are made if appropriate.

ELECTIVE CARDIOVERSION (⊙**92960**, ⊙**92961**)

⊙**92960** Cardioversion, elective, electrical conversion of arrhythmia; external
CPT Assistant Summer 93:13, Nov 99:49, Jun 00:5, Nov 00:9, Jul 01:11; *CPT Changes: An Insider's View* 2000

⊙**92961**   internal (separate procedure)
CPT Assistant Summer 93:13, Nov 99:49, Jun 00:5, Jul 00:5, Nov 00:9; *CPT Changes: An Insider's View* 2000

Intent and Use of Code ⊙**92960**

Code **92960** describes elective external cardioversion. This service should be reported as an isolated procedure and not in the context of critical care or when it is an integral part of a procedure such as an electrophysiology study or coronary artery bypass graft (CABG) surgery.

Code **92960** specifically describes elective (non-emergency) external electrical cardioversion. Elective cardioversion is most often used to treat atrial fibrillation and atrial flutter if antiarrhythmic drugs fail to convert the heart back to normal sinus rhythm or if the patient is hemodynamically unstable. The electric shock given in cardioversion is synchronized (ie, timed to occur during the R wave of the electrocardiogram). The patient will have his or her heart rhythm monitored for several hours after the procedure to ensure the rhythm remains stable.

This procedure can be performed in an intensive care unit, a coronary care unit, emergency department, or in any room in an outpatient area that houses the necessary equipment (eg, cardiac monitor, crash cart).

Questions are often raised regarding use of the cardioversion codes to report defibrillation. Defibrillation is the delivery of an electrical impulse to the heart. This impulse is intended to interrupt life-threatening abnormal rhythms (eg, ventricular fibrillation, pleiomorphic ventricular tachycardia, or ventricular tachycardia associated with shock) and allow the normal sinus impulse and electrical conduction to resume. The electrical impulse must be strong enough to cause depolarization (neutralization of the positive and negative electrical charges) of a large percentage of the myocardium. The timing of the defibrillation shock is not synchronized to the cardiac cycle (ie, it is not delivered during an R wave).

CHAPTER 5

There is no CPT code to report defibrillation as a procedure performed in isolation. Defibrillation may be performed as part of critical care services, at the end of open heart surgery, during cardiac catheterization and coronary angiography, or during an electrophysiological procedure. Defibrillation is often a component of cardiac resuscitation, especially in adults. In all of these situations, defibrillation is not a separately reportable service.

Pharmacologic cardioversion (the use of drugs to convert the heart back to normal sinus rhythm) is reported based on the specific services provided. For example, the use of prolonged services, critical care, E/M services, or codes describing therapeutic or diagnostic infusion or injection procedures may also be reported, depending on the specific services provided.

> **CODING TIP** Code **92960** is used to report the physician services related to the elective cardioversion. There is no separate CPT code to use to report defibrillation.

Description of Service for Code ⊙92960

Informed consent is obtained for the patient, and medical records are reviewed to be sure adequate precautions against systemic embolization have been taken. Defibrillator pads are placed, and the patient's cardiac rhythm is monitored. Sedation or anesthesia and airway patency are managed appropriately. (Services provided by an anesthesiologist are reported separately.) Synchronized shocks are provided with increasing energy until the arrhythmia is converted or maximum doses of energy are used. The patient's rhythm is observed, and the patient is closely monitored until consciousness is fully regained. A 12-lead ECG may be obtained and is reported separately. A report of the cardioversion procedure is generated.

Intent and Use of Code ⊙92961

Code **92961** is used to describe internal cardioversion. Internal cardioversion may be undertaken as a separate procedure to treat atrial flutter or fibrillation that is refractory to transthoracic cardioversion. Internal cardioversion requires vascular access with electrode catheters positioned in the heart and/or great vessels under fluoroscopic guidance. This code should not be reported in conjunction with an electrophysiology study or other intracardiac procedures. Code **92961** should not be reported with codes **93282-93284**, **93287**, **93289**, **93295**, **93296**, **93618-93624**, **93631**, **93640-93642**, **93650-93652**, or **93662**.

Description of Service for Code ⊙92961

The patient is brought to the procedure room where he or she is sterilely prepared and draped. Blood pressure, ECG, and pulse oximetry are monitored. Local anesthesia is administered, and an electrode catheter is place in a vein using standard percutaneous techniques. The electrode catheter is advanced to the right atrium under fluoroscopic guidance and connected electrically to an external cardioverter-defibrillator. A second electrode is placed in the coronary sinus or pulmonary artery and also connected to the external cardioverter-defibrillator. Conscious sedation is then administered to the patient, and synchronized cardioversion is performed. The electrode catheters are then removed, hemostasis obtained, and the patient is observed until the effect of sedation has cleared. The results of the procedure are carefully documented by the physician and explained to the patient, the patient's family, and the referring physician.

> **PAYMENT POLICY ALERT** Currently there is no CPT code to specifically describe pharmacological cardioversion. To report a therapeutic, prophylactic, or diagnostic intravenous (IV) infusion or injection, use CPT codes **96365-96379** (other than hydration) for the administration of substances or drugs. The fluid used to administer the drug(s) is incidental hydration and is not separately reportable. These services typically require direct physician supervision for any or all patient assessment, provision of consent, safety oversight, and intraservice supervision of staff. Typically, such infusions require special consideration to prepare, dose, or dispose of; practice training and competency for staff who administer the infusions; and periodic patient assessment with vital sign monitoring during the infusion.
>
> Intravenous or intra-arterial push is defined as:
>
> - an injection in which the health care professional who administers the substance or drug is continuously present to administer the injection and observe the patient, or
> - an infusion of 15 minutes or less.
>
> Private insurers may differ in their payment policies.

EXTERNAL COUNTERPULSATION THERAPY (HCPCS LEVEL II **G0166**)

Intent and Use of HCPCS Level II Code G0166

External counterpulsation (ECP) is a noninvasive treatment involving sequential compression (inflation and deflation) of cuffs wrapped around the patient's calves, thighs, and buttocks. By timing the compression sequence to the patient's cardiac cycle, ECP is intended to increase diastolic aortic pressure, thereby increasing coronary perfusion pressure, which possibly enhances the development of coronary collateral circulation and reduces the workload of the heart. ECP was developed for treatment of end-stage angina pectoris that is refractory to conventional therapy (ie, surgery or angioplasty). Treatment sessions are usually held for one hour, five days a week, for a duration of seven weeks. Currently there is no CPT code to report ECP. For Medicare patients, this procedure should be reported using the Healthcare Common Procedure Coding System (HCPCS) Level II code **G0166**, *External counterpulsation, per treatment session.*

PAYMENT POLICY ALERT The Centers for Medicare & Medicaid Services (CMS) has approved limited coverage of ECP for stable angina pectoris only. See section 20.20 of the Medicare National Coverage Determination (NCD) manual, which is available at www.cms.hhs.gov/transmittals/downloads/R898CP.pdf.

CMS has stated that it will not allow services designated by CPT codes **92971**, **93000**, **93005**, **93010**, **93720**, **93721**, **93722**, **93922**, and **97016** to be reported on the same day as ECP, unless they are medically necessary and delivered in a clinical setting not involving ECP treatment. If patients undergoing ECP require significant E/M services during the period of treatment, these services should be reported with **modifier 25**. (Refer to Chapter 6 for further discussion regarding the use of **modifier 25**.)

CORONARY THROMBECTOMY (⊙+92973)

⊙**+92973** Percutaneous transluminal coronary thrombectomy (List separately in addition to code for primary procedure)
CPT Assistant Mar 02:2,10, Mar 04:10; CPT Changes: An Insider's View 2002

Intent and Use of Code ⊙+92973

Add-on code **92973** describes a process of motorized mechanical thrombectomy wherein removal of thrombus within the lumen of a coronary vessel occurs, differing from the coronary atherectomy procedures (**92995**, **92996**) that alter the anatomy of the coronary artery by modifying the arterial wall or removing a portion of plaque. Add-on code **92973** describes a different procedure using a unique method

of fragmenting and removing clots from the coronary artery. Currently, the only device that meets this requirement for coronary thrombectomy is Angioget®. Note that the reference to *"Angioget® or similar catheter"* is intended neither to endorse any specific proprietary catheter type nor to exclude the use of any new procedurally similar catheter system.

All other devices (eg, Export™, Diver CE™, Fetch™, Pronto™) do not mechanically fragment clot but work to break up the clot by advancing the aspiration catheter in a back and forth manner. The technique used with these types of catheters does not meet the criteria as outlined in the American Medical Association Specialty Society Relative Value System Update Committee (RUC) Description of Procedure for code **92973** wherein the system includes a drive unit, pump, and foot pedal. Code **92973** involves the physician stepping on a foot pedal to activate the catheter which is then withdrawn across the lesion in order to remove the intracoronary thrombus. The use of Export™, Diver CE™, Fetch™, or Pronto™ catheters for aspiration of thrombus performed in conjunction with a percutaneous coronary intervention is not separately reportable. To further clarify, it would not be appropriate to report code **92973** to represent the use of a Fogarty catheter, as this type of catheter is not used in the coronary arteries.

Code **92973** has been designated as an add-on code, as percutaneous transluminal coronary thrombectomy is performed at the same session as percutaneous intracoronary stent placement or percutaneous intracoronary balloon angioplasty. A stand-alone mechanical catheter aspiration thrombectomy independent of another percutaneous coronary intervention is very rare but may occur. In this circumstance, code **93799**, *Unlisted cardiovascular service or procedure,* may be reported.

CODING TIP Code **92973** is used to report mechanical thrombectomy using an *Angiojet® or similar catheter* that mechanically fragments and removes clots. Other procedures using catheters (eg, Diver CE™, Fetch™, Pronto™) that aspirate thrombus but do not mechanically fragment thrombus are not reportable with code **92973**. Code **92973** is an add-on code and should be reported when thrombectomy is used as part of a percutaneous coronary intervention. Code **92973** should be used in conjunction with codes **92980** and **92982**. Code **92973** should be reported one time per vessel, regardless of the number of sites treated in the same vessel.

CHAPTER 5

Description of Service for Code ⊙+92973

After defining the relevant anatomy by coronary angiography, a guiding catheter is introduced into the ostium of the coronary artery or vein graft being treated. Through the guiding catheter, a guidewire is used to cross the lesion and thrombus, and the thrombectomy catheter is advanced over the guidewire to a position distal to the thrombotic lesion. The catheter is activated by depressing a foot pedal and manually withdrawn slowly across the lesion in order to remove the intracoronary thrombus. After deactivation, the thrombectomy catheter is again advanced distal to the initial lesion, and a repeat withdrawal pass is made. After several passes have been performed with adequate reduction in the thrombus burden, the catheter is removed. Following the removal of the catheter, definitive treatment of the original stenosis is performed, usually requiring additional balloon angioplasty or stent placement (**92980, 92982**).

INTRAVASCULAR RADIATION DELIVERY DEVICE (⊙+92974)

⊙+92974   Transcatheter placement of radiation delivery device for subsequent coronary intravascular brachytherapy (List separately in addition to code for primary procedure)
CPT Assistant Mar 02:2; CPT Changes: An Insider's View 2002

Intent and Use of Code ⊙+92974

Add-on code **92974** describes transcatheter placement of a radiation delivery device for coronary intravascular brachytherapy. Intravascular brachytherapy uses catheter-based radiation (Gamma or Beta) to treat patients with restenosis of previously placed coronary stents. Prior to intravascular brachytherapy, the pertinent vessel must first be recanalized by conventional methods, such as intravascular coronary balloon angioplasty (**92982**), atherectomy (**92995**), and/or stent placement (**92980**). Intravascular brachytherapy is reported separately, as this service requires insertion and positioning of a separate catheter system and significantly more

time and skill. The radiation physicist's calculation of the dosage or placement of the radioelement is not included in add-on code **92974**.

CODING TIP Intravascular radioelement application is reported with codes **77785-77787** when performed in conjunction with add-on code **92974**.

Description of Service for Code ⊙+92974

Radiation therapy may be used to treat patients with restenosis occurring within a previously placed intracoronary stent (in-stent restenosis). The procedure used to perform brachytherapy is complex. Coronary angiography is performed first, often using quantitative angiographic techniques. The interventional cardiologist may then proceed with a balloon angioplasty of the in-stent restenosis and then repeat the angiographic studies. Intravascular ultrasound may also be used to image the lesion from the arterial lumen to assist the interventional cardiologist and the radiation oncologist in choosing the appropriate kind of radiation source and in determining the needed radiation dose. The interventional cardiologist then advances the radiation delivery device through the guiding catheter in the coronary artery ostium to a position spanning the lesion to be treated. The radiation source is then maneuvered to the target lesion by the interventional cardiologist, radiation oncologist, or other appropriately licensed physician. It is left in place for a period of time (usually minutes) determined by the radiation oncologist as part of the calculation of the radiation dose. While the radiation source is deployed, the cardiologist monitors the status of the patient and the catheter position. At the end of the treatment period, the radiation source is removed, the guiding catheter and intra-arterial sheath are removed, and hemostasis is obtained.

CORONARY THROMBOLYSIS (⊙92975-92977)

⊙92975   Thrombolysis, coronary; by intracoronary infusion, including selective coronary angiography

92977   by intravenous infusion

Intent and Use of Code ⊙92975

Code **92975** designates selective coronary angiography and coronary thrombolysis by intracoronary infusion.

Intent and Use of Code 92977

Code **92977** is reported for this procedure when intravenous infusion of a thrombolytic agent is administered by the physician.

CODING TIP For thrombolysis of vessels other than the coronaries, see codes **37201** and **75896**. For cerebral thrombolysis, use code **37195**.

PAYMENT POLICY ALERT Although considered a covered service for Medicare beneficiaries, intravenous coronary thrombolysis has been assigned zero physician work units in the Medicare fee schedule, as CMS maintains that this service is most often performed by nursing personnel in the hospital setting. The physician work of monitoring a patient who has received intravenous thrombolytic therapy is captured in the E/M service provided to the patient.

INTRAVASCULAR ULTRASOUND (⊙+92978, ⊙+92979)

⊙+**92978** Intravascular ultrasound (coronary vessel or graft) during diagnostic evaluation and/or therapeutic intervention including imaging supervision, interpretation and report; initial vessel (List separately in addition to code for primary procedure)
CPT Assistant Nov 97:43-44, Nov 99:49, Mar 02:2, Jan 07:28; *CPT Changes: An Insider's View* 2000

⊙+**92979** each additional vessel (List separately in addition to code for primary procedure)
CPT Assistant Nov 97:43-44, Nov 99:49; *CPT Changes: An Insider's View* 2000

Intent and Use of Code ⊙+92978

Add-on code **92978** is used to report intravascular ultrasound (of a coronary vessel or graft) during diagnostic evaluation and/or therapeutic intervention, including imaging supervision, interpretation, and report; initial vessel.

Intravascular ultrasound services include all transducer manipulations and repositioning within the specific vessel being examined, both before and after therapeutic intervention (eg, stent placement [92980, 92981]).

Description of Service for Code ⊙+92978

Through a coronary guiding catheter, a wire is advanced across the coronary lesion of interest. The ultrasound device is advanced over the wire to the site. Ultrasound images are obtained and recorded as the device is pulled back across the segment of interest. This process is repeated as needed to ensure adequate imaging. Using the ultrasound imaging console, quantitative measurements are performed on the images obtained to guide therapeutic decisions.

Intent and Use of Code ⊙+92979

Add-on code **92979** is used to report the ultrasound procedure on each additional coronary artery when more than one coronary artery is evaluated with intravascular ultrasound as part of a diagnostic or therapeutic procedure.

Add-on codes **92978** and **92979** can be used only once per interventional session for each artery. For example, when three stents are placed in one coronary artery, intracoronary ultrasound might be used to check the deployment after each stent is placed. Although rare, should the ultrasound catheter be introduced into the artery three separate times, add-on code **92978** would be used only once.

Description of Service for Code ⊙+92979

The guide catheter used for first intracoronary ultrasound procedure (**92978**) may be left in place, or a new guide catheter may be introduced to engage a new coronary ostium/graft as needed. A wire is advanced through the guide into the new coronary artery or graft (a separate vessel from the original vessel imaged and reported with code **92978**) and then across the coronary lesion of interest. The ultrasound device is advanced over the wire to the site. Ultrasound images are obtained and recorded as the device is pulled back across the segment of interest. This process is repeated as needed to ensure adequate imaging. Using the ultrasound imaging console, quantitative measurements are performed on the images obtained to guide therapeutic decisions.

CHAPTER 5

INTRACORONARY STENT PLACEMENT (⊙**92980**, ⊙**+92981**)

⊙**92980** Transcatheter placement of an intracoronary stent(s), percutaneous, with or without other therapeutic intervention, any method; single vessel
CPT Assistant Aug 96:2, Dec 96:11, Apr 98:9, Aug 98:3, Aug 00:11, Mar 01:11, Apr 01:10, Mar 02:2, Aug 03:10, Apr 05:14

⊙**+92981** each additional vessel (List separately in addition to code for primary procedure)
CPT Assistant Mar 01:11, Apr 01:10, Aug 03:10

Intent and Use of Codes ⊙**92980** and ⊙**+92981**

Codes **92980** and **92981** are used to report coronary artery stenting. Four main coronary vessels are recognized: (1) left main coronary artery (LMCA); (2) left anterior descending coronary artery; (3) left circumflex; and (4) right coronary artery. If one or more stents is placed in the same vessel or in any number of its branches, code **92980** or code **92981** is reported only once. For example, stenting of the left circumflex and its obtuse marginal branch would be coded once using code **92980**. Modifier 22 may be added, with supporting documentation, to indicate the procedure was more complex than a standard stent because of involvement of the obtuse marginal branch. These same coding paradigms are applied to coronary angioplasty (**92982**, **92984**) or atherectomy (**92995**, **92996**) procedures. See Coding Solutions and Examples under Percutaneous Transluminal Coronary Angioplasty (**92982**, **92984**) later in this chapter.

Coronary angioplasty (**92982**, **92984**) or atherectomy (**92995**, **92996**) in the same vessel is considered part of the stenting procedure and is not reported separately. If additional vessels are treated with angioplasty or atherectomy but not with stenting, use code **92984** or code **92996** as appropriate.

Codes **92973** (percutaneous transluminal coronary thrombectomy) and **92974** (coronary brachytherapy) are add-on codes for reporting procedures performed in addition to coronary stenting, atherectomy, and angioplasty, and are not included in the "therapeutic intervention" of code **92980**. Codes **92978** and **92979** are add-on codes for reporting intravascular ultrasound procedures performed in addition to coronary and bypass graft diagnostic and interventional services and are not included in the "therapeutic intervention" of code **92980**.

Codes **93454-93461** should be reported when formal diagnostic coronary angiography services are performed for appropriate clinical indications at the same session as percutaneous coronary intervention(s) (**92980-92984**, **92995**, **92996**). When percutaneous coronary intervention(s) are performed at a different session from the supporting diagnostic coronary angiogram, the diagnostic angiogram has already been reported separately, and there is not an appropriate clinical indication to repeat formal diagnostic coronary angiography (eg, as documented in the medical record, inadequate or unavailable prior coronary angiography, or a relevant change in the patient's clinical condition); all catheter placement and angiography services associated with the intervention are inherent to the procedure; and the diagnostic angiography codes (**93454-93461**) should not be utilized again. For example, the stent placement code (**92980**) is valued by the AMA's Relative Value Update Committee (RUC) to include all catheter placement and angiography services inherent to the procedure. As a result, when coronary stenting is performed based on the findings of a prior diagnostic cardiac catheterization done at a separate setting, code **93454** should not be reported to describe the coronary injections performed to guide stent placement.

PAYMENT POLICY ALERT The CPT descriptor for code **92980** contains the phrase "transcatheter placement of intracoronary stent(s)," indicating that the code is used only once, no matter how many stents are placed in the same vessel. The service described by code **92980** was valued in the Medicare Fee Schedule to include the possibility of placing more than one stent in a vessel. However, if a second stent is placed in a different vessel, add-on code **92981** should be reported as well.

CMS states that it is not appropriate to report supervision and imaging (S&I) separately for therapeutic coronary artery procedures. The placement of all catheters, as well as all angiography performed during the course of the therapeutic procedure, are included in code **92980**. However, when a diagnostic cardiac catheterization is performed and immediately followed by a therapeutic procedure such as stenting, all of the appropriate cardiac catheterization codes should be reported in addition to the code for the therapeutic procedure. For Medicare beneficiaries, CMS will reimburse the stent at 100% of the allowable charge and the diagnostic catheterization at 50%.

Description of Service for Code ⊙92980

The decision is made to place a stent after full discussion with the patient and/or family. The patient is prepared for the procedure, which includes sterilization of the access site and cannulation with an indwelling sheath. (Typically the femoral artery is used.) A guide catheter is positioned in the appropriate coronary ostium, and baseline arteriograms are obtained. Usually the lesion is predilated with a conventional angioplasty balloon. The stent delivery system is loaded on the guidewire.

Both are then inserted into the guide catheter and advanced into the coronary artery using fluoroscopic guidance. The operator positions the stent in the target vessel, reconfirming the location by fluoroscopy and comparison to previous contrast injections. When the operator is confident that the stent is in the correct location, the balloon is inflated to expand and secure the stent. The balloon is then deflated and the catheter removed. Frequently, a second, high-pressure balloon catheter is inserted and inflated to more fully expand the stent. Antithrombotics and antiplatelet drugs are used to prevent thrombosis of the newly placed stent.

The CPT Editorial Panel has made an important change in the coding convention for reporting different therapeutic coronary artery procedures performed in multiple vessels. Now the most highly valued service is reported with the initial vessel code, while any other therapeutic coronary artery procedures employed in different vessels are reported using the appropriate "each additional vessel" code(s). If a stent is placed in one vessel, and atherectomy without stenting is performed in a separate vessel, report codes **92980**, **92996**. If a stent is placed in one vessel and angioplasty without stenting is performed in a separate vessel, report codes **92980**, **92984**.

From a CPT coding perspective, therapeutic cardiovascular procedures such as balloon angioplasty (**92982**), atherectomy (**92984**), and intracoronary stent placement (**92980**) do not include a preceding diagnostic cardiac catheterization, nor do they describe any particular angiography procedure. These distinct procedures (diagnostic catheterization and therapeutic procedures), therefore, should be reported separately when performed at the same session or on the same day at a different session.

Description of Service for Code ⊙+92981

An additional stent (loaded on a separate carrying catheter) is inserted through a guiding catheter and advanced into the separate coronary vessel using fluoroscopic guidance. The operator positions the stent in the target vessel and confirms the location by fluoroscopy and comparison to previous contrast injections. When the operator is confident that the stent is in the correct location, the balloon is inflated to expand and secure the stent. The balloon is then deflated and the catheter removed. Frequently, a second, high-pressure balloon catheter is inserted and inflated to more fully expand the stent. Note: At the time of initial stent (**92980**) placement, it is determined that an additional stent is required in a separate vessel. This additional service (**92981**) represents only the intraservice work of placing the additional stent. It does not include any pre- or postwork, as these portions of the service are captured in the initial stent placement code.

PERCUTANEOUS TRANSLUMINAL CORONARY ANGIOPLASTY (⊙92982, ⊙+92984)

⊙**92982** Percutaneous transluminal coronary balloon angioplasty; single vessel
CPT *Assistant* Winter 92:15, Aug 96:2, Apr 97:10, Mar 02:2, Apr 05:14

⊙**+92984** each additional vessel (List separately in addition to code for primary procedure)
CPT *Assistant* Winter 92:15, Aug 96:2, Dec 96:11, Apr 97:10, Apr 05:14

Intent and Use of Codes ⊙92982 and ⊙+92984

Code **92982** is used to describe percutaneous transluminal coronary angioplasty (PTCA) of a single vessel. Add-on code **92984** is used to describe PTCA for each additional vessel. These procedures include the placement of catheters for the purpose of coronary angioplasty, the injection of dye to determine catheter and balloon placement, and the interpretation of the therapeutic results. Code **92982** is used as a collective code that indicates one service when two or more blockages in the same major coronary artery or its branches are treated with PTCA. If blockages are treated in two or more separate coronary arteries at the same session, the service is coded using the single-vessel code (**92982**) to identify the first vessel and the "each additional vessel" code (**92984**) to identify each additional vessel treated.

Add-on code **92984** (each additional vessel) refers only to four main coronary vessels: (1) right coronary artery; (2) left main coronary artery (LMCA); (3) left anterior descending coronary artery; and (4) left circumflex. Angioplasty performed on one of these

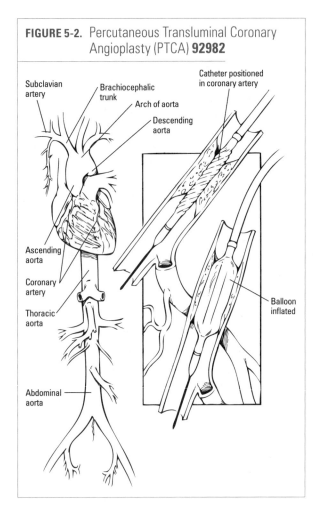

FIGURE 5-2. Percutaneous Transluminal Coronary Angioplasty (PTCA) **92982**

arteries and any number of its branches would be coded as a single angioplasty. In this case, angioplasty on the left circumflex and its obtuse marginal branch would be coded once using code **92982**. **Modifier 22** may be added, with supporting documentation, to indicate the procedure was more complex than a standard angioplasty because of involvement of the obtuse marginal branch.

EXAMPLE 1: PTCA is performed in a patient's left anterior descending artery (LAD) and right coronary artery (RCA).

Coding Solution: Use add-on codes **92982** (coronary angioplasty—single vessel) and **92984** (coronary angioplasty—each additional vessel).

EXAMPLE 2: Angioplasty is performed in three separate lesions using two separate guidewires in the first and second diagonal branches of the LAD.

Coding Solution: Use add-on code **92982** (coronary angioplasty—single vessel). In this case, all interventions involved only the LAD or its branches, so only one intervention can be coded.

EXAMPLE 3: Angioplasty is performed in the RCA; the left circumflex coronary (LCX), first and second obtuse marginal branches; and the LAD.

Coding Solution: Use add-on codes **92982** and **92984**. In this case, angioplasty is performed in all three major vessels, so the first code is for "coronary angioplasty—single vessel," and the code for "coronary angioplasty—each additional vessel" is used once for the second and again for the third major artery treated. Because the two marginal branches are both part of the circumflex system, they constitute only a single vessel.

Intent and Use

A single bypass graft may be connected into only one coronary artery or connected to two or more coronary arteries. Several local Medicare carriers have defined rules for coding coronary graft interventions.

A bypass graft and the native artery to which it connects are considered a single major artery.

Many details of coding for percutaneous coronary interventions are not well defined and may be interpreted differently by various insurance carriers. Send documentation of the procedure with the claim. This documentation should clearly specify:

- all coronary or graft ostia that were cannulated;
- details of which ostia and vessels were used to approach each lesion;
- the highest level (most complex) procedure in each major coronary artery; and
- details about anatomic variations that qualify as branches of, or physiologic equivalents to, one of the defined major coronary arteries.

EXAMPLE 1: A patient undergoes angioplasty of a distal LAD lesion through a vein graft, and a lesion in the same vein graft is stented.

Coding Solution: Code **92980** is used to describe the stenting procedure. The angioplasty in the LAD supplied by this graft is not coded because it involves the same major vessel.

Intent and Use

A bypass graft connecting to two major native vessels (eg, a graft that connects first to the LAD and continues on to connect to the LCX) is analogous to the LMCA. If it is used to perform a coronary angioplasty on two major native vessels (eg, the LAD and the LCX), these procedures are reported with code **92982** (initial vessel) and add-on code **92984** (additional vessel).

EXAMPLE 2: A patient has a saphenous vein graft anastomosed to the circumflex obtuse marginal, after which the graft jumps to the RCA posterolateral branch. Through the vein graft, the circumflex obtuse marginal lesion is treated with angioplasty, and a second lesion in the RCA posterolateral branch is treated with angioplasty.

Coding Solution: Code **92982** is used to describe angioplasty, initial vessel, and add-on code **92984** for angioplasty, each additional vessel. Even though the procedure was performed through one vein graft ostium, blockages in two major coronary arteries were dilated. The vein graft is analogous to the LMCA, and each artery is coded separately.

Intent and Use

Coronary interventions requiring guiding catheter placement into more than one coronary or graft ostium are coded as multiple procedures.

EXAMPLE 3: The patient has a saphenous vein graft anastomosed to the RCA posterolateral branch. Through the vein graft, the RCA posterolateral branch lesion is treated with angioplasty. Using a separate guiding catheter and wire, a lesion in the proximal RCA is stented.

Coding Solution: Code **92980** is used to describe the stenting procedure in the proximal RCA.

Intent and Use

Add-on code **92984** (angioplasty, each additional vessel) is used to describe the angioplasty in the distal RCA through the vein graft. In this case, it is appropriate to code two procedures in one major coronary artery because separate approaches were used for each of the two lesions.

EXAMPLE 4: The patient undergoes the following procedures: PTCA of the distal LAD via a graft from the left internal mammary artery, stenting of the proximal LAD via the LMCA; then atherectomy of the circumflex, angioplasty of the RCA proximally, and angioplasty of the distal RCA via a saphenous vein graft.

Coding Solution: In this case, each intervention deserves a separate code, because each is performed through separate approaches. The most complex procedure, stenting of the LAD, requires use of code **92980**. All other procedures are coded using the

"each additional vessel" codes as follows: **92996** for atherectomy of the circumflex, and **92984** a total of three times for all three angioplasties.

EXAMPLE 5: The patient undergoes PTCA of the circumflex first obtuse marginal branch via a saphenous vein graft and angioplasty of the second circumflex obtuse marginal via a separate saphenous vein graft.

Coding Solution: In this case, because two different ostia are cannulated, it is appropriate to use code **92982** (angioplasty, single vessel) for angioplasty on one left circumflex branch and add-on code **92984** (angioplasty, each additional vessel) for angioplasty of the second left circumflex branch.

PAYMENT POLICY ALERT CMS states that it is not appropriate to report S&I separately for therapeutic coronary artery procedures. The placement of all catheters, as well as all angiography performed during the course of the therapeutic procedure, are included in code **92982**. However, when a diagnostic cardiac catheterization is performed and immediately followed by a therapeutic procedure such as PTCA, all the appropriate cardiac catheterization codes should be reported in addition to the code for the therapeutic procedure. For Medicare beneficiaries, CMS will reimburse the PTCA at 100% of the allowable charge and the diagnostic catheterization at 50%.

PAYMENT POLICY ALERT The cutting balloon is a type of balloon catheter used to perform PTCA. There is no specific CPT code to describe the use of this particular catheter. The American College of Cardiology Coding Task Force, as well as the Cardiac Catheterization and Intervention Committee, have reviewed this procedure and device. There is a consensus among these clinicians that the use of a cutting balloon is similar to that of other PTCA balloons, and the procedure should be reported using the existing PTCA codes. However, there exists variation among Medicare carrier medical directors about payment policy for cutting balloon procedures. Interventional cardiologists should check with local carrier medical directors for accurate advice regarding local payment policy, coding, and documentation requirements.

PERCUTANEOUS BALLOON VALVULOPLASTY (⊙**92986-92990**)

⊙**92986** Percutaneous balloon valvuloplasty; aortic valve

⊙**92987**   mitral valve

92990   pulmonary valve
       CPT Assistant Winter 91:3

Intent and Use of Codes ⊙**92986-92990**

Codes **92986**, **92987**, and **92990** describe percutaneous balloon valvuloplasty of the aortic, mitral, and pulmonary valves, respectively.

Description of Service for Code ⊙**92987**

After an assessment of the severity of mitral stenosis, the decision is made to proceed with balloon catheter dilation, which is discussed fully with the patient and family, as well as with the referring physician. Oral anticoagulation is discontinued prior to this procedure. In some cases hospitalization a day or more prior to the procedure is necessary for intravenous heparin therapy. The patient is taken to the catheterization laboratory where the right and left femoral areas are prepared and the left femoral artery and vein and the right femoral vein are cannulated. If diagnostic cardiac catheterization has not been performed previously, a complete right and left heart catheterization, coronary angiography, and left ventriculography are performed when indicated (coded separately). Via the left femoral artery, a pigtail catheter is placed in the left ventricle, and a right heart catheter with cardiac output measurement capability is placed via the left femoral vein into the pulmonary artery. From the right femoral venous puncture, transseptal cannulation of the left atrium via puncture of the intra-atrial septum is performed. A .025-inch spring tip guidewire is placed through the transseptal catheter into the left atrium, and the left atrial sheath is removed. A 14-French dilator is passed over the wire to dilate the subcutaneous area at the right femoral puncture in the intra-atrial septum. The dilator is removed over the exchange wire, and the Inoue catheter is elongated (stretched) and passed over the guidewire and into the left atrium through the transseptal puncture. The balloon is unstretched, and the guidewire removed. The operator introduces a steering stylet into the shaft of the balloon catheter, inflates the distal portion of the balloon, and manipulates the catheter across the mitral valve into the left ventricle. The balloon is withdrawn until the partially inflated distal portion engages the mitral valve. Full inflation of the balloon is accomplished using

a solution containing saline-contrast to expand the balloon. The balloon is then deflated by withdrawing the saline-contrast solution. The catheter is withdrawn into the left atrium, and left atrial pressure is again measured through the balloon catheter. Left ventricular pressure is measured via the left femoral arterial pigtail catheter. If sufficient diminution of the pressure gradient has not occurred, an assessment is made of any potential resultant mitral regurgitation using either left ventriculography or Doppler echocardiography in the catheterization laboratory. The process of crossing the mitral valve, inflating the balloon to a large diameter, and then assessing the resultant improvement in transmittal pressure gradient and potential for mitral regurgitation is repeated in a stepwise fashion with increasingly larger volumes of solution until either optimal opening of the mitral valve is accomplished or evidence of mitral valve regurgitation begins to appear. When the operator is confident that an optimal result has been achieved, the deflated balloon is stretched and withdrawn from the left atrium and removed from the vascular system. The pigtail and pulmonary artery catheters are removed. The vascular sheaths are removed, usually within a few hours after the procedure is completed, and hemostasis of the puncture sites is performed. Bed rest for at least six hours after sheath removal, and predischarge monitoring is necessary. Hospital and office visits related to the procedure for 90 days following the procedure are included in this code.

BALLOON ATRIAL SEPTOSTOMY (**92992**, **92993**)

92992 Atrial septectomy or septostomy; transvenous method, balloon (eg, Rashkind type) (includes cardiac catheterization)
       CPT Assistant Nov 97:44, Apr 98:3, 10, Nov 07:9

92993   blade method (Park septostomy) (includes cardiac catheterization)
       CPT Assistant Apr 98:10

Intent and Use of Codes 92992 and 92993

Code **92992** or code **92993** reports this therapeutic service, depending on the method used.

Code **92992** (Rashkind-type balloon septostomy) and code **92993** (Park-type blade septostomy) describe therapeutic techniques that also intrinsically include left and right heart catheterization. Code **92992** should be reported for accessing the right atrium and crossing through the interatrial septum to the left atrium to place a balloon catheter for enlargement of an atrial septal communication. Code **92993** is used to report a similar procedure in which a blade is used to enlarge the atrial septal communication. Left and right heart catheterization is intrinsic to these procedures. If additional diagnostic cardiac catheterization procedures are performed for clinical reasons, this warrants additional reporting using the appropriate cardiac catheterization procedure code(s).

No additional radiological supervision and interpretation coding is warranted for the septostomy procedures (**92992** or **92993**), as these codes also include the radiological supervision and interpretation of filming required.

Cardiac catheterization procedure codes **93462**, **93532**, and **93533** include an atrial septal puncture for passage of a catheter to access the left heart through the septum without enlarging the hole for therapeutic purposes (described by codes **92992** or **92993**). Therefore, it is not appropriate to additionally report codes **92992** or **92993**.

> **CODING TIP** Code **92992** should be reported by appending **modifier 52**, Reduced Services, for atrial septostomy performed in the intensive care unit (ICU) setting under echocardiographic guidance, without pressure monitoring.

PERCUTANEOUS TRANSLUMINAL CORONARY ATHERECTOMY (⊙**92995**, ⊙**+92996**)

⊙**92995** Percutaneous transluminal coronary atherectomy, by mechanical or other method, with or without balloon angioplasty; single vessel
CPT Assistant Winter 92:15

⊙**+92996** each additional vessel (List separately in addition to code for primary procedure)
CPT Assistant Winter 92:15, Apr 98:3

Intent and Use of Codes ⊙**92995** and ⊙**+92996**

Code **92995** and add-on code **92996** include laser atherectomy. Before 1997, the three types of atherectomy catheters approved by the Food and Drug Administration were the directional atherectomy catheter (Atherocath™); the transluminal extraction atherectomy catheter (TEC™); and the rotational atherectomy catheter (Rotablator™). All these catheters remove plaque by cutting, suctioning, and/or abrading it. At present, rotational atherectomy catheter

(Rotablator™) is the predominant atherectomy approach for coronary intervention.

In some cases, atherectomy alone may achieve adequate results. In other cases, atherectomy and balloon angioplasty are both needed to adequately reduce the degree of blockage in the artery. This is reflected in the coding language, which includes the phrase, "with or without balloon angioplasty." This language refers only to the situation in which atherectomy is insufficient to clear the blockage and balloon angioplasty must be performed in the same vessel. When multiple coronary arteries are treated at the same setting using different techniques, the service must be identified with multiple codes.

> **PAYMENT POLICY ALERT** There is no CPT code for distal embolic protection. Distal protection should not be reported separately.

EXAMPLE 1: The patient undergoes treatment of a calcified lesion in the left anterior descending artery (LAD) using rotational atherectomy, followed by balloon angioplasty, followed by coronary stent placement.

Coding Solution: In this case, report code **92980**, as the balloon angioplasty and atherectomy are included in the single-vessel stent procedure.

EXAMPLE 2: The patient undergoes treatment of a calcified lesion in the mid-LAD using rotational atherectomy, followed by balloon angioplasty, followed by coronary stent placement. A distal LAD lesion is treated with balloon angioplasty followed by stenting. Next a calcified lesion in the LCX is treated with rotational atherectomy followed by balloon angioplasty.

Coding Solution: In this case, report code **92980** for the LAD as the balloon angioplasty and atherectomy are included in the stent procedure. No additional code is reported for stenting the distal lesion in the LAD, as this is the same vessel. Add-on code **92996** is reported for the atherectomy of the LCX, which includes the balloon angioplasty.

PERCUTANEOUS TRANSLUMINAL PULMONARY ARTERY BALLOON ANGIOPLASTY (**92997**, **+92998**)

92997 Percutaneous transluminal pulmonary artery balloon angioplasty; single vessel
CPT Assistant Nov 97:44

+92998 each additional vessel (List separately in addition to code for primary procedure)
CPT Assistant Nov 97:44

Intent and Use of Code 92997

Code **92997** is used to report percutaneous transluminal pulmonary artery angioplasty, single vessel. This is in contradistinction to code **92986**, which describes balloon dilation of the pulmonary valve.

Intent and Use of Code +92998

Code **92998** reports this procedure for each additional vessel. It is intended for use in reporting angioplasty to each separate branch or sub-branch of the left or right pulmonary artery.

CATEGORY III CODES: PROSTHETIC AORTIC HEART PROCEDURES (**0256T-0259T**)

0256T Implantation of catheter-delivered prosthetic aortic heart valve; endovascular approach
CPT Changes: An Insider's View 2011

0257T open thoracic approach (eg, transapical, transventricular)
CPT Changes: An Insider's View 2011

0258T Transthoracic cardiac exposure (eg, sternotomy, thoracotomy, subxiphoid) for catheter-delivered aortic valve replacement; without cardiopulmonary bypass
CPT Changes: An Insider's View 2011

0259T with cardiopulmonary bypass
CPT Changes: An Insider's View 2011

Intent and Use of Codes 0256T and 0257T

Codes **0256T** and **0257T** are used to report implantation of a catheter-delivered prosthetic aortic heart valve. Code **0256T** describes the endovascular approach. Code **0257T** describes the open thoracic approach. Codes **0256T** and **0257T** do not include cardiac catheterization (**93451-93572**) when performed at the time of the procedure for diagnostic purposes. Therefore, when performed, diagnostic cardiac catheterization should be reported separately from the **93451-93572** series of codes. Codes **0256T** and **0257T** do include all other catheterization(s), temporary pacing, intraprocedural contrast injection(s), fluoroscopic radiological supervision and interpretation, and imaging guidance, which are not reported separately when performed to complete the aortic valve procedure. When reporting code **0257T** for open thoracic implantation, transthoracic cardiac exposure is reported separately using code **0258T** or code **0259T** as appropriate.

Clinical Example for Code 0256T

A 75-year-old female presents with a history of diabetes mellitus, chronic kidney disease, and chronic obstructive lung disease on home oxygen. She has well-documented critical valvular aortic stenosis with estimated aortic valve orifice area of 0.5 cm². She has noted progressively worsening dyspnea on exertion despite stable lung disease. Of late she has become intermittently lightheaded when exerting herself and had one syncopal episode. Her cardiologist has recommended aortic valve replacement. She has been rejected for conventional open heart aortic valve replacement by two cardiovascular surgeons citing operative risks that outweigh the benefit. Implantation of catheter-delivered prosthetic aortic heart valve is performed using an endovascular approach.

Clinical Example for Code 0257T

A patient similar to the one described in the example for code **0256T** has been rejected for conventional open heart surgery for aortic valve replacement by two cardiovascular surgeons citing operative risks that outweigh the benefit. Significant aortoiliac disease precludes transfemoral or transiliac vascular access. Implantation of a catheter-delivered prosthetic aortic heart valve is performed using a transapical approach.

Intent and Use of Codes 0258T and 0259T

Codes **0258T** and **0259T** are used to report transthoracic cardiac exposure for the purpose of transcatheter-delivered aortic valve replacement. Code **0258T** describes the procedure without cardiopulmonary bypass. Code **0259T** describes the procedure with cardiopulmonary bypass.

Clinical Example for Code 0258T

A patient similar to the one described in the example for code **0256T** has been rejected for conventional open heart surgery for aortic valve replacement by two cardiovascular surgeons citing operative risks that outweigh the benefit. Significant aortoiliac disease precludes transfemoral or transiliac vascular access. Transthoracic cardiac exposure (0258T) is performed, which allows for implantation of a catheter-delivered prosthetic aortic heart valve using a transapical approach (0257T).

Clinical Example for Code 0259T

A patient similar to the one described in the example for code 0256T has been rejected for conventional open heart surgery for aortic valve replacement by two cardiovascular surgeons citing operative risks that outweigh the benefit. Significant aortoiliac disease precludes transfemoral or transiliac vascular access. Transthoracic cardiac exposure with cardiopulmonary bypass (0259T) is performed, which allows for implantation of a catheter-delivered prosthetic aortic heart valve using a transapical approach (0257T).

CATHETER-DELIVERED PROSTHETIC PULMONARY VALVE (●0262T)

●0262T Implantation of catheter-delivered prosthetic pulmonary valve, endovascular approach
CPT Changes: An Insider's View 2012

Intent and Use of Code ●0262T

Category III code 0262T includes all congenital cardiac catheterization(s), intraprocedural contrast injection(s), fluoroscopic radiological supervision and interpretation, and imaging guidance performed to complete the pulmonary valve procedure. Do not report code 0262T in conjunction with codes 76000, 76001, 93563, 93566-93568, 93530. Code 0262T includes stent deployment within the pulmonary conduit; therefore, do not report code 0262T in conjunction with code 92990. Do not report codes 37205, 37206, 75960 for stent placement within the pulmonary conduit. Report codes 92980, 92981, 37205, 37206, 75960 separately when cardiovascular stent placement is performed at a site separate from the prosthetic valve delivery site. Report code 92997 and 92998 separately when pulmonary artery angioplasty is performed at a site separate from the prosthetic valve delivery site.

Clinical Example for Code ●0262T

A 16-year old patient with a history of total repair of Tetralogy of Fallot has developed shortness of breath and extreme weakness upon exertion believed to be due to a failing pulmonary conduit; cardiac MRI finds severe pulmonary regurgitation and right ventricular dilatation. The patient is found to be a candidate for endovascular pulmonary valve implantation.

Description of Service for Code ●0262T

General anesthesia is induced; the patient is intubated and connected to a mechanical ventilator. The patient is further positioned to allow biplanar fluoroscopic capability.

Potential impact to the coronary artery from implantation is accessed. A stiff guidewire is placed across the RV to PA conduit. Under fluoroscopic guidance, an angiographic catheter of choice is placed in position to assess the appropriate site for valve implantation and quantification of pulmonary valve stenosis and/or regurgitation. The angiographic catheter is withdrawn.

A balloon angioplasty catheter is passed over the guidewire and positioned within the RV to PA conduit at the appropriate level, crossing the existing valve within the conduit. Pre-dilation of the conduit and existing valve using the balloon angioplasty/valvuloplasty catheter is performed. Assessment is then undertaken of the size of the newly dilated conduit, waist of the existing valve, and compliance of the conduit to ensure a suitable valve delivery site. Angiography of the area may also be performed at this time to rule out conduit rupture.

When anatomically indicated, the conduit is reinforced by inserting a balloon-expandable stent. Fluoroscopy/angiography may be performed to confirm stent placement.

In preparation for implantation, the percutaneous pulmonary valve is repeatedly rinsed per protocol. The delivery catheter system is vigorously flushed to remove air. The stented valve is crimped onto the delivery catheter system. Correct orientation of the valve on the delivery catheter system is confirmed by the operator and another staff member in the room. Depending on the system, the valve may then be covered with an outer sheath while flushing with saline.

After confirming anti-coagulation, the femoral vein or other venous access is sequentially dilated to accept the delivery catheter. Over the guidewire, the delivery system is advanced under fluoroscopy into the right ventricular outflow tract, to the target position within the conduit. Position is confirmed by fluoroscopy and/or by injection of contrast. The stented valve is implanted by successive inflation of balloons on the delivery catheter system. The balloons are deflated and the delivery system is withdrawn.

Repeat angiography and pressure measurements are done to confirm placement. If clinically indicated, an additional high-pressure angioplasty balloon may be used to post-dilate the newly implanted stented valve within the conduit.

After confirming satisfactory position and function of the valve, as well as assessing the degree of any para-valvular regurgitation, the guide wire and sheath are removed from the patient. The opening of the access artery is closed via blind closure, manual compression, or a closure device. The venous access may also be closed.

HOME PROTHROMBIN TIME TESTING (INR MONITORING) (HCPCS LEVEL II **G0248**, **G0249**, **G0250**)

Three G-codes are used to report home monitoring of the International Normalized Ratio (INR): **G0248**, **G0249**, and **G0250**.

G0248   Demonstration, prior to initial use, of home INR monitoring for patient with either mechanical heart valve(s), chronic atrial fibrillation, or venous thromboembolism who meets Medicare coverage criteria, under the direction of a physician; includes: face-to-face demonstration of use and care of the INR monitor, obtaining at least one blood sample, provision of instructions for reporting home INR test results, and documentation of patient ability to perform testing prior to its use

G0249   Provision of test materials and equipment for home INR monitoring of patient with either mechanical heart valve(s), chronic atrial fibrillation, or venous thromboembolism who meets Medicare coverage criteria; includes provision of materials for use in the home and reporting of test results to physician; not occurring more frequently than once a week

G0250   Physician review, interpretation, and patient management of home INR testing for a patient with either mechanical heart valve(s), chronic atrial fibrillation, or venous thromboembolism who meets Medicare coverage criteria; includes face-to-face verification by the physician that the patient uses the device in the context of the management of the anticoagulation therapy following initiation of the home INR monitoring; not occurring more frequently than once a week

Intent and Use of Code G0248

Code **G0248** applies to demonstration of the use and care of the INR monitor, collection of at least one blood sample, provision of instructions for reporting home INR test results, and documentation of a patient's ability to perform testing. The testing unit and its supplies will likely be billed by a durable medical equipment provider.

Intent and Use of Code G0249

Code **G0249** includes the provision of materials for use in the home and reporting of test results to physician (per four tests).

Intent and Use of Code G0250

Code **G0250** is used to report physician review and interpretation and patient management (per four tests).

PAYMENT POLICY ALERT Medicare covers the use of home prothrombin time and INR monitoring as part of anticoagulation management for patients with mechanical heart valves, atrial fibrillation, or venous thromboembolism who are prescribed warfarin therapy. The monitoring and home testing must be prescribed by a physician and three patient requirements met. The patient:

- must have been anticoagulated for at least 3 months prior to use of the home INR;
- must undergo an educational program on anticoagulation management and the use of the device prior to its use in the home; and
- must limit self-testing with the device to a frequency of once per week.

(Refer to Chapter 2 for further information related to anticoagulant management services [**99363**, **99364**].)

CARDIOGRAPHY (**93000**, **93005**, **93010**)

93000   Electrocardiogram, routine ECG with at least 12 leads; with interpretation and report
CPT Assistant Aug 97:9, Feb 05:9, Mar 05:1,11, Jul 08:3

93005   tracing only, without interpretation and report
CPT Assistant Aug 97:9, Mar 05:1

93010   interpretation and report only
CPT Assistant Aug 97:9, Mar 05:1, Apr 07:1

Intent and Use of Code 93000

Code **93000** describes an electrocardiographic service and identifies the complete service, which includes the reading (complete with hookup, tracing, and monitoring); the interpretation of the procedure; and the report. This procedure is carried out by attaching electrodes to the patient's limbs. Unipolar electrodes are then placed at appropriate locations on the chest to detect depolarization and repolarization of the heart. The resultant information enables the physician to determine certain irregularities regarding the heartbeat and heart function. The data can be obtained by a nonphysician provider, but the analysis and report require a physician's interpretation to perform.

Code **93000** is used in offices where the physician provides the complete service (ie, the physician owns the equipment and employs the personnel). If only the tracing or the interpretation and report are performed, separate codes should be used to identify the specific component provided (**93005** or **93010**).

Description of Service for Code 93000

During the ECG, electrodes are attached to the limbs, and unipolar electrodes are positioned at appropriate thoracic interspace for recording electrical voltage shifts at the skin surface, representing cardiac depolarization and repolarization. The tracing is reviewed by the physician; appropriate measurements are made (including axis, intervals, and voltages); an overall interpretation is made; and a report is prepared, signed, and transmitted to the patient's medical record. This service may be accomplished by editing, reviewing, and signing a computer-generated report.

Intent and Use of Code 93005

Code **93005** describes the performance of the technical component only (tracing) and does not include the interpretation and report. This service is typically performed by a nonphysician health care professional. Code **93005** should be used when only this specific component of the electrocardiographic service is provided.

Intent and Use of Code 93010

Code **93010** is for hospitalized patients. The physician is generally not involved in obtaining the tracing and would report code **93010** for the professional service only. It is also reported when the tracing is acquired in the outpatient setting with equipment and personnel not owned or employed by the physician (ie, when the physician is providing only the interpretation).

As implied by the parenthetical note following code **93010**, if extended ECG monitoring is performed, the prolonged service codes (**99354-99359**) should be appended to the appropriate E/M code to identify the additional service provided.

CODING TIP Vector-cardiograms may be reported using ECG codes **93000-93010**. Phonocardiograms should be reported by using the "unlisted services" code **93799**. Provide documentation.

CODING TIP Codes **93012** and **93014** have been deleted. Telephonic transmission of postsymptom electrocardiogram rhythm strips is reported with codes **93268-93272**.

CARDIOVASCULAR STRESS TESTING (93015-93018)

93015 Cardiovascular stress test using maximal or submaximal treadmill or bicycle exercise, continuous electrocardiographic monitoring, and/or pharmacological stress; with physician supervision, with interpretation and report
CPT Assistant Apr 96:11, Jun 96:10, Aug 02:10, Jul 08:3, Jan 10:8, May 10:5

93016 physician supervision only, without interpretation and report
CPT Assistant Apr 96:11, Aug 02:10, Jul 08:3, Jan 10:8, May 10:5

93017 tracing only, without interpretation and report
CPT Assistant Aug 02:10, Jul 08:3, Jan 10:8, May 10:5

93018 interpretation and report only
CPT Assistant Apr 96:11, Jun 96:10, Jul 08:3, Jan 10:8

Intent and Use of Codes 93015-93018

CPT coding for the stress test consists of three components:

- physician supervision of the test (**93016**);
- the ECG tracing (the technical component) (**93017**); and
- the physician interpretation and report (**93018**).

Code **93015** is used to report the complete cardiac stress test procedure, which includes all three components. Because code **93015** includes the technical component, supervision, and interpretation, this code is properly reportable only by a physician in a nonfacility setting (eg, office, clinic, or diagnostic testing center).

When a complete procedure (**93015**) is not performed, stress testing codes **93016-93018** are reported in conjunction with code **93350** to capture the cardiovascular stress portion of the study.

In a facility setting (eg, hospital), the facility reports the technical component of the service, and the physician(s) report the applicable component codes (**93016, 93018**). Each physician should take care to report only those components of the stress test that he or she actually provides, as defined earlier.

Intent and Use of Code 93015

Code **93015** is used to report cardiovascular stress testing. Code **93015** describes the complete service, including physician supervision of the test and interpretation and report of the results provided after the administration of the test. It is used to report stress testing by a physician in an office or other setting with physician-owned equipment. Set-up of the equipment and application of the electrodes for monitoring are inherently included in the procedure. Code **93015** should be used if all three components of this procedure are performed by a single physician in a nonfacility setting.

This procedure combines the use of a stressing agent or device (such as a treadmill, stationary cycle, or chemical stressor of the heart) with some type of ECG monitoring. For this procedure, the physician places monitoring leads for information retrieval during the test. In addition to the ECG leads, the physician is also responsible for monitoring the heart rate, blood pressure, and any symptoms that may occur as a result of the testing. Once monitoring and data retrieval devices have been applied, the physician can apply stress to the heart in any number of methods including physical exercise by using a mechanical apparatus (eg, exercise bike, treadmill, etc) or by administering a pharmacologic agent (eg, beta-1 agonist). At this point, the patient is monitored for irregularity in heart function, as well as for any other symptomatic responses to the stress (eg, labored breathing) to ensure the safety of the patient during the testing, as well as to obtain pertinent information regarding possible pathology. Once the desired results are achieved, the patient is monitored to ensure safe return of the heart to a nonstressed state. The ECG recording and other information can then be analyzed by the physician.

Code **93015** includes all the component codes **93016**, **93017**, and **93018**. This code should be used if all three components of this procedure are performed by a single physician. If the complete procedure is not performed, the provider should report codes **93016-93018** according to the specific procedures actually provided.

> **CODING TIP** Set up of the equipment and application of the electrodes for monitoring are inherent in cardiac stress testing and not additionally reportable by any CPT code.

Description of Service for Code 93015

Cardiovascular stress testing is performed using one of a variety of protocols and methods. This may involve exercise on a treadmill, an upright or supine bicycle ergometer, or an arm ergometer. Nonexercise stress testing is commonly accomplished by administering a pharmacologic agent such as a beta-1 agonist (dobutamine) or a coronary vasodilator (adenosine or dipyridamole). Other less-common methods for nonexercise stress testing include cold pressor testing or atrial pacing. Stress testing may be performed to symptom-limited endpoints or to a submaximal endpoint. Heart rate, blood pressure, symptoms, and the electrocardiogram are monitored during the stress testing, with recording of 12-lead ECG tracings before, during, and after stress testing. If imaging modalities are used, such as radionuclide (planar or tomographic) or echocardiographic (transthoracic or transesophageal) methods, the imaging procedures are coded separately. Physician supervision of the actual stress testing, review of the data, interpretation, and preparation of a report are all included in this code.

Intent and Use of Code 93016

Code **93016** is used alone to report supervision of a stress test in circumstances in which another physician provides the interpretation and report. Codes **93016** and **93018** are both used to report provision of the complete stress testing service by a physician in a hospital or other setting with institution-owned equipment.

Intent and Use of Code 93017

Code **93017** reports only the technical component (tracing or recording) of a stress test.

Intent and Use of Code 93018

Code **93018** reports only the interpretation and report of an exercise stress test.

> **CODING TIP** Code **93799**, *Unlisted cardiovascular service or procedure,* should be reported for inert gas rebreathing for cardiac output measurement during rest and during exercise.

> **POLICY PAYMENT ALERT** The professional component of a stress test is reported using codes **93016** and **93018** together. Medicare no longer accepts code **93015** with **modifier 26** appended to designate the professional component of a service provided in a setting where the physician does not own the equipment.

ERGONOVINE PROVOCATION TESTING (**93024**)

93024   Ergonovine provocation test

Intent and Use of Code 93024

Code **93024** describes an ergonovine provocation test. Currently, ergonovine is not performed often but may be used if angina is thought to be caused by coronary artery spasm.

MICROVOLT T-WAVE ALTERNANS TESTING (**93025**)

93025   Microvolt T-wave alternans for assessment of ventricular arrhythmias
CPT Assistant Mar 02:3; CPT Changes: An Insider's View 2002

Intent and Use of Code 93025

Code **93025** is used to report this noninvasive cardiac diagnostic test designed to identify patients at risk of life-threatening ventricular arrhythmias and sudden cardiac death.

> **PAYMENT POLICY ALERT** CMS has determined that there is sufficient evidence to conclude that Microvolt T-Wave Alternans (MTWA) diagnostic testing is reasonable and necessary for the evaluation of patients at risk of sudden cardiac death only when the spectral analytic method is used. In March 2006, CMS issued a national coverage determination (NCD) for this indication. An updated version, implemented in August 2008, states that Microvolt T-Wave Alternans diagnostic testing is covered for the evaluation of patients at risk for sudden cardiac death only when the spectral analysis method is used. For more information on this NCD, go to www.cms.hhs.gov/mcd/viewncd.asp.

Description of Service for Code 93025

The patient's skin is prepared meticulously, and seven specialized alternans sensors are applied in addition to seven conventional ECG leads. The sensor's electrical impedance is assessed to ensure good electrical contact. Baseline sampling at rest is monitored and displayed. Careful selection of the exercise protocol is crucial to ensure that the heart rate increases gradually between 90 and 110 beats per minute (bpm), preferably over 3 to 4 minutes (this is the heart rate range in which T-wave alternans is measured). The treadmill speed and grade are slowly increased to achieve a gradual ramp up of the patient's heart rate from between 90 and 110 bpm to over 110 bpm.

After the start of exercise, if the heart rate increases too rapidly, the workload must be decreased to allow the heart rate to fall within the 90 to 110 bpm range for a few minutes. Alternatively, the test can be stopped and restarted using a different exercise protocol with a more gradual increase in workload. For the purposes of measuring T-wave alternans, the target heart rate (after the patient has exercised for a few minutes with heart rates between 90 and 110 bpm) is 120 bpm. Throughout the text, the noise level of each sensor is monitored carefully to ensure sufficiently low noise levels. If the noise levels are too high, then the sensor placement may need to be readjusted and/or patient instruction given. T-wave alternans is monitored throughout the diagnostic test to ensure that complete data are collected and artifacts will not obscure the interpretation.

After the heart rate reaches 120 bpm, the T-wave alternans portion of the stress test is completed. At times, the stress test will be done for multiple reasons. In addition to the measurement of T-wave alternans, the stress test may be used as a symptom-limited stress test to detect myocardial ischemia, or it may be used as a maximal exercise test to measure functional capacity and VO_2 max. After the patient reaches a heart rate of 120 bpm, the workload can then be increased as necessary to complete the additional portions of the stress test.

After the exercise portion of the test, the patient is monitored during recovery from exercise. An alternans trend report is then produced, and a determination is made of the presence of sustained alternans and the onset heart rate of this event. The results are classified as positive, negative, or indeterminate. The sensors are then removed, and the test report is completed.

RHYTHM ECG (**93040-93042**)

93040   Rhythm ECG, 1-3 leads; with interpretation and report
CPT Assistant Apr 04:8, Oct 10:10

93041   tracing only without interpretation and report
CPT Assistant Apr 04:8, Oct 10:10

93042   interpretation and report only
CPT Assistant Apr 04:8

Intent and Use of Code 93040

Code **93040** describes the acquisition of a rhythm ECG (one to three leads), interpretation, and report as a complete service.

Code **93040** includes the component codes **93041** and **93042**. Codes **93040-93042** are appropriate when an order for the test is triggered by an event, the rhythm strip is used to help diagnose the presence or absence of an arrhythmia, and a written report is generated and signed by the interpreting physician. It is not appropriate to use these codes for reviewing the telemetry monitor strips taken from a monitoring system in the hospital. The need for an electrocardiogram or rhythm strip should be supported by documentation in the patient medical record.

Intent and Use of Code 93041

Code **93041** is used to report the technical component only.

Intent and Use of Code 93042

Code **93042** is used to report the professional component only (in this case, the interpretation).

CODING TIP Codes **93040-93042** (rhythm ECG, one to three leads) are not to be used for rhythm monitoring. The American College of Cardiology provided this clarification and added that codes **93040-93042** should not be used to report electrocardiographic rhythm monitoring. For ECG monitoring, see codes **99354-99360**.

PAYMENT POLICY ALERT Most insurers also consider the EGG rhythm strip (**93040-93042**) and the intravenous (IV) infusion (**96365-96366**) to be bundled into this service and not separately reportable.

CARDIOGRAPHY CARDIOVASCULAR MONITORING SERVICES (**93224-93229, 93268, 93270-93272**)

According to CPT guidelines, cardiovascular monitoring services are diagnostic medical procedures using in-person and remote technology to assess cardiovascular rhythm (eg, ECG) data. Holter monitors (**93224-93227**) include up to 48 hours of continuous recording. Mobile cardiac telemetry monitors (**93228, 93229**) have the capability of transmitting a tracing at any time, always have internal ECG analysis algorithms designed to detect major arrhythmias, and transmit to an attended surveillance center. Event monitors (**93268-93272**) record segments of ECGs with recording initiation triggered either by patient activation or by an internal automatic, preprogrammed detection algorithm (or both) and transmit the recorded electrocardiographic data when requested (but cannot transmit immediately based upon the patient or algorithmic activation rhythm) and do not require attended surveillance.

Attended surveillance: The immediate availability of a remote technician to respond to rhythm or device alert transmissions from a patient, either from an implanted or wearable monitoring or therapy device, as they are generated and transmitted to the remote surveillance location or center.

Electrocardiographic rhythm–derived elements: Elements derived from recordings of the electrical activation of the heart, including, but not limited to, heart rhythm, rate, ST analysis, heart rate variability, and T-wave alternans.

Mobile cardiovascular telemetry (MCT): Continuously records the electrocardiographic rhythm from external electrodes placed on the patient's body. Segments of the ECG data are automatically (ie, without patient intervention) transmitted to a remote surveillance location by cellular or landline telephone signal. The segments of the rhythm, selected for transmission, are triggered automatically (MCT device algorithm) by rapid and slow heart rates or by the patient during a symptomatic episode. There is continuous real-time data analysis by preprogrammed algorithms in the device and attended surveillance of the transmitted rhythm segments by a surveillance center technician to evaluate any arrhythmias and to determine signal quality. The surveillance center technician reviews the data and notifies the physician depending on the prescribed criteria.

ECG rhythm–derived elements are distinct from physiologic data, even when the same device is capable of producing both. Implantable cardiovascular monitor (ICM) device services are always separately reported from implantable cardioverter-defibrillator (ICD) services.

EXTERNAL ELECTROCARDIOGRAPHIC RECORDING/MONITORING (**93224-93227**)

93224   External electrocardiographic recording up to 48 hours by continuous rhythm recording and storage; includes recording, scanning analysis with report, physician review and interpretation
CPT Assistant Oct 05:14, Apr 07:3, Mar 08:4, Mar 09:5; CPT Changes: An Insider's View 2009, 2011

93225   recording (includes connection, recording, and disconnection)
CPT Assistant Oct 05:14, Apr 07:3, Mar 09:5; CPT Changes: An Insider's View 2009, 2011

93226   scanning analysis with report
CPT Assistant Oct 05:14, Apr 07:3, Mar 09:5; CPT Changes: An Insider's View 2009, 2011

93227   physician review and interpretation
CPT Assistant Apr 07:3, Mar 09:5, Apr 09:7; CPT Changes: An Insider's View 2009, 2011

Intent and Use of Codes 93224-93227

Codes **93224-93227** describe complete, technical, and professional components of the use of various electrocardiographic monitoring devices (eg, Holter monitors) by continuous original ECG waveform. Code **93224** includes all the component codes **93225**, **93226**, and **93227**. Codes **93224-93227** describe external electrocardiographic recording for up to 48 hours. For 12 hours or less of continuous recording, **modifier 52** should be appended.

Description of Service for Code 93224

Electrodes are attached to the skin and connected to a device that records ECG waveforms continuously, often capturing two ECG leads and storing the data on recording tape or in computer chip memory. These data are then processed (typically by computerized superimposition scanning, which looks for and prints variations from the baseline waveform). The data are then reviewed, measured, interpreted, and reported by the physician. Sometimes, initial data scanning and review are performed by specially trained nonphysician personnel. However, these data are then reviewed, analyzed, and interpreted by the physician, and a report is prepared and transmitted to the patient's medical record.

The monitoring system is received by the clinic. The data are downloaded and scanning analysis is performed. (The process takes up to 2 hours on average.) A technician is required to compile and print relevant data and arrhythmias (including logged diary events) to be interpreted by the physician. Scanned arrhythmias meeting "immediate notification criteria" are promptly brought to the physician's attention.

EXTERNAL MOBILE CARDIOVASCULAR TELEMETRY/RECORDING (**93228**, **93229**)

93228   External mobile cardiovascular telemetry with electrocardiographic recording, concurrent computerized real time data analysis and greater than 24 hours of accessible ECG data storage (retrievable with query) with ECG triggered and patient selected events transmitted to a remote attended surveillance center for up to 30 days; physician review and interpretation with report
CPT Changes: An Insider's View 2009, 2011

93229   technical support for connection and patient instructions for use, attended surveillance, analysis and physician prescribed transmission of daily and emergent data reports
CPT Changes: An Insider's View 2009, 2011

Intent and Use of Codes 93228 and 93229

Mobile cardiovascular telemetry (MCT) services include a device capable of continuously recording the ECG rhythm from external electrodes. MCT continuously records the electrocardiographic rhythm from external electrodes placed on the patient's body. The system monitors the patient 24 hours a day via the wearable device as he or she continues with a normal daily routine. Periodically, and as events occur, patient activity is automatically transmitted to a remote surveillance location.

Segments of the ECG data are automatically (ie, without patient intervention) transmitted to a remote surveillance center via cellular or landline telephone signal. There is an MCT device algorithm that determines the segments of the rhythm that are triggered automatically and selected for transmission; this may be a rapid and/or slow heart rate or may be triggered by the patient when various symptoms are experienced. Physician analysis of the data is reported with code **93228**. The surveillance center services are reported with code **93229**.

Key to the technical portion of this service is the attended surveillance and immediate availability of a technician to respond to the rhythm or device alert transmissions from the patient as they are generated and transmitted to the surveillance location.

This technology provides for continuous real-time data analysis by preprogrammed algorithms in the device, as well as attended surveillance of the transmitted rhythm segments. A surveillance center technician evaluates any arrhythmias, reviews the data, and may notify the physician depending on the prescribed criteria.

Codes **93228** and **93229** describe external mobile telemetry with ECG-triggered transmissions to an attended surveillance center. Codes **93224-93227** and **93268-93272** differ from codes **93228** and **93229** in that these codes represent services associated with external cardiovascular monitoring devices that do not perform automatic ECG-triggered transmissions to an attended surveillance center. Therefore, it is not appropriate to report code **93228** in addition to codes **93224** and **93227**, nor is it appropriate to report code **93229** in addition to codes **93224** or **93226**.

Code **93228** represents the physician's review and interpretation along with a report of the events transmitted for physician review during a 30-day time frame. The code is reported only once per 30 days regardless of the number of transmissions the physician may receive on that particular patient during that period.

The physician's staff may also be involved in providing some basic information about the service prescribed by the physician to the patient and may also have a role in organizing and prioritizing the information sent to the physician for review. Services of this nature provided by the physician's staff are included in the reimbursement for the physician's work (review and interpretation) and do not justify the submission of code **93229**.

As described previously in this section, MCT requires the attended surveillance of a remote monitoring center, as well as the capabilities of the device as described by the code definition. Code **93229** was developed to describe the technical support provided in conjunction with MCT by the attended surveillance center and is to be billed only once per 30 days.

Description of Service for Codes 93228 and 93229

Algorithm determined automatic ECG-triggered and patient-triggered events are transmitted to a remote attended surveillance center. The remote attended surveillance center transmits recordings to the physician's office during business hours. During business hours, arrhythmia events meeting "immediate notification criteria" are promptly brought to the interpreting physician's attention. After business hours, arrhythmia events meeting "immediate notification criteria" are promptly brought to the on-call physician's attention. Services include all transmissions for up to 30 days.

EXTERNAL ECG RHYTHM-DERIVED EVENT RECORDING (93268-93272)

93268   External patient and, when performed, auto activated electrocardiographic rhythm derived event recording with symptom-related memory loop with remote download capability up to 30 days, 24-hour attended monitoring; includes transmission, physician review and interpretation
CPT Assistant Jun 96:2, Nov 99:49-50, Oct 05:14, Apr 07:3, Mar 08:4, Mar 09:5; *CPT Changes: An Insider's View* 2003, 2009, 2011

93270   recording (includes connection, recording, and disconnection)
CPT Assistant Jun 96:2, Oct 05:14, Apr 07:3, Mar 09:5; *CPT Changes: An Insider's View* 2009, 2011

93271   transmission download and analysis
CPT Assistant Jun 96:2, Oct 05:14, Apr 07:3, Mar 09:5; *CPT Changes: An Insider's View* 2009, 2011

93272   physician review and interpretation
CPT Assistant Jun 96:2, Apr 98:14, Nov 99:49-50, Oct 05:14, Apr 07:3, Mar 09:5, Apr 09:7; *CPT Changes: An Insider's View* 2009, 2011

Intent and Use of Codes 93268-93272

The **93268-93272** series of codes should be reported for event recorders that include presymptom "memory loop technology" for heart rhythm transmission. These recorders provide physicians with a rhythm strip of a patient's cardiac rhythm "prior" (presymptom) and/or "subsequent" (postsymptom) to the symptomatology that prompted the patient to activate the device. These codes require 24-hour attended monitoring of a wearable device.

Intent and Use of Code 93268

Code **93268** represents the overall service of hooking up the device, recording, monitoring, receiving transmission, analyzing, and disconnecting the device, and the reviewing physician's interpretation of the rhythm strips and preparation of a report within a 30-day period. Arrhythmia monitoring services may be provided by clinics, hospitals, or independent laboratories that are staffed by technicians or nurses to receive and respond to the transmission of the electrocardiographic rhythm strip.

Code **93268** is used to report the complete service for patient-demand, single- or multiple-event recording devices using memory loop technology. Code **93268** includes all the component codes **93270**, **93271**, and **93272**. When the entire (global) service is provided, report code **93268**, not the individual component codes. The interpretation of all rhythm strips received during the 30-day period is included in this service and should not be reported separately (eg, do not additionally report code **93042**).

Description of Service for Codes 93268-93272

Algorithm-determined automatic ECG-triggered, symptomatic patient-triggered events, or routinely scheduled rhythm recordings are transmitted to a surveillance center. The surveillance center receives and produces a report, which is sent to the physician's office, typically during business hours. Arrhythmia events meeting "immediate notification criteria" are promptly brought to the interpreting physician's attention. After business hours, arrhythmia events meeting "immediate notification criteria" are promptly brought to the on-call physician's attention. Services include all transmissions up to 30 days.

CODING TIP If less than 24-hour attended monitoring is performed, code **93799** (unlisted cardiovascular service) may be used. Check with your local carrier or payer for its payment policy. If a physician is providing attended monitoring during office hours only, do not report codes **93268**, **93270**, **93271**, and **93272**.

PAYMENT POLICY ALERT Many physicians contract with various types of arrhythmia services to supply devices, receive transmissions, and/or provide reports. Under these circumstances, Holter monitor and patient event recorder services should not be reported by the physician as a global service. Check with your Medicare carriers and commercial payers to determine appropriate reporting when purchasing all or part of these services from a supplier.

Intent and Use of Code 93270

Code **93270** represents connection, recording, and disconnection services.

CODING TIP Codes **93270** and **93271** together represent the technical component of the service.

Intent and Use of Code 93271

Code **93271** represents transmission, download receipt, and analysis services.

Intent and Use of Code 93272

Code **93272** is used to report the professional component only.

SIGNAL-AVERAGED ECG (**93278**)

93278   Signal-averaged electrocardiography (SAECG), with or without ECG

Intent and Use of Code 93278

Code **93278** is used to report the complete signal-averaged ECG (SAECG) service. The professional component only would be reported by adding **modifier 26** to code **93278**.

Description of Service for Code 93278

Multiple-surface electrodes are placed on the patient's limbs and chest, and an electrocardiogram is recorded over a period of 10 to 20 minutes (sufficient to obtain 100 to 400 cycles) and "averaged." Sophisticated computer analysis follows, in either the time domain or the frequency domain. The resulting data are then summarized and interpreted by the physician. A report is prepared, signed, and transmitted to the patient's medical record.

IMPLANTABLE AND WEARABLE CARDIAC DEVICE EVALUATIONS (**93279-93299**)

According to the CPT guidelines, cardiac device evaluation services are diagnostic medical procedures using in-person and remote technology to assess device therapy and cardiovascular physiologic data.

Codes **93279-93299** describe this technology and technical/professional physician and service center practice. Codes **93279-93292** are reported per procedure.

The pacemaker and ICD interrogation device evaluations, periprocedural device evaluations and programming, and programming device evaluations may not be reported in conjunction with pacemaker or ICD device and/or lead insertion or revision services by the same physician. The following definitions and instructions apply to codes **93279-93299**.

Attended surveillance: The immediate availability of a remote technician to respond to rhythm or device alert transmissions from a patient, either from an implanted or wearable monitoring or therapy device, as they are generated and transmitted to the remote surveillance location or center.

Device, single lead: A pacemaker or implantable cardioverter-defibrillator with pacing and sensing function in only one chamber of the heart.

Device, dual lead: A pacemaker or implantable cardioverter-defibrillator with pacing and sensing function in only two chambers of the heart.

Device, multiple lead: A pacemaker or implantable cardioverter-defibrillator with pacing and sensing function in three or more chambers of the heart.

Electrocardiographic rhythm–derived elements: Elements derived from recordings of the electrical activation of the heart including, but not limited to, heart rhythm, rate, ST analysis, heart rate variability, and T-wave alternans.

Implantable cardiovascular monitor (ICM): An implantable cardiovascular device used to assist the physician in the management of non-rhythm related cardiac conditions such as heart failure. The device collects longitudinal physiologic cardiovascular data elements from one or more internal sensors (such as right ventricular pressure, left atrial pressure, or an index of lung water) and/or external sensors (such as blood pressure or body weight) for patient assessment and management. The data are stored and transmitted to the physician either by local telemetry or remotely to an Internet-based file server or surveillance technician. The function of the ICM may be an additional function of an implantable cardiac device (eg, implantable cardioverter-defibrillator) or a function of a stand-alone device. When ICM functionality is included in an ICD device or pacemaker, the ICM data and the ICD or pacemaker heart rhythm data such as sensing, pacing, and tachycardia detection therapy are distinct and, therefore, the monitoring processes are distinct.

Implantable cardioverter-defibrillator (ICD): An implantable device that provides high-energy and low-energy stimulation to one or more chambers of the heart to terminate rapid heart rhythms called tachycardia or fibrillation. ICDs also have pacemaker functions to treat slow heart rhythms called bradycardia. In addition to the tachycardia and bradycardia functions, the ICD may or may not include the functionality of an implantable cardiovascular monitor or an implantable loop recorder.

Implantable loop recorder (ILR): An implantable device that continuously records the electrocardiographic rhythm triggered automatically by rapid and slow heart rates or by the patient during a symptomatic episode. The ILR function may be the only function of the device or it may be part of a pacemaker or implantable cardioverter-defibrillator device. The data are stored and transmitted to the physician either by local telemetry or remotely to an Internet-based file server or surveillance technician. Extraction of data and compilation or report for physician interpretation are usually performed in the office setting.

Pacemaker: An implantable device that provides low-energy localized stimulation to one or more chambers of the heart to initiate contraction in that chamber.

Physiologic cardiovascular data elements: Data elements from one or more internal sensors (such as right ventricular pressure, left atrial pressure, or an index of lung water) and/or external sensors (such as blood pressure or body weight) for patient assessment and management. It does not include ECG rhythm–derived data elements.

Codes **93293-93296** are reported no more than once every 90 days. Do not report codes **93293-93296** if the monitoring period is less than 30 days. Codes **93297** and **93298** are reported no more than once every 30 days. Do not report codes **93297-93299** if the monitoring period is less than 10 days.

A service center may report code **93296** or code **93299** during a period in which a physician performs an in-person interrogation device evaluation. A physician may not report an in-person and remote interrogation of the same device during the same period. Report only remote services when an in-person interrogation device evaluation is performed during a period of remote interrogation device evaluation. A period is established by the initiation of the remote monitoring or the 91st day of a pacemaker or implantable cardioverter-defibrillator (ICD) monitoring or the 31st day of an implantable loop recorder (ILR) or implantable cardiovascular monitor (ICM) monitoring and extends for the subsequent 90 or 30 days, respectively, for which remote monitoring is occurring. Programming device evaluations and in-person interrogation device evaluations may not be reported on the same date by the same physician. Programming device evaluations and remote interrogation device evaluations may both be reported during the remote interrogation device evaluation period.

ECG rhythm–derived elements are distinct from physiologic data, even when the same device is capable of producing both. ICM device services are always separately reported from ICD services. When ILR data are derived from an ICD or pacemaker, do not report ILR services with pacemaker or ICD services.

CODING TIP Do not report codes **93268-93272** when performing the procedures described by codes **93279-93289**, **93291-93296**, or **93298-93299**. Do not report codes **93040-93042** when performing the procedures described by codes **93279-93289**, **93291-93296**, or **93298-93299**.

PROGRAMMING DEVICE EVALUATION (IN PERSON) (**93279-93285**)

93279 Programming device evaluation (in person) with iterative adjustment of the implantable device to test the function of the device and select optimal permanent programmed values with physician analysis, review and report; single lead pacemaker system
CPT Changes: An Insider's View 2009, 2010

93280 dual lead pacemaker system
CPT Changes: An Insider's View 2009, 2010

93281 multiple lead pacemaker system
CPT Changes: An Insider's View 2009, 2010

93282 single lead implantable cardioverter-defibrillator system
CPT Changes: An Insider's View 2009, 2010

93283 dual lead implantable cardioverter-defibrillator system
CPT Changes: An Insider's View 2009, 2010

93284 multiple lead implantable cardioverter-defibrillator system
CPT Changes: An Insider's View 2009, 2010

93285 implantable loop recorder system
CPT Changes: An Insider's View 2009, 2010

Intent and Use of Codes 93279-93285

A programming evaluation (**93279-93285**) is a customized evaluation in which the physician prescribes the appropriate behavior of the device for the patient and evaluates both the patient's condition and the device's function. Use the programming evaluation codes when all device functions, including battery, programmable settings, and lead(s), when present, are evaluated. A programming evaluation is also used for assessment of capture thresholds, iterative adjustments (ie, progressive changes in the pacing output of a lead), and programmable parameters. Evaluation allows the operator to assess and select the most appropriate parameters to provide for appropriate therapy and verify device function. The final program parameters may or may not change as a result of the evaluation.

Components to be evaluated include all of the interrogation evaluation and a selection of specific programmed parameters.

CPT guidelines indicate that programming device evaluation (in person) (**93279-93285**) is a procedure performed for patients with a pacemaker, implantable cardioverter-defibrillator, or implantable loop recorder. All device functions, including the battery, programmable settings, and lead(s), when present, are evaluated. To assess capture thresholds, iterative adjustments (eg, progressive changes in pacing output of a pacing lead) of the programmable parameters are conducted. The iterative adjustments provide information that permits the operator to assess and select the most appropriate final program parameters to provide for consistent delivery of the appropriate therapy and to verify the function of the device. The final program parameters may or may not change after evaluation.

The programming device evaluation includes all the components of the interrogation device evaluation (remote) or the interrogation device evaluation (in person), and it includes the selection of patient-specific programmed parameters depending on the type of device. The components that must be evaluated for the various types of programming device evaluations are listed as follows.

Pacemaker: Programmed parameters, lead(s), battery, capture and sensing function, and heart rhythm. Often, but not always, the sensor rate response, lower and upper heart rates, AV intervals, pacing voltage and pulse duration, sensing value, and diagnostics will be adjusted during a programming evaluation.

Implantable cardioverter-defibrillator (ICD): Programmed parameters, lead(s), battery, capture and sensing function, presence or absence of therapy for ventricular tachyarrhythmias, and underlying heart rhythm. Often, but not always, the sensor rate response, lower and upper heart rates, AV intervals, pacing voltage and pulse duration, sensing value, and diagnostics will be adjusted during a programming evaluation. In addition, ventricular tachycardia detection and therapies are sometimes altered depending on the interrogated data, patient's rhythm, symptoms, and condition.

Implantable loop recorder (ILR): Programmed parameters and the heart rhythm during recorded episodes from both patient-initiated and device algorithm–detected events. Often, but not always, the tachycardia and bradycardia detection criteria will be adjusted during a programming evaluation.

Description of Service for Code 93279

After verbal consent is obtained from the patient to proceed, the patient is connected to a single- or multi-lead, free-running electrocardiogram monitor. A communication link is obtained between the pacemaker and the programmer. The current rhythm is assessed and recorded. The magnet mode response is assessed and recorded. An attempt to obtain and record the patient's underlying rhythm is performed. The appropriate safety techniques are given to the patient who is pacemaker dependent.

A full interrogation of the stored pacemaker data is obtained and reviewed for alert conditions. The current interrogated measurements are compared to the extensive stored and trended data. These data are reviewed for device alerts in regard to battery and lead function including voltage, impedance, and current. Additional measurements are made when necessary to assess the status of the insulation and conductors of the leads. The appropriate lead polarity for sensing and capture parameters are identified. Stored summary and

recorded rhythm information are reviewed for evidence of atrial fibrillation, premature ventricular contractions, and nonsustained and sustained ventricular tachycardia. The appropriate rhythm alerts and recording parameters are identified. The pacing capture threshold is measured in a single chamber by varying the voltage output and pulse width in a step-wise fashion to determine the appropriate safety margin for final device parameters and to optimize pacemaker device longevity. The appropriate voltage and pulse width parameters are identified.

The sensing threshold is measured by recording the signal from a single lead and chamber and by iterative (step-wise) adjustment of pacemaker sensing value to determine the appropriate sensing safety margin. The appropriate mode and threshold for sensing are identified. Heart rate adaptation to exercise or physiologic stress data are reviewed and adjusted in an iterative (step-wise) technique. Data considered to select the appropriate final programmed values include multiple heart rate histograms and trended activity levels. When necessary, in-office assessment is completed through the patient's exercise activity to establish adequate heart rate response to exercise. The appropriate rate response parameters are identified.

After detailed analysis of each of these parameters, a decision is made about the adequacy of the initial programmed pacemaker parameters and any identified changes that need to be made to optimize the device performance relative to the patient's clinical condition. These device programming changes are made, and any additional recommendations for further cardiac evaluation or treatment are given.

Description of Service for Code 93280

After verbal consent is obtained from the patient to proceed, the patient is connected to a single- or multi-lead, free-running electrocardiogram monitor. A communication link is obtained between the pacemaker and the programmer. The current rhythm is assessed and recorded. The magnet mode response is assessed and recorded. An attempt to obtain and record the patient's underlying rhythm is performed with appropriate safety considerations given to the patient who is pacemaker dependent.

A full interrogation of the stored pacemaker data is obtained and reviewed for alert conditions. Current interrogated measurements are compared to the extensive stored data. Trended data are reviewed for device alerts in regard to battery and lead function, including voltage, impedance, and current. Additional measurements are made when necessary to assess the status of the insulation and conductors of the leads. The appropriate lead polarity for sensing and capture parameters is identified. Stored summary and recorded rhythm information is reviewed for evidence of atrial fibrillation, premature ventricular contractions, and nonsustained and sustained ventricular tachycardia. The appropriate rhythm alerts and recording parameters are identified.

The pacing capture threshold is measured in a single chamber by varying the voltage output and pulse width in a step-wise fashion to determine the appropriate safety margin for final device parameters and to optimize pacemaker device longevity. The appropriate voltage and pulse width parameters are identified. The sensing threshold is measured by recording the signal from a single lead and chamber and by iterative (step-wise) adjustment of pacemaker sensing value to determine the appropriate sensing safety margin. The appropriate mode and threshold for sensing are identified. Heart rate adaptation to exercise or physiologic stress data are reviewed and adjusted in an iterative (step-wise) technique. Data considered to select the appropriate final programmed values include multiple heart rate histograms and trended activity levels. When necessary, in-office assessment is completed through patient exercise activity to establish adequate heart rate response to exercise. The appropriate rate response parameters are identified.

After the detailed analysis of each of these parameters, a decision is made about the adequacy of the initial programmed pacemaker parameters and any identified changes that need to be made to optimize the device performance relative to the patient's clinical condition. These device programming changes are made, and any additional recommendations for further cardiac evaluation or treatment are given.

Description of Service for Code 93281

After verbal consent is obtained from the patient to proceed, the patient is connected to a single- or multi-lead, free-running electrocardiogram monitor. A communication link is obtained between the pacemaker and the programmer. The current rhythm is assessed and recorded. The magnet mode response is assessed and recorded. An attempt to obtain and record the patient's underlying rhythm is performed with appropriate safety considerations given to the patient who is pacemaker dependent.

A full interrogation of the stored pacemaker data is obtained, and results are reviewed for alert conditions. The current interrogated measurements are compared to the extensive stored data. Trended data are reviewed

for device alerts with regard to battery and lead function, including voltage, impedance, and current. Additional measurements are made when necessary to assess the status of the insulation and lead conductors. The appropriate lead polarity for sensing and capture parameters is identified. Appropriate sensing of chamber-specific electrical activity and adjustment of pacemaker device parameters to accommodate for interim changes in the patient's status are performed. Stored summary and recorded rhythm information is reviewed for evidence of atrial fibrillation, premature ventricular contractions, and nonsustained and sustained ventricular tachycardia. The appropriate rhythm alerts and recording parameters are identified.

The pacing capture threshold is measured separately in three or more chambers (usually the right atrium, right ventricle, and left ventricle) by varying the voltage output and pulse width in a step-wise fashion to determine the appropriate safety margin for final device parameters and to optimize pacemaker device longevity. Care is taken to appropriately identify the capture of the ventricular chamber of interest (right, left, or both) to avoid incorrect conclusions about capture safety margins. The appropriate voltage and pulse width parameters are identified. The sensing threshold is measured separately in both chambers (usually the right atrium and right ventricle) by recording the signal from each lead and chamber and by iterative (step-wise) adjustment of the pacemaker sensing value to determine the appropriate sensing safety margin. The appropriate mode and threshold for sensing are identified. Influence of the stimulation of one chamber on the sensing and activation of the other chamber are evaluated for atrial to right and left ventricular, ventricular to atrial, right ventricle to left ventricle, and left ventricle to right ventricle conduction; cross-talk sensing between the chambers; and far-field electrogram detection. The potential influence of these issues for permanent programming is identified.

Anodal right ventricular stimulation during left ventricular pacing is assessed, and the presence or absence of phrenic nerve (diaphragmatic) stimulation in regard to pacing output and pacing polarity configuration is identified for permanent programming. Iterative (step-wise) programming of arteriovenous interval timing, whether fixed or dynamic, and determination of its influence on the percentage of ventricular pacing and hemodynamics or limitation of heart rate response are completed. Heart rate adaptation to exercise or physiologic stress data are reviewed and adjusted using an iterative (step-wise) technique. Data considered to select the appropriate final programmed values include multiple heart rate histograms and trended activity levels. When necessary, in-office assessment is completed through patient's exercise activity to establish adequate heart rate response to exercise. The appropriate rate response parameters are identified.

After detailed analysis of each of these parameters, a decision is made about the adequacy of the initial programmed pacemaker parameters and any identified changes that need to be made to optimize the device performance relative to the patient's clinical condition. These device programming changes are made, and any additional recommendations for further cardiac evaluation or treatment are given.

Description of Service for Code 93282

After verbal consent is obtained from the patient to proceed, the patient is connected to a single- or multi-lead electrocardiogram recording system. A communication link is established between the device and the programmer.

A full interrogation of the stored device parameters is obtained. The current rhythm is assessed and recorded. The stored pacing and tachyarrhythmia episode data are retrieved, and detailed physician analysis of these data is performed.

The stored summary and recorded rhythm data are reviewed. Pacing capture threshold data and lead impedance are measured within the ventricular chamber. Based on this information, the physician identifies any pacing or integrity issues with the existing lead and determines the appropriate pacing output settings. Sensing threshold data are obtained by recording the signal from the ventricular chamber and utilizing iterative (step-wise) adjustment of ICD sensing level. Based on this information, the physician identifies the appropriate ICD sensing settings. Ventricular stimulation and the presence or absence of phrenic nerve (diaphragmatic) stimulation are assessed in regard to pacing output, and pacing polarity configuration is made.

After detailed analysis of the data, a decision is made regarding the appropriateness of the initial programmed pacing and antitachycardia parameters and therapies relative to the patient's clinical status. If indicated, the device's programming is altered at this time.

Description of Service for Code 93283

After verbal consent is obtained from the patient to proceed, the patient is connected to a single- or multi-lead electrocardiogram recording system. A communication link is established between the device and the programmer.

A full interrogation of the stored device parameters is obtained. The current rhythm is assessed and recorded to include the differentiation between the presence of an underlying native rhythm (if present). Stored pacing and tachyarrhythmia episode data are retrieved, and detailed physician analysis of these data is performed. The stored summary and recorded rhythm data are reviewed for evidence of interval arrhythmias. The pacing capture threshold data and lead impedance are measured separately in both chambers (usually the right atrium and ventricle). Based on this information, the physician identifies any pacing or integrity issues within the existing leads and determines the appropriate pacing output settings (eg, voltage, pulse width duration) individually for each chamber. The sensing threshold data are obtained in each chamber by recording the signal from the atrial and the ventricular chambers individually. Influence of the stimulation of one chamber on the sensing and activation of the other chambers (cross talk) is evaluated. Atrial and ventricular stimulation individually in each chamber is assessed to confirm the presence or absence of phrenic nerve (diaphragmatic) stimulation.

Iterative programming of the arteriovenous interval timing, whether fixed or dynamic, is completed. The heart rate adaptation to exercise or physiologic stress data are reviewed and adjustments are made in an iterative fashion. Based on this information, the physician identifies the appropriate ICD sensing settings to allow for appropriate sensing safety margins.

After a detailed analysis of the data, a decision is made regarding the appropriateness of the initial programmed pacing and antitachycardia parameters. The therapies relative to the patient's clinical status are evaluated, and, if indicated, alteration in the device's programming is performed at this time.

Description of Service for Code 93284

After verbal consent is obtained from the patient to proceed, the patient is connected to a single- or multi-lead electrocardiogram recording system. A communication link is established between the device and the programmer.

A full interrogation of the stored device parameters is obtained and reviewed. The current rhythm is assessed and recorded to include the differentiation between the presence of an underlying native rhythm (if present) in each chamber. Stored pacing and tachyarrhythmia episode data are retrieved. Detailed physician analysis of these data is performed. The stored summary and recorded rhythm data are reviewed for evidence of interval arrhythmias. Pacing capture threshold data and lead impedance are measured separately in all chambers (usually the right atrium and ventricle and the left ventricle).

Based on this information, the physician identifies any pacing or integrity issues within the existing leads and determines the appropriate pacing output settings (eg, voltage, pulse width duration) individually for each chamber.

The sensing threshold data are obtained in each chamber by recording the signal from atrial (sensed P waves) and ventricular (sensed R waves) activity, if present. Influence of the stimulation of one chamber on the sensing and activation of the other chambers (cross talk) is evaluated.

Atrial and ventricular stimulation individually in each chamber is assessed to confirm the presence or absence of phrenic nerve (diaphragmatic) stimulation in regard to pacing output and pacing polarity configuration. Iterative programming of the arteriovenous interval timing, whether fixed or dynamic, and its influence on the percentage of ventricular pacing and hemodynamics or limitation of heart rate response are completed. Heart rate adaptation to exercise or physiologic stress data are reviewed and adjusted in an iterative fashion.

After detailed analysis of the data, a decision is made regarding the appropriateness of the initial programmed pacing and antitachycardia parameters. The therapies relative to the patient's clinical status are evaluated, and, if indicated, alteration in the device's programming is performed at this time.

Description of Service for Code 93285

After verbal consent is obtained from the patient to proceed, a communication link is created between the ILR and the programmer. Programmed parameters are obtained. Stored ILR data are obtained and downloaded for physician review.

A full interrogation of the stored ILR data is obtained and reviewed for alert conditions. The current interrogated measurements are compared to the extensive stored and trended data and reviewed for device alerts with regard to battery function, including voltage and impedance. The underlying signal strength is assessed. The sensing threshold is measured by recording the signal from the ILR and by iterative (step-wise) adjustment of the sensing value to determine the appropriate sensing safety margin. The appropriate threshold for sensing is identified. The sensing and gain parameters are programmed as appropriate to ensure optimal device sensing.

The patient-activated recorded rhythm episodes are reviewed for evidence of tachycardia, bradycardia, and cardiac rhythm pauses. Specific rhythm waveforms are downloaded and reviewed for atrial fibrillation, premature atrial contractions (PACs), supraventricular tachycardia (SVT), premature ventricular contractions (PVCs), nonsustained ventricular tachycardia, sustained ventricular tachycardia, sinus pauses, evidence of cardiac arteriovenous (AV) block, and recording system artifact. The appropriate rhythm alerts and recording parameters are identified.

The automatically recorded rhythm episodes (based on previously programmed detection parameters) are reviewed for evidence of tachycardia, bradycardia, and cardiac rhythm pauses. Specific rhythm waveforms are downloaded and reviewed for atrial fibrillation, PACs, SVT, PVCs, nonsustained ventricular tachycardia, sustained ventricular tachycardia, sinus pauses, evidence of cardiac AV block, and recording system artifact. The appropriate rhythm alerts and recording parameters are identified. Parameters describing the criteria for automatic rhythm detection are reviewed for appropriateness and programmed for optimal rhythm detection. Parameters describing the device memory capacity as well as the recording capacity of the number of patient-activated and automatically detected episodes are reviewed. The amount of pre- and postdetection electrocardiographic recording time is assessed. Programmed changes to these values are made as appropriate to optimize ILR recording function.

After detailed analysis of each of these parameters, a decision is made about the adequacy of the initial programmed ILR parameters and any identified changes that need to be made to optimize the device performance relative to the patient's clinical condition. These device programming changes are made, and any additional recommendations for further cardiac evaluation or treatment are given.

PERI-PROCEDURAL DEVICE EVALUATION AND PROGRAMMING (**93286, 93287**)

93286   Peri-procedural device evaluation (in person) and programming of device system parameters before or after a surgery, procedure, or test with physician analysis, review and report; single, dual, or multiple lead pacemaker system
CPT Changes: An Insider's View 2009, 2010

93287   single, dual, or multiple lead implantable cardioverter-defibrillator system
CPT Changes: An Insider's View 2009, 2010

Intent and Use of Codes 93286 and 93287

Codes **93286** and **93287** describe the evaluation of a pacemaker or ICD to adjust settings prior to and after a surgery, procedure, or test. No codes were previously available to report these services. They are also used when device system data are interrogated to evaluate lead(s), sensor(s), and battery, and a review of stored information, including patient and system measurements. In addition, physicians should use these codes when a device is programmed to a setting appropriate for a surgery, procedure, or test, as needed, and when a second evaluation and programming are performed after the surgery, procedure, or test to re-establish the appropriate therapeutic settings.

According to CPT guidelines, if one provider performs both the pre- and postevaluation and programming service, the appropriate code, either **93286** or **93287**, would be reported two times. If one provider performs the presurgical service and a separate provider performs the postsurgical service, each provider reports either code **93286** or code **93287** only one time.

> **CODING TIP** Report code **93286** once before and once after the surgery, procedure, or test, when device evaluation and programming is performed before and after the surgery, procedure, or test. Do not report code **93286** in conjunction with codes **93279-93281** or code **93288**.

Description of Service for Code 93286

After verbal consent is obtained from the patient to proceed, a communication link is created between the pacemaker and the programmer. The doctor-specified parameter(s) is changed and device reinterrogation completed to confirm programming. The patient's stability is assessed after the preprocedural (test, surgery) programming. The patient is informed about temporary changes that have been made and the expected timing of postprocedure (test, surgery) restoration to baseline settings. An initial note is placed in the patient's chart documenting the temporary changes.

After intervention (test, surgery), an interim history is obtained, and the appropriateness of returning the pacemaker to the original programmed settings is determined. After obtaining verbal consent from the patient to proceed, a communication link is obtained between the pacemaker and the programmer. The doctor-specified parameter(s) is changed and device reinterrogation completed to confirm programming. The patient's stability is assessed after

the postprocedural (test, surgery) programming. The patient is informed about the permanent changes (restoration of programming) that have been made and the expected timing of their next pacemaker evaluation. A second note is placed in the patient's chart documenting the changes.

Description of Service for Code 93287

After verbal consent from the patient to proceed is obtained, a communication link is established between the device and the programmer. The doctor-specified changes in the device's programmed pacing are made, antitachycardia parameters based upon the preprocedural evaluation are performed, and the device reinterrogated to confirm programming changes. The changes made to the device, including expected timing of postprocedure restoration or reprogramming of settings, are explained to the patient. An initial report documenting the device issues and the changes made prior to the procedure is placed in the patient's chart.

After intervention (test, surgery), stability of the patient is assessed. An interim history is obtained, and the appropriateness of returning the device to its original settings is determined. After verbal consent is obtained from the patient to proceed, a communication link is established between the ICD and the programmer. Physician-specified changes in the device programming are made, and the device is interrogated to confirm programming. Stability of the patient is assessed. The patient is informed of any changes or restoration of the original programmed settings. A second report is placed in the patient's chart.

INTERROGATION DEVICE EVALUATION (IN PERSON) (**93288-93292**)

93288   Interrogation device evaluation (in person) with physician analysis, review and report, includes connection, recording and disconnection per patient encounter; single, dual, or multiple lead pacemaker system
CPT Changes: An Insider's View 2009

93289   single, dual, or multiple lead implantable cardioverter-defibrillator system, including analysis of heart rhythm derived data elements
CPT Changes: An Insider's View 2009

93290   implantable cardiovascular monitor system, including analysis of 1 or more recorded physiologic cardiovascular data elements from all internal and external sensors
CPT Changes: An Insider's View 2009

93291   implantable loop recorder system, including heart rhythm derived data analysis
CPT Changes: An Insider's View 2009

93292   wearable defibrillator system
CPT Changes: An Insider's View 2009

Intent and Use of Codes 93288-93292

The distinction between in-person (**93288-93292**) and remote (**93294-93296**) interrogation is an important aspect of the new CPT codes. The previous coding structure did not recognize the value of the information obtained and presented for physician review, independent of whether it was derived directly from the implanted device or from remote sensors in contact with the device and its telemetry system. Remote interrogation network systems have become important to current practice. This technology merges outpatient monitoring, device and arrhythmia detection, wireless communications, and the Internet to allow device- and cardiac rhythm–related problems to be quickly identified, analyzed, and communicated to the prescribing physician. Correctly describing and valuing the work provided by the physician, including complex data collection; the effort of the physician and independent testing facilities (IDTF), when present; and office personnel required a new strategic approach to coding.

Key differences between remote and in-person codes include:

- In-person codes (**93288-93292**) are billed per incident.

- Remote services codes (**93294-93296**) are billed once per 90-day period.

- A physician or practice may not report an in-person and remote interrogation of the same device during the same service period.

- During the remote interrogation, it is acceptable to pull the data as often as needed; however, billing is allowed only once per 90-day period.

- A physician or practice may not report codes **93294-93296** if service is less than 30 days.

- Programming device evaluations and in-person interrogation device evaluations may not be reported on the same date of service by the same physician, as the programming device evaluation includes all elements of the interrogation device evaluation.

- Programming device evaluations and remote interrogation device evaluation may be reported during the same remote period.

- Use code **93290** for monitoring physiologic cardiovascular data elements derived from an ICD. For heart-derived data elements use code **93289**. Do not report code **93290** in addition to code **93297** or code **93299**.

For interrogation device evaluation, CPT guidelines instruct an evaluation of an implantable device such as a cardiac pacemaker, implantable cardioverter-defibrillator, implantable cardiovascular monitor, or implantable loop recorder. Stored and measured information about the lead(s), when present; sensor(s), when present; battery; and the implanted device function, as well as data collected about the patient's heart rhythm and heart rate, are retrieved using an office, hospital, or emergency room instrument or via a remote interrogation system. The retrieved information is evaluated to determine the current programming of the device and to evaluate certain aspects of the device function such as battery voltage, lead impedance, tachycardia detection settings, and rhythm treatment settings.

The components that must be evaluated for the various types of implantable cardiac devices are listed as follows. (The required components for both remote and in-person interrogations are the same.)

Pacemaker: Programmed parameters, lead(s), battery, capture, sensing function, and heart rhythm.

Implantable cardioverter-defibrillator (ICD): Programmed parameters, lead(s), battery, capture, sensing function, presence or absence of therapy for ventricular tachyarrhythmias, and underlying heart rhythm.

Implantable cardiovascular monitor (ICM): Programmed parameters and analysis of at least one recorded physiologic cardiovascular data element from either internal or external sensors.

Implantable loop recorder (ILR): Programmed parameters and the heart rate and rhythm during recorded episodes from both patient initiated and device algorithm detected events, when present.

> **CODING TIP** Do not report code **93291** in addition to implantation of an event recorder (**33282**) or device interrogation procedures (**93288-93290**, **93298**, **93299**). Do not report code **93292** in addition to initial set-up and programming of a wearable cardioverter-defibrillator (**93745**).

Description of Service for Code 93288

The information from the pacemaker is interrogated by telemetric communication and either printed for review or reviewed on the programmer or computer monitor. Critical review of the interrogated data with assessment of normal pacemaker function and safety of the current programmed parameters are completed.

Data from an electrogram for appropriateness or presence of arrhythmia and appropriate sensing and capture are reviewed. The stored episodes of data are reviewed for appropriate sensing, capture, magnet reversion, and noise reversions.

Alerts generated from the pacemaker device are reviewed, if required. Battery voltage and impedance, pacing lead impedance, and sensed electrogram voltage amplitude for each lead are reviewed. Counts of paced and sensed events from each chamber for which there are leads located are provided for review. The stored episodes of sensed events including arrhythmias, ectopic beats, nonsustained and sustained atrial and ventricular arrhythmias, and, when appropriate, mode switch episodes are evaluated. The frequency, rate, and duration are noted for heart rate response during activities, rate histograms, and indicators of patient activity level.

Description of Service for Code 93289

The information from the pacemaker is interrogated by telemetric communication and either printed for review or reviewed on the programmer or computer monitor. The interrogated data are critically reviewed in order to assess the appropriateness of the pacemaker's function and the safety of the current programmed parameters and to determine if device function is normal.

The data reviewed includes the presenting electrogram for appropriateness or presence of arrhythmia and appropriate sensing and capture; stored episodes of data for appropriate sensing, capture, magnet reversion, and noise reversions; alerts generated from the pacemaker device; battery voltage and impedance, pacing lead impedance, and sensed electrogram voltage amplitude for each lead; counters of paced and sensed events from each chamber for which there are leads located; stored episodes of sensed events including arrhythmias, ectopic beats, nonsustained and sustained atrial and ventricular arrhythmias, and, when appropriate, mode switch episodes, with the frequency, rate, and duration noted; and the heart rate response during activities, rate histograms, and indicators of patient activity level.

Description of Service for Code 93290

The information from the ICM is interrogated by telemetric communication and either printed for review or reviewed on the programmer or computer monitor. The interrogated data, with assessment of the appropriateness of the function of the ICM and appropriateness of the current programmed parameters, are critically reviewed.

Data reviewed may include, but are not limited to: (1) weight; (2) systemic blood pressure; (3) right atrial, right ventricular, left atrial, left ventricular, pulmonary arterial pressures; (4) intrathoracic impedance measurements; and (5) other measures of physiologic parameters.

In addition, stored episodes of data are reviewed to assess the history and trends identified by any of the collected data. Further, alerts generated from the ICM are reviewed along with battery voltage and sensor information to validate the integrity of the ICM system.

Description of Service for Code 93291

Verbal consent is obtained from the patient to proceed. A communication link is created between the ILR and the programmer. Programmed parameters are obtained. Stored ILR data are obtained and downloaded for physician review.

A full interrogation of the stored ILR data is obtained and reviewed for alert conditions. The current interrogated measurements are compared to the extensive stored and trended data and reviewed for device alerts with regard to battery function, including voltage, and impedance. The underlying signal strength is assessed. If sensing is inadequate, instructions are given to the patient for further follow-up and potential reprogramming. Patient-activated recorded rhythm episodes are reviewed for evidence of tachycardia, bradycardia, and cardiac rhythm pauses. Specific rhythm waveforms are downloaded and reviewed for atrial fibrillation, premature atrial contractions (PACs), supraventricular tachycardia (SVT), premature ventricular contractions (PVCs), nonsustained ventricular tachycardia, sustained ventricular tachycardia, sinus pauses, evidence of cardiac arteriovenous (AV) block, and recording system artifact. The appropriate rhythm alerts and recording parameters are identified. Automatically recorded rhythm episodes (based on previously programmed detection parameters) are reviewed for evidence of tachycardia, bradycardia, and cardiac rhythm pauses. Specific rhythm waveforms are downloaded and reviewed for atrial fibrillation, PACs, SVT,

PVCs, nonsustained ventricular tachycardia, sustained ventricular tachycardia, sinus pauses, evidence of cardiac AV block, and recording system artifact. The appropriate rhythm alerts and recording parameters are identified. Parameters describing the criteria for automatic rhythm detect are reviewed for appropriateness. Parameters describing the device memory capacity and the recording capacity of the number of patient-activated and automatically detected episodes are reviewed. The amount of pre- and postdetection electrocardiographic recording time is assessed.

After detailed physician analysis of each of these parameters, recommendations for further cardiac evaluation or treatment are given.

Description of Service for Code 93292

The information from the wearable device is interrogated by telemetric communication and either printed for review or reviewed on the programmer or computer monitor. The interrogated data, with assessment of the appropriateness of the wearable device's function and appropriateness of the current programmed parameters, are critically reviewed.

The data reviewed may include, but are not limited to, presenting electrograms; stored episodes of data; alerts generated from the device; battery voltage and impedance; pacing and shocking lead impedance and sensed electrogram voltage amplitude; and histogram and/or counters of paced and sensed events from each chamber. Stored episodes of sensed arrhythmia events including the type, frequency, rate, and duration are noted.

Heart rate response during activities, rate histograms, and indicators of patient activity level are evaluated. A rhythm strip is recorded for 30 seconds and evaluated for heart rate and capture, sensing of each lead, and for atrial or ventricular arrhythmias. A second rhythm strip may be recorded, with a magnet located over the device, and evaluated for capture and sensing of each lead for atrial or ventricular arrhythmias and the magnet response including paced rate. Physician review of these data produces an assessment of the adequacy of each lead's sensing and capture and of battery function. In addition, stored episodes of data are reviewed to assess the history and trends identified by any of the collected data.

TRANSTELEPHONIC RHYTHM STRIP EVALUATIONS (TTM) (93293)

93293	Transtelephonic rhythm strip pacemaker evaluation(s) single, dual, or multiple lead pacemaker system, includes recording with and without magnet application with physician analysis, review and report(s), up to 90 days *CPT Changes: An Insider's View 2009*

Intent and Use of Code 93293

The CPT guidelines differentiate code **93293** from the in-person evaluation codes **93040**, **93041**, and **93042**. Transtelephonic rhythm strip pacemaker evaluation involves service of transmission of an electrocardiographic rhythm strip over the telephone by the patient using a transmitter and recorded by a receiving location using a receiver/recorder (also commonly known as transtelephonic pacemaker monitoring). The electrocardiographic rhythm strip is recorded both with and without a magnet applied over the pacemaker. The rhythm strip is evaluated for heart rate and rhythm, atrial and ventricular capture (if observed), and atrial and ventricular sensing (if observed). In addition, the battery status of the pacemaker is determined by measuring the paced rate on the electrocardiographic rhythm strip recorded with the magnet applied.

> **CODING TIP** Report code **93293** only once per 90 days.

Description of Service for Code 93293

A rhythm strip is recorded for 30 seconds and evaluated for heart rate and capture, sensing of each lead, and for atrial or ventricular arrhythmias. A second rhythm strip is recorded, with a magnet located over the pacemaker, and evaluated for capture and sensing of each lead, for atrial or ventricular arrhythmias, and for the magnet response including paced rate. Physician review of these data produces an assessment of the adequacy of each lead's sensing, capture, and battery function.

The technician receives the rhythm strip data with a second rhythm strip after application of a magnet to the pacemaker. The technician reviews the rhythm strips for sensing, capture, and intrinsic and paced heart rates. The parameters are reviewed and analyzed by the technician.

CHAPTER 5

If presented to the technician, the technician documents any patient symptoms that are patient-reported during the interrogation. The technician reports to the physician on any parameters that are designated by the physician. The technician enters findings into the monitoring center or local independent diagnostic testing facility's database. The technician validates function by assessing if the lead data and arrhythmia events are normal or abnormal. After the data are entered and evaluated, the technician generates a comprehensive report of all evaluated parameters, which is then delivered to the physician. The physician reviews the data and confirms the function of each lead, the battery, capture, and sensing. An assessment is made of the adequacy of the function and the time interval to the next analysis as well as the type of device evaluation that should be done at that time.

INTERROGATION DEVICE EVALUATION (REMOTE) (**93294-93299**)

93294   Interrogation device evaluation(s) (remote), up to 90 days; single, dual, or multiple lead pacemaker system with interim physician analysis, review(s) and report(s)
CPT Changes: An Insider's View 2009

93295   single, dual, or multiple lead implantable cardioverter-defibrillator system with interim physician analysis, review(s) and report(s)
CPT Changes: An Insider's View 2009

93296   single, dual, or multiple lead pacemaker system or implantable cardioverter-defibrillator system, remote data acquisition(s), receipt of transmissions and technician review, technical support and distribution of results
CPT Changes: An Insider's View 2009

93297   Interrogation device evaluation(s), (remote) up to 30 days; implantable cardiovascular monitor system, including analysis of 1 or more recorded physiologic cardiovascular data elements from all internal and external sensors, physician analysis, review(s) and report(s)
CPT Changes: An Insider's View 2009

93298   implantable loop recorder system, including analysis of recorded heart rhythm data, physician analysis, review(s) and report(s)
CPT Changes: An Insider's View 2009

93299   implantable cardiovascular monitor system or implantable loop recorder system, remote data acquisition(s), receipt of transmissions and technician review, technical support and distribution of results
CPT Changes: An Insider's View 2009

Intent and Use of Codes 93294-93299

Per CPT guidelines, interrogation device evaluation (remote) is a procedure performed for patients with pacemakers, implantable cardioverter-defibrillators, or implantable loop recorders using data obtained remotely. All device functions, including the programmed parameters, lead(s), battery, capture and sensing function, presence or absence of therapy for ventricular tachyarrhythmias (for ICDs), and underlying heart rhythm are evaluated.

The components that must be evaluated for the various types of implantable cardiac devices are listed as follows. (The required components for both remote and in-person interrogations are the same.)

Pacemaker: Programmed parameters, lead(s), battery, capture and sensing function, and heart rhythm.

Implantable cardioverter-defibrillator (ICD): Programmed parameters, lead(s), battery, capture and sensing function, presence or absence of therapy for ventricular tachyarrhythmias, and underlying heart rhythm.

Implantable cardiovascular monitor (ICM): Programmed parameters and analysis of at least one recorded physiologic cardiovascular data element from either internal or external sensors.

Implantable loop recorder (ILR): Programmed parameters and the heart rate and rhythm during recorded episodes from both patient-initiated and device algorithm–detected events, when present.

CODING TIP   Codes **93293-93296** are reported no more than once every 90 days. Do not report codes **93293-93296** if the monitoring period is less than 30 days.

Description of Service for Code 93294

The information from the pacemaker is interrogated by telemetric communication and either printed for review or reviewed on the programmer or computer monitor. The interrogated data are critically reviewed for assessment of the appropriateness of the pacemaker's function and safety of the current programmed parameters and to assess if the device function is normal.

The data reviewed include the presenting electrogram for appropriateness or presence of arrhythmia and appropriate sensing and capture; stored episodes of data for appropriate sensing, capture, appropriate magnet reversion, and noise reversions; alerts generated from the pacemaker device; battery voltage and impedance, pacing lead impedance, and sensed electrogram voltage amplitude for each lead; and counters of paced and sensed events from each chamber for which there are leads located. Stored episodes of sensed events including arrhythmias, ectopic beats, nonsustained and sustained atrial and ventricular arrhythmias, and, when appropriate, mode switch episodes, frequency, rate, and duration are noted. Heart rate response during activities, rate histograms, and indicators of patient activity level are evaluated.

Description of Service for Code 93295

The information from the ICD is interrogated by telemetric communication and either printed for review or reviewed on the programmer or computer monitor. The interrogated data, with assessment of the appropriateness of the function of ICD, safety of the current programmed pacing, and antitachycardia parameters and assessment of device function, are critically assessed.

The data reviewed include the presenting electrograms for appropriateness of pacing and sensing; stored episodes of data; alerts generated from the device; battery voltage and impedance; pacing and shocking lead impedance; and sensed electrogram voltage amplitude for each lead. Histogram and/or counters of paced and sensed events from each chamber and stored episodes of sensed arrhythmia events including the type, frequency, rate, and duration are noted. Adequacy of heart rate response is evaluated.

Description of Service for Code 93296

Remote ICD device evaluation includes monitoring of all programmed parameters, leads, battery, capture and sensing function, presence or absence of therapy for ventricular tachyarrhythmias, and underlying heart rhythm. Based on the physician's order, a patient with an ICD is registered for remote interrogation at a monitoring facility. The monitoring facility delivers the equipment to the patient with instructions for connection to the telephone system. The provider provides additional telephone support to help the patient complete the connections. The provider establishes a schedule for device interrogations based on the physician's order.

The interrogated data are assembled and sent to the provider by an electrodiagnostic technician. It is then reviewed by the nurse for device alerts and is compared to the physician-directed parameters for

communication to the patient's physician. The interrogated data are both scheduled and triggered by the patient and/or device alarm–initiated episodes.

The technician receives data through the device information system and inputs that data into the provider's database. The technician then reviews all the data generated from the system. The data are then incorporated into the provider's system. The parameters are reviewed and analyzed by the technician and, if present, patient symptoms are documented. The technician reports to the physician if any parameters designated by the physician are exceeded. The technician enters findings into the provider's database and validates function by assessing if the lead data and arrhythmia events are normal or abnormal. After the data are entered and evaluated, the technician generates a comprehensive report of all evaluated parameters, which is then delivered to the physician. There is an average of 1.25 events per patient per quarter.

Description of Service for Code 93297

The information from the ICM is interrogated by telemetric communication and either printed for review or reviewed on the programmer or computer monitor. The interrogated data, with assessment of the appropriateness of the function of the ICM and appropriateness of the current programmed parameters, are critically reviewed.

Data reviewed may include, but are not limited to: (1) weight; (2) systemic blood pressure; (3) right atrial, right ventricular, left atrial, left ventricular, pulmonary arterial pressures; (4) intrathoracic impedance measurements; and (5) other measures of physiologic parameters.

In addition, stored episodes of data are reviewed to assess the history and trends identified by any of the collected data. Further, alerts generated from the ICM are reviewed along with battery voltage and sensor information to validate the integrity of the ICM system.

Description of Service for Code 93298

Verbal consent is obtained from the patient to proceed. A communication link is created between the ILR and the programmer. Programmed parameters are obtained. Stored ILR data are obtained and downloaded for physician review.

A full interrogation of the stored ILR data is obtained and reviewed for alert conditions. The current interrogated measurements are compared to the extensive stored and trended data and reviewed for device alerts with regard to battery function, including voltage and impedance. The underlying signal strength is assessed. Sensing threshold is measured by recording the signal from the ILR and by iterative (step-wise) adjustment of the sensing value to determine the appropriate sensing safety margin. The appropriate threshold for sensing is identified. The sensing and gain parameters are programmed as appropriate to ensure optimal device sensing. Patient-activated recorded rhythm episodes are reviewed for evidence of tachycardia, bradycardia, and cardiac rhythm pauses. Specific rhythm waveforms are downloaded and reviewed for atrial fibrillation, premature atrial contractions (PACs), supraventricular tachycardia (SVT), premature ventricular contractions (PVCs), nonsustained ventricular tachycardia, sustained ventricular tachycardia, sinus pauses, evidence of cardiac arteriovenous (AV) block, and recording system artifact. The appropriate rhythm alerts and recording parameters are identified. Automatically recorded rhythm episodes (based on previously programmed detection parameters) are reviewed for evidence of tachycardia, bradycardia, and cardiac rhythm pauses. Specific rhythm waveforms are downloaded and reviewed for atrial fibrillation, PACs, SVT, PVCs, nonsustained ventricular tachycardia, sustained ventricular tachycardia, sinus pauses, evidence of cardiac AV block, and recording system artifact. The appropriate rhythm alerts and recording parameters are identified. Parameters describing the criteria for automatic rhythm detection are reviewed for appropriateness and programmed for optimal rhythm detection. Parameters describing the device memory capacity and the recording capacity of the number of patient-activated and automatically detected episodes are reviewed. The amount of pre- and postdetection electrocardiographic recording time is assessed. Programmed changes to these values are made as appropriate to optimize ILR recording function.

After the physician performs a detailed analysis of each parameter, a decision is made about the adequacy of the initial programmed ILR parameters and any identified changes that need to be made to optimize the device performance relative to the patient's clinical condition. These device programming changes are made, and any additional recommendations for further cardiac evaluation or treatment are given.

Description of Service for Code 93299

An ILR is an implantable device that continuously records ECG rhythm triggered automatically by rapid and slow heart rates or by the patient during a symptomatic episode. It is designed to detect transient symptoms, most significantly syncope, which may not be detected by other types of cardiac monitoring. After implantation, the ECG segments data are automatically stored for those episodes when the R-R interval falls outside of predetermined limits. The patient can also trigger storage, when symptoms are experienced.

A patient with an ILR is referred by the physician to the testing facility for around-the-clock ECG monitoring. The facility enrolls the patient and educates the patient on the use of the service. An assessment of the underlying signal strength is made, and if sensing is inadequate, instructions are given to the patient for further follow-up and potential reprogramming. The facility furnishing this service transmits the data via modem. Interrogated ECG data, which includes automatically recorded (trending samples) rhythm episodes (based on previously programmed detection parameters) as well as patient-activated rhythm (symptomatic and asymptomatic transmissions) episodes, are transmitted to the monitoring center and reviewed by the electrodiagnostic technician (a certified cardiographic technician) for device alerts and compared to physician-directed parameters for possible communication to the physician if the criteria is met. The interrogated data are transmitted to the physician for review with the frequency of delivery determined by the physician based upon the patient's condition. An average of six trending samples is transmitted each day (ie, every 4 hours) in addition to an average of 300 asymptomatic transmissions per month and approximately four symptomatic transmissions generated by the patient. These data are compiled into a monthly report and distributed to the physician.

TRANSTHORACIC ECHOCARDIOGRAPHY (**93303-93308, 93350-+93352**)

93303   Transthoracic echocardiography for congenital cardiac anomalies; complete
          CPT Assistant Nov 97:44, Dec 97:5, Sep 05:10-11, Mar 08:4; *Clinical Examples in Radiology* Fall 06:9-10

93304   follow-up or limited study
          CPT Assistant Nov 97:44, Dec 97:5, Jan 10:8; *Clinical Examples in Radiology* Fall 06:9-10

93306   Echocardiography, transthoracic, real-time with image documentation (2D), includes M-mode recording, when performed, complete, with spectral Doppler echocardiography, and with color flow Doppler echocardiography
          CPT Changes: An Insider's View 2009

93307   Echocardiography, transthoracic, real-time with image documentation (2D), includes M-mode recording, when performed, complete, without spectral or color Doppler echocardiography

CPT Assistant Dec 97:5, Sep 05:11; *CPT Changes: An Insider's View* 2009; *Clinical Examples in Radiology* Fall 06:9-10

93308 Echocardiography, transthoracic, real-time with image documentation (2D), includes M-mode recording, when performed, follow-up or limited study

CPT Assistant Dec 97:5, Sep 05:11, Jan 10:8; *CPT Changes: An Insider's View* 2009; *Clinical Examples in Radiology* Fall 06:9-10

93350 Echocardiography, transthoracic, real-time with image documentation (2D), includes M-mode recording, when performed, during rest and cardiovascular stress test using treadmill, bicycle exercise and/or pharmacologically induced stress, with interpretation and report;

CPT Assistant Aug 02:11, Jan 10:8; *CPT Changes: An Insider's View* 2009

93351 including performance of continuous electrocardiographic monitoring, with physician supervision

CPT Changes: An Insider's View 2009

+93352 Use of echocardiographic contrast agent during stress echocardiography (List separately in addition to code for primary procedure)

CPT Changes: An Insider's View 2009

Intent and Use of Codes 93303-93308, 93350-+93352

Transthoracic echocardiography is a procedure in which ultrasound transducer is placed at various locations on the precordium and upper abdomen and used to image the cardiac chambers, valves, and great vessels. Coupling gel is used to improve ultrasonic transmission. The operator adjusts the transducer position and orientation, as well as the instrument controls, to optimize structure visualization. Two-dimensional images are recorded in dynamic format, typically onto videotape, but sometimes also in digital format. Time-motion (M-mode) records may also be made, typically by positioning an examining cursor across the relevant cardiovascular structures using two-dimensional images as an anatomic reference. The recorded data are then reviewed, measured, analyzed, and interpreted by the physician. A report is prepared and transmitted to the patient's medical record.

According to CPT guidelines, echocardiography includes obtaining ultrasonic signals from the heart and great vessels, with real time image and/or Doppler ultrasonic signal documentation, with interpretation

and report. When interpretation is performed separately, use **modifier 26**. (Refer to Chapter 6 for further information regarding use of **modifier 26**.) A complete transthoracic echocardiogram without spectral or color flow Doppler (**93307**) is a comprehensive procedure that includes two-dimensional and, when performed, selected M-mode examination of the left and right atria, left and right ventricles, the aortic, mitral, and tricuspid valves, the pericardium, and adjacent portions of the aorta. Multiple views are required to obtain a complete functional and anatomic evaluation, and appropriate measurements are obtained and recorded. Despite significant effort, identification and measurement of some structures may not always be possible. In such instances, the reason that an element could not be visualized must be documented. Additional structures that may be visualized (eg, pulmonary veins, pulmonary artery, pulmonic valve, inferior vena cava) would be included as part of the service.

A limited or a follow-up transthoracic echocardiogram (two-dimensional with or without M-mode recordings, **93308**), in contrast, is a focused study performed to evaluate one specific cardiac problem or region of the heart. Spectral (add-on code **93321**) and color flow Doppler (add-on code **93325**) provide additional information to morphologic images obtained by two-dimensional echocardiography, by depicting blood flowing through cardiac chambers, arteries, veins, and valves, as well as detecting and localizing any abnormal regions of blood flow (ie, valvular regurgitation, localized obstructions, or shunts). Color flow velocity and direction are mapped onto two-dimensional echocardiographic images. Spectral Doppler uses pulsed wave and/or continuous wave ultrasound that quantifies hemodynamic information about cardiac structures in a clinically meaningful way.

A complete transthoracic echocardiogram (**93306**) is bundled with spectral Doppler and color flow Doppler in a comprehensive procedure to provide information on cardiac structure, morphology, and function. When a follow-up or limited echocardiographic study (**93308**) requires focused spectral Doppler information, then the limited or follow-up spectral Doppler add-on code is used (**93321**). Code **93325** can be also be used with the limited echocardiographic study if color flow information is required as there is no limited or focused color Doppler code.

In stress echocardiography, echocardiographic images are recorded from multiple cardiac windows before, after, and in some protocols, during stress. The stress is achieved by: (1) walking on a treadmill; (2) using a bicycle (supine or upright); or (3) the administration of pharmacological agents that either simulate exercise (by increasing heart rate, blood pressure, or myocardial contractility) or alter coronary flow (vasodilation). The patient's ECG, heart rate, and blood pressure are monitored at baseline, throughout the procedure, and during recovery. Reports are prepared to evaluate: (1) the duration of stress, the reason for stopping, and the hemodynamic response to stress; (2) the electrocardiographic response to stress; and (3) the echocardiographic response to stress.

When a stress echocardiogram is performed with a complete cardiovascular stress test (continuous electrocardiographic monitoring, physician supervision, interpretation, and report), use code **93351**. When only the professional components of a complete stress test and a stress echocardiogram are provided (eg, in a facility setting) by the same physician, use code **93351** with **modifier 26**. When all professional services of a stress test are not performed by the same physician performing the stress echocardiogram, use code **93350** in conjunction with the appropriate codes (**93016-93018**) for the components of the cardiovascular stress test that are provided. When left ventricular endocardial borders cannot be adequately identified by standard echocardiographic imaging, echocardiographic contrast may be infused intravenously both at rest and with stress to achieve that purpose. Code **93352** is used to report the administration of echocardiographic contrast agent in conjunction with the stress echocardiography codes (**93350** or **93351**). Supply of contrast agent and/or drugs used for pharmacological stress is reported separately in addition to the procedure code.

Report of an echocardiographic study, whether complete or limited, includes an interpretation of all obtained information, documentation of all clinically relevant findings including quantitative measurements obtained, plus a description of any recognized abnormalities. Pertinent images, videotape, and/or digital data are archived for permanent storage and are available for subsequent review. Use of echocardiography not meeting these criteria is not separately reportable.

Use of ultrasound, without thorough evaluation of each anatomic region, image documentation, and a final written report cannot be reported using the above CPT codes. Studies obtained from handheld devices that can provide all of the elements described above, including storing of echocardiographic data for archiving and later retrieval are acceptable, provided a final, written report is generated.

CODING TIP Code **93351** includes stress echocardiogram with a complete cardiovascular stress test (continuous electrocardiographic monitoring) using physician-owned equipment and also includes physician supervision, interpretation, and report. When the equipment is not physician owned, such as in a facility setting, then only the professional components of the exercise test and echocardiogram can be reported. It is no longer proper coding to combine code **93350** or code **93350 26** with codes **93016** and **93018** in a facility setting. Instead, use **modifier 26** in conjunction with code **93351** (**93351 26**). In situations when one provider supervises, but another provider interprets separate parts of the services, then code **93350** would be used in conjunction with the appropriate exercise electrocardiogram physician codes (**93016-93018**) for the professional components of the cardiovascular stress test when the physician owns the echocardiographic equipment, and code **93350 26** when the physician does not.

Intent and Use of Code 93303

Code **93303** is used to report complete transthoracic echocardiographic imaging for morphology of complex congenital cardiac anomalies. When pulsed wave and/or continuous wave with spectral display and/or Doppler color flow velocity mapping is performed in conjunction with code **93303**, add-on codes **93320**, **93321**, and **93325** should also be reported, as appropriate.

Intent and Use of Code 93304

Code **93304** is used for a follow-up or limited study for morphology of complex congenital heart disease, usually during or after a surgical or interventional repair procedure (eg, pulmonary artery banding of systemic to pulmonary artery shunt). When spectral and/or Doppler color flow velocity mapping is performed in conjunction with code **93304**, add-on codes **93320**, **93321**, and **93325** should also be reported, as appropriate.

CODING TIP Codes **93303**, **93304**, and **93315-93317** should not be used for "simple" congenital anomalies such as patent foramen ovale (PFO), bicuspid aortic valve, or when complex congenital heart disease is suspected but not found on echocardiographic evaluation. In this case, the noncongenital echocardiography codes should be used. As a general rule, when a congenital procedure code is used, it should be "linked" to a congenital ICD-9-CM diagnosis code in order to ensure appropriate claims processing.

Intent and Use of Code 93306

Code **93306** is used to report a transthoracic two-dimensional echocardiogram that includes both spectral Doppler and color flow Doppler. Prior to 2009 when this code was added to the CPT codebook, physicians reported this service with code **93307** plus add-on codes **93320** (spectral Doppler) and **93325** (color flow Doppler). Reporting component services is inappropriate and will result in improper claims processing.

Intent and Use of Code 93307

Code **93307** describes a transthoracic echocardiogram that does not include spectral or color flow Doppler. All cardiac anatomic structures, including the atria, the ventricles, the valves, the pericardium, and adjacent portions of the aorta are included as described in CPT guidelines. Spectral or color flow Doppler codes (**93320**, **93321**, and/or **93325**) cannot be reported in conjunction with code **93307**.

> **CODING TIP** Code 96374, *Therapeutic, prophylactic, or diagnostic injection (specify substance or drug); intravenous push, single or initial substance/drug,* may be reported in addition to code 93306, 93307, or 93308 for injection of contrast media for imaging during contrast echocardiography with resting echocardiography. **Modifier 59** should be appended to code 96374. Based on payer requirements, the appropriate HCPCS Level II code should also be reported for the contrast material used.

Description of Service for Code 93307

An ultrasound transducer is placed at various locations on the precordium and upper abdomen and used to image the cardiac chambers, valves, and great vessels. Coupling gel is used to improve ultrasonic transmission. The operator adjusts the transducer position and orientation, as well as the instrument controls to optimize structure visualization. Two-dimensional images are recorded in dynamic format, typically onto videotape, but sometimes also in digital format. Time-motion (M-mode) records may also be made, typically by positioning an examining cursor across the relevant cardiovascular structures using two-dimensional images as an anatomic reference. The recorded data are then reviewed, measured, analyzed, and interpreted by the physician. A report is prepared and transmitted to the patient's medical record.

> **PAYMENT POLICY ALERT** Carriers vary considerably in their use of clinical indications and guidelines for the frequency of diagnostic services. Contact your local carrier to ascertain which International Classification of Diseases, 9th Revision, Clinical Modification (ICD-9-CM) codes can be used to justify the need for echocardiography.

Intent and Use of Code 93308

Code **93308** refers to the use of echocardiographic imaging (two-dimensional only, or two-dimensional with M-mode recordings) when a study is performed to evaluate one specific cardiac problem or region of the heart. Examples include the evaluation of progression or resolution of a pericardial effusion, or a serial evaluation of left ventricular function during antineoplastic chemotherapy. When spectral and/or Doppler color flow velocity mapping is performed in conjunction with code **93308**, the limited spectral Doppler add-on code (**93321**) or the color flow mapping add-on code (**93325**) should also be reported.

Intent and Use of Codes 93350 and 93351

Code **93350** is used to report the performance and interpretation of a stress echocardiogram when all professional services of a stress test are not performed by the same physician performing the stress echocardiogram. This code is to be used in conjunction with the appropriate stress test codes (**93016-93018**) for the components of the cardiovascular stress test that are provided. Code **93350** should never be reported with the complete stress test code **93015**.

Code **93351** is used when a stress echocardiogram is performed with a complete cardiovascular stress test (continuous electrocardiographic monitoring, physician supervision, interpretation, and report). This code would be used when the physician owns the equipment.

Code **93351** with **modifier 26** is used for a stress echocardiogram when the physician does not own the equipment as in a hospital or facility setting but still interprets the stress test as well as the stress echocardiogram. (Refer to Chapter 6 for further information regarding the use of **modifier 26**.) Code **93351 26** should never be used in conjunction with code **93350 26**, code **93016** (stress ECG physician supervision only, without interpretation or report), and code **93018** (stress ECG interpretation and report only) since these are inclusive of **93351 26**. However, when one physician provides the interpretation of the stress echocardiogram and the interpretation of the exercise test,

CHAPTER 5

but the exercise test is supervised by another provider, then code **93350 26** in conjuction with code **93018** would be appropriate.

Intent and Use of Code +93352

Add-on code **93352** is only to be used with stress echocardiography. A contrast agent may be administered with a stress echocardiogram to improve the delineation of the left ventricular endocardial borders in a patient whose noncontrast echocardiography study is inadequate or suboptimal and for whom the LV function information is essential to the management of the patient. Neither code **93350** nor code **93351** includes administration of a contrast agent.

Add-on code **93352** is used to report the administration of echocardiographic contrast agent in conjunction with the stress echocardiography codes (**93350**, **93351**). Supply of contrast agent and/or drugs used for pharmacological stress are reported separately in addition to the procedure code.

> **CODING TIP** Do not report code **93351** in conjunction with codes **93015-93018**, **93350**. Do not report code **93351 26** in conjunction with codes **93016**, **93018**, **93350 26**.

TRANSESOPHAGEAL ECHOCARDIOGRAPHY (⊙**93312**-⊙**93318**)

⊙**93312** Echocardiography, transesophageal, real-time with image documentation (2D) (with or without M-mode recording); including probe placement, image acquisition, interpretation and report
CPT Assistant Dec 97:5, Jan 00:10, Jan 10:8

⊙**93313**   placement of transesophageal probe only
CPT Assistant Dec 97:5, Mar 08:4, Jan 10:8

⊙**93314**   image acquisition, interpretation and report only
CPT Assistant Dec 97:5, Jan 00:10, Jan 10:8

⊙**93315** Transesophageal echocardiography for congenital cardiac anomalies; including probe placement, image acquisition, interpretation and report
CPT Assistant Nov 97:44, Dec 97:5, Jan 10:8

⊙**93316**   placement of transesophageal probe only
CPT Assistant Nov 97:44, Dec 97:5, Jan 10:8

⊙**93317**   image acquisition, interpretation and report only
CPT Assistant Nov 97:44, Dec 97:5, Jan 10:8

⊙**93318** Echocardiography, transesophageal (TEE) for monitoring purposes, including probe placement, real time 2-dimensional image acquisition and interpretation leading to ongoing (continuous) assessment of (dynamically changing) cardiac pumping function and to therapeutic measures on an immediate time basis
CPT Assistant Mar 08:4, Jan 10:8, Apr 10:6; *CPT Changes: An Insider's View* 2001

Intent and Use of Codes ⊙93312 and ⊙93315

Code **93312** (noncongenital) and code **93315** (complex congenital) is used to report the complete transesophageal echocardiography (TEE), that is, probe placement, image acquisition, and report for service performed in the physician's office when the physician owns the equipment. Codes **93313-93314** and codes **93316-93317** are used to report components of the service performed in a hospital or other setting when the physician does not own the equipment. Add-on spectral Doppler codes **93320** (comprehensive) and **93321** (limited) and/or color flow Doppler (**93325**) are separately billable when performed.

Intent and Use of Code ⊙93313

Code **93313** is used to report placement of the transesophageal probe only.

Intent and Use of Code ⊙93314

Code **93314** is used to report the image acquisition, interpretation, and report only or when the probe is placed by a different physician. When spectral and/or Doppler color flow velocity mapping is performed in conjunction with code **93304**, add-on codes **93320**, **93321**, and **93325**, as appropriate, should also be reported.

Intent and Use of Code ⊙93316

Code **93316** is used to report placement of the transesophageal probe only in patients with complex congenital heart disease.

Intent and Use of Code ⊙93317

Code **93317** is used for image acquisition, interpretation, and report only in complex congenital heart disease or when the probe is placed by a different physician. When spectral and/or Doppler color flow velocity mapping is performed in conjunction with code **93317**, add-on codes **93320**, **93321**, and **93325**, as appropriate, should also be reported.

Intent and Use of Code ⊙93318

Code **93318** describes transesophageal echocardiography (TEE) monitoring to assess cardiovascular function and assist with therapeutic decisions performed intraoperatively. This code includes placement of a transesophageal echocardiography probe and the use of TEE technology for continuous monitoring purposes during surgical operations and other types of interventions that produce acute and dynamic changes in cardiovascular function (eg, abdominal/thoracic aneurysm repair or open cardiac procedures).

Description of Service for Code ⊙93318

The initial application of the aortic cross-clamp produces an immediate increase in peripheral vascular resistance and impedance to left ventricular ejection. While marked increases in blood pressure proximal to the aortic cross-clamp are usually observed, some patients exhibit a fall in blood pressure due to sudden cardiac failure. This is evident in TEE images as left ventricular distention and impaired cardiac contractility, which would lead the anesthesiologist to: (1) ask the surgeon to release the aortic cross-clamp at least partially; (2) administer a vasodilator; and (3) administer an inotrope (eg, digitalis, dopamine, dobutamine, amrinone). When the aortic cross-clamp is removed after the aortic graft is in place, hypotension usually ensues due to the sudden decrease in peripheral vascular resistance and reperfusion of tissues distal to the clamp with the entry of vasodilating metabolites that have accumulated from anaerobic metabolism during the ischemic period of aortic cross-clamping. Because many of these patients have coronary artery disease, the hypotension may reflect cardiac dysfunction in addition to the sudden decrease in vascular resistance occasioned by removal of the aortic cross-clamp. In such patients, there is an optimal degree of intravascular volume and cardiac filling (ie, preload), and the TEE images can guide the intravenous administration of fluid and blood products. Ventricular wall motion abnormalities are indicative of myocardial ischemia, which can be treated by administration of coronary vasodilators, adjustments in intravascular blood volume, and, if necessary, administration of either an inotrope or a vasopressor or both in order to provide systemic blood pressure sufficient to perfuse the heart.

DOPPLER ECHOCARDIOGRAPHY (+93320-+93325)

+93320 Doppler echocardiography, pulsed wave and/or continuous wave with spectral display (List separately in addition to codes for echocardiographic imaging); complete
CPT Assistant Nov 97:44, Dec 97:5, Mar 08:4; *Clinical Examples in Radiology* Fall 06:9-10

+93321 follow-up or limited study (List separately in addition to codes for echocardiographic imaging)
CPT Assistant Nov 97:44, Dec 97:5, Jan 10:8; *Clinical Examples in Radiology* Fall 06:9-10

+93325 Doppler echocardiography color flow velocity mapping (List separately in addition to codes for echocardiographic imaging)
CPT Assistant Nov 97:44, Dec 97:5; *Clinical Examples in Radiology* Fall 06:9-10

Intent and Use of Code +93320

Add-on code **93320** describes a complete spectral Doppler study using pulsed wave and/or continuous wave Doppler that is listed separately in addition to codes for echocardiographic morphologic imaging. These codes include **93303**, **93304**, **93312**, **93314**, **93315**, **93317**, **93350**, and **93351**, but never the limited two-dimensional echocardiograhic code **93308**.

Intent and Use of Code +93321

Add-on code **93321** describes follow-up or limited studies for spectral Doppler echocardiography or a focused clinical purpose. An example includes the recording of tricuspid regurgitant velocity for estimating pulmonary artery systolic pressure in a limited study. Re-evaluation of the transmitral velocity profile in a patient with mitral stenosis to assess a change in gradient or valve area would similarly represent a focused follow-up study. Such studies are always done in conjunction with another two-dimensional imaging study for an anatomic reference, in which case the appropriate code would also be listed. These codes include **93303**, **93304**, **93308**, **93312**, **93314**, **93315**, **93317**, **93350**, and **93351**, but never code **93307**.

Intent and Use of Code +93325

Add-on code **93325** describes color flow velocity mapping. This code is separately reported in addition to the appropriate code for echocardiography including fetal echocardiography: **76825-76828** and **93303**, **93304**, **93308**, **93312**, **93314**, **93315**, **93317**, **93350**, and **93351**, but never code **93306** or code **93307**.

CHAPTER 5

Description of Service for Code +93325

An ultrasound transducer is placed at various locations on the precordium and upper abdomen (or transesophageally) and used to image blood flowing through the cardiac chambers and valves, as well as to detect and localize any abnormal regions of blood flow (ie, valvular regurgitation, localized obstructions, or shunts). Typically, data describing blood flow velocity and direction are mapped onto two-dimensional echocardiographic images to demonstrate flowstreams in relation to accompanying anatomic structures. The operator records dynamic color Doppler images onto videotape and/or digital format. The recorded data are then reviewed, measured, analyzed, and interpreted by the physician. A report is prepared, signed, and transmitted to the patient's medical record.

CARDIAC CATHETERIZATION FOR THE PATIENT WITH NONCONGENITAL HEART DISEASE (⊙93451-⊙+93462)

⊙⊘**93451** Right heart catheterization including measurement(s) of oxygen saturation and cardiac output, when performed
CPT Changes: An Insider's View 2011

⊙**93452** Left heart catheterization including intraprocedural injection(s) for left ventriculography, imaging supervision and interpretation, when performed
CPT Changes: An Insider's View 2011

⊙**93453** Combined right and left heart catheterization including intraprocedural injection(s) for left ventriculography, imaging supervision and interpretation, when performed
CPT Changes: An Insider's View 2011

⊙**93454** Catheter placement in coronary artery(s) for coronary angiography, including intraprocedural injection(s) for coronary angiography, imaging supervision and interpretation;
CPT Changes: An Insider's View 2011

⊙**93455** with catheter placement(s) in bypass graft(s) (internal mammary, free arterial venous grafts) including intraprocedural injection(s) for bypass graft angiography
CPT Changes: An Insider's View 2011

⊙⊘**93456** with right heart catheterization
CPT Changes: An Insider's View 2011

⊙**93457** with catheter placement(s) in bypass graft(s) (internal mammary, free arterial, venous grafts) including intraprocedural injection(s)

for bypass graft angiography and right heart catheterization
CPT Changes: An Insider's View 2011

⊙**93458** with left heart catheterization including intraprocedural injection(s) for left ventriculography, when performed
CPT Changes: An Insider's View 2011

⊙**93459** with left heart catheterization including intraprocedural injection(s) for left ventriculography, when performed, catheter placement(s) in bypass graft(s) (internal mammary, free arterial, venous grafts) with bypass graft angiography
CPT Changes: An Insider's View 2011

⊙**93460** with right and left heart catheterization including intraprocedural injection(s) for left ventriculography, when performed
CPT Changes: An Insider's View 2011

⊙**93461** with right and left heart catheterization including intraprocedural injection(s) for left ventriculography, when performed, catheter placement(s) in bypass graft(s) (internal mammary, free arterial, venous grafts) with bypass graft angiography
CPT Changes: An Insider's View 2011

⊙**+93462** Left heart catheterization by transseptal puncture through intact septum or by transapical puncture (List separately in addition to code for primary procedure)
CPT Changes: An Insider's View 2011

⊙**+93463** Pharmacologic agent administration (eg, inhaled nitric oxide, intravenous infusion of nitroprusside, dobutamine, milrinone, or other agent), including assessing hemodynamic measurements before, during, after, and repeat pharmacologic agent administration, when performed (List separately in addition to code for primary procedure)
CPT Changes: An Insider's View 2011

⊙**+93464** Physiologic exercise study (eg, bicycle or arm ergometry) including assessing hemodynamic measurements before and after (List separately in addition to code for primary procedure)
CPT Changes: An Insider's View 2011

Intent and Use of Codes ⊙**93451**-⊙**93461**

The coding structure of the cardiac catheterization procedure/service codes differentiates between noncongenital heart disease (**93451-93464**) and congenital heart disease (**93530-93533**). Right heart catheterization includes introduction of a cardiac catheter into the venous system that is then directed into the right atrium, right ventricle, and pulmonary artery. Because right heart catheterization does not include right ventricular or right atrial angiography (**93566**), pulmonary angiography (**93567**), or supravalvular aortography (**93568**), a catheter placement code (**93451, 93453, 93456,** or **93457**) and one or more contrast injection procedure add-on code(s) (**93566, 93567,** or **93568**) should be reported, when performed.

Left heart catheterization (**93452, 93453, 93458-93461**) involves insertion of a catheter into the arterial system and then into a left-sided cardiac chamber(s) (left ventricle or left atrium) and includes intraprocedural injection(s) for left ventricular/left atrial angiography, imaging supervision, and interpretation, when performed. Therefore, differing from the right heart catheterization instruction, it would not be appropriate to report the injection procedure add-on codes **93563-93565** in addition to codes **93452-93461**.

The use of the noncongenital heart disease cardiac catheterization procedure codes is comprehensively outlined in the CPT guidelines. Cardiac catheterization is a diagnostic medical procedure that includes introduction, positioning, and repositioning, when necessary, of catheter(s), within the vascular system; recording of intracardiac and/or intravascular pressure(s); and final evaluation and report of the procedure. There are two code families for cardiac catheterization: one for congenital heart disease and one for all other conditions. Anomalous coronary arteries, patent foramen ovale, mitral valve prolapse, and bicuspid aortic valve are not considered congenital abnormalities for coding purposes and are to be reported with the non-congenital catheterization codes **93451-93464, 93566-93568.**

Right heart catheterization includes catheter placement in one or more right-sided cardiac chamber(s) or structures (ie, the right atrium, right ventricle, pulmonary artery, pulmonary wedge), obtaining blood samples for measurement of blood gases, and cardiac output measurements (Fick or other method), when performed.

Left heart catheterization involves catheter placement in a left-sided (systemic) cardiac chamber(s) (left ventricle or left atrium) and includes left ventricular injection(s) when performed. Do not report code **93503** in conjunction with other diagnostic cardiac catheterization codes. When right heart catheterization is performed in conjunction with other cardiac catheterization services, report code **93453, 93456, 93457, 93460,** or **93461.** For placement of a flow-directed

catheter (eg, Swan-Ganz) performed for hemodynamic monitoring purposes not in conjunction with other catheterization services, report code **93503.**

Right heart catheterization does not include right ventricular or right atrial angiography (**93566**). When left heart catheterization is performed using either transapical puncture of the left ventricle or transseptal puncture of an intact septum, report code **93462** in conjunction with codes **93452, 93453, 93458-93461, 93651,** and **93652.** Catheter placement(s) in coronary artery(ies) involves selective engagement of the origins of the native coronary artery(ies) for the purpose of coronary angiography. Catheter placement(s) in bypass graft(s) (venous, internal mammary, free arterial graft[s]) involve selective engagement of the origins of the graft(s) for the purpose of bypass angiography. It is typically performed only in conjunction with coronary angiography of native vessels.

The cardiac catheterization codes (**93452-93461**), other than those for congenital heart disease, include contrast injection(s), imaging supervision, interpretation, and report for imaging typically performed. Codes for left heart catheterization (**93452, 93453, 93458-93461**), other than those for congenital heart disease, include intraprocedural injection(s) for left ventricular/ left atrial angiography, imaging supervision, and interpretation, when performed. Codes for coronary catheter placement(s) (**93454-93461**), other than those for congenital heart disease, include intraprocedural injection(s) for coronary angiography, imaging supervision, and interpretation. Codes for catheter placement(s) in bypass graft(s) (**93455, 93457, 93459, 93461**), other than those for congenital heart disease, include intraprocedural injection(s) for bypass graft angiography, imaging supervision, and interpretation. Do not report codes **93563-93565** in conjunction with codes **93452-93461.**

Cardiac catheterization (**93451-93461**) includes all roadmapping angiography in order to place the catheters, including any injections and imaging supervision, interpretation, and report. It does not include contrast injection(s) and imaging supervision, interpretation, and report for imaging that is separately identified by specific procedure code(s).

When right ventricular or right atrial angiography is performed at the time of heart catheterization, use code **93566** with the appropriate catheterization code (**93451, 93453, 93456, 93457, 93460,** or **93461**). Use code **93567** when supravalvular ascending aortography is performed at the time of heart catheterization. Use code **93568** with the appropriate right heart catheterization code when pulmonary angiography is performed. Separately reported injection procedures do not include introduction of catheters but do include repositioning of catheters when necessary and use of automatic power injectors, when performed.

Injection procedures (**93563-93568**) represent separate identifiable services and may be coded in conjunction with one another when appropriate. The technical details of angiography, supervision of filming and processing, interpretation, and report are included. Therefore, it is not appropriate to report radiology codes **75605**, **75625**, **75741**, or **75743** to represent the radiological supervision and interpretation and report when performing the services described by add-on codes **93563-93568**. Add-on code **93568** is reported for treatment of ventricular tachycardia in addition to codes **93530-93533** and codes **93451, 93453, 93456, 93457, 93460,** and **93461.**

For angiography of noncoronary arteries and veins performed as a distinct service, use appropriate codes from the Radiology section and the Vascular Injection Procedures section of the CPT codebook. (For further information pertaining to the reporting of noncoronary selective/nonselective catheterization reporting and nonselective renal and iliac angiography at the time of cardiac catheterization, refer to the coding examples provided in this chapter and in Chapter 3.) When cardiac catheterization is combined with pharmacologic agent administration with the specific purpose of repeating hemodynamic measurements to evaluate hemodynamic response, use code **93463** in conjunction with codes **93451-93453** and codes **93456-93461.** Do not report code **93463** for intracoronary administration of pharmacologic agents during percutaneous coronary interventional procedures; during intracoronary assessment of coronary pressure, flow, or resistance; or during intracoronary imaging procedures. Do not report code **93463** in conjunction with codes **92975, 92977, 92980, 92982,** or **92995.**

When cardiac catheterization is combined with exercise (eg, walking or arm or leg ergometry protocol) with the specific purpose of repeating hemodynamic measurements to evaluate hemodynamic response, report code **93464** in conjunction with codes **93451-93453, 93456-93461,** and **93530-93533.**

Contrast injection to image the access site(s) for the specific purpose of placing a closure device is inherent to the catheterization procedure and not separately reportable.

Closure device placement at the vascular access site is inherent to the catheterization procedure and not separately reportable. However, in 2003 the Centers for

Medicare and Medicaid Services (CMS) established HCPCS Level II **code G0269**, *Placement of occlusive device into either a venous or aterial access site, post surgical or interventional procedure (eg, angioseal plug, vascular plug)* to report this procedure. The CMS has assigned a physician work RVU of 0 (zero) for this code and placement of vascular closure devices remains a non-payable service. While providers are not required to report code **G0269** it may be reported in the hospital setting under the Outpatient Prospective Payment System (OPPS) or for tracking purposes.

> **CODING TIP** **Modifier 51** should not be appended to codes **93451, 93456,** and **93503.**

Moderate sedation codes (**99143-99150**) may not be submitted by the same physician who performs a noncongenital cardiac catheterization procedure or a congenital cardiac catheterization reported by code **93530.** If the presence of an additional physician is necessary to provide such services, the appropriate anesthesia service codes may be utilized as indicated. (Refer to Appendix G for further information related to the use of the moderate sedation codes.)

Codes **93451-93464** and **93530** are assigned the CPT moderate sedation symbol indicating that moderate sedation is an inherent part of the procedure. However, assignment of this symbol does not prevent separate reporting of an associated anesthesia procedure/service (CPT codes **00100-02999**) when performed by a physician other than the health care professional performing the diagnostic or therapeutic procedure. In such cases the person providing anesthesia services shall be present for the purpose of continuously monitoring the patient and shall not act as a surgical assistant. When clinical conditions of the patient require such anesthesia services, or in the circumstances when the patient does not require sedation, the operating physician is not required to report the procedure as a reduced service using **modifier 52.**

It is appropriate to append **modifier 26** to the codes for noncongenital and congenital cardiac catheterization codes when the procedure was performed in a hospital or institutional setting and the physician is reporting his or her professional services only. The institution will be reporting to insurance carriers technical charges associated with the use of its equipment and personnel. Private insurance may have a different policy regarding the use of this modifier, and coders and billers should contact each insurance company with which they work to ascertain its policy. (Refer to Chapter 6 for further information regarding the use of the HCPCS Level II **modifier TC** and CPT **modifier 26**.)

> **CODING TIP** There is currently no CPT code to report the use of mechanical devices (ie, Perclose®, ProGlide™, AngioSeal™, VasoSeal™) for closure of the femoral artery following cardiac catheterization. Any means of achieving hemostasis following cardiac catheterization, whether manual or mechanical, is an integral part of the catheterization procedure. HCPCS Level II code **G0269** is used to report in the hospital setting and does not include separate payment.

> **CODING TIP** The American College of Cardiology Coding Task Force indicates that although not typically studied "in preparation" for bypass surgery, should angiography be performed to evaluate the right or left internal mammary artery, for example, due to prior thoracic surgery or radiation, the appropriate diagnostic cardiac catheterization with angiography code (**93455**, **93457**, **93459**, or **93461**) should be reported, based on the catheterization approach performed. This guideline may, however, differ from third-party payer guidelines. Eligibility for payment, as well as coverage policy, is determined by each individual insurer or third-party payer. For reimbursement or third-party payer policy issues, please contact your local third-party payer.

Description of Service for Code ⊙93451

Moderate sedation is administered, and adequate moderate sedation monitoring is verified. Percutaneous venous access is obtained, typically through the internal jugular, subclavian, or femoral vein. A thin-walled needle is inserted percutaneously into the vein, through which a flexible guidewire is inserted into the vein. The needle is removed over the wire, a sheath/dilator system is inserted over the guidewire, the dilator is removed, and the sidearm of the sheath is flushed to remove any clot or air. A pulmonary artery catheter is inserted through the sheath, the balloon on the tip of the catheter is inflated, and the catheter is passed through the right atrium and right ventricle and into the pulmonary artery. Fluoroscopic guidance is used throughout the procedure. As the catheter tip passes through the heart into the lungs, pressure measurements are obtained within each cardiac chamber and then the main pulmonary artery. The catheter is advanced further to a point that the balloon tip occludes the pulmonary artery. The pressure transduced from the tip of the catheter in this position represents a pulmonary wedge pressure, an indirect

measurement of left atrial and left ventricular end diastolic pressure. Oxygen saturation measurements are obtained in the various cardiac chambers to assess for intracardiac shunts and to assess cardiac output. Serial injections may be performed through the catheter to measure thermodilution cardiac output. Angiography of the peripheral vessel is performed as needed to assess problems with retrograde passage of the sheath, wire, or catheters, and longer sheaths or stiffer wires are used when necessary.

Hypertension, hypotension, and oxygen desaturation are common and are treated appropriately with medications and/or oxygen as needed during the procedure. The catheter is either sewn in place for ongoing monitoring in an appropriate hospital setting or it is removed and hemostasis is achieved by appropriate means by the physician or technician under the physician's supervision.

Description of Service for Code ⊙93452

Moderate sedation is administered, and adequate moderate sedation monitoring is verified. A thin-walled needle is inserted percutaneously into a peripheral artery, through which a flexible guidewire is inserted into the artery. (See Figure 5-3.) The needle is removed over the wire, a sheath/dilator system is inserted over the guidewire, the dilator is removed, and the sidearm of the sheath is flushed to remove any clot or air. An appropriate catheter is inserted over the wire through the sheath into the arterial system under fluoroscopic guidance throughout the procedure. The catheter is advanced retrograde through the arterial system to the ascending aorta. The wire is removed, and the catheter is attached to the pressure manifold. Pressure is measured in the aortic root. The catheter is then used to cross the aortic valve retrograde into the left ventricle. Left ventricular pressure is measured. The catheter is then attached to a power injector, with careful removal of any air from the tubing. Power injection is then performed to fill the ventricle, allowing examination of systolic function and the competence of the mitral valve in an appropriate angiographic view. The power injector is disconnected from the catheter, the catheter is reattached to the manifold, all air is removed, and a careful pullback is performed across the aortic valve to assess for a transaortic valve gradient. The patient's arterial pressure, electrocardiogram, and oxygen saturation are constantly monitored throughout the procedure. All catheters are removed once angiography is completed. Angiography of the peripheral vessel is performed as needed to assess problems with retrograde passage of the sheath, wire, or catheters, and longer sheaths or stiffer wires are used when necessary.

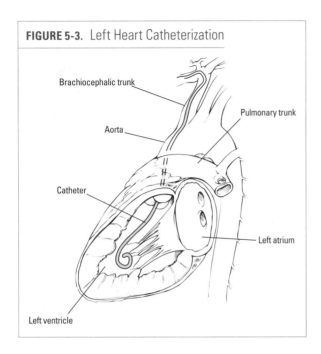

FIGURE 5-3. Left Heart Catheterization

Brachiocephalic trunk

Pulmonary trunk

Aorta

Catheter

Left atrium

Left ventricle

Hypertension, hypotension, and oxygen desaturation are common and are treated appropriately with medications and/or oxygen as needed during the procedure. Images are reviewed to ensure no additional views are required before leaving the procedure suite. Angiography of the access site may be performed to assess for any complications and suitability for a percutaneous closure device. The catheter and sheath are removed, and hemostasis is achieved by appropriate means by the physician or technician under the physician's supervision.

Description of Service for Code ⊙93453

Moderate sedation is administered, and adequate moderate sedation monitoring is verified. Percutaneous venous access is obtained, typically through the internal jugular, subclavian, or femoral vein. A thin-walled needle is inserted percutaneously into the vein, through which a flexible guidewire is inserted into the vein. (See Figure 5-4.) The needle is removed over the wire, a sheath/dilator system is inserted over the guidewire, the dilator is removed, and the sidearm of the sheath is flushed to remove any clot or air. A pulmonary artery catheter is inserted through the sheath, a balloon on the tip of the catheter is inflated, and the catheter is passed through the right atrium and right ventricle and into the pulmonary artery. Fluoroscopic guidance is used throughout the procedure. As the catheter tip passes through the heart into the lungs, pressure measurements are obtained within each cardiac chamber and the main pulmonary artery. The catheter is advanced further to a point that the balloon tip occludes the pulmonary artery. The pressure transduced from the tip of the catheter in this

position represents a pulmonary wedge pressure, an indirect measurement of left atrial and left ventricular end diastolic pressure. Oxygen saturation measurements are obtained to assess for intracardiac shunts and to assess cardiac output. Serial injections may be performed through the catheter to measure thermodilution cardiac output.

A thin-walled needle is inserted percutaneously into a peripheral artery, through which a flexible guidewire is inserted into the artery. The needle is removed over the wire, a sheath/dilator system is inserted over the guidewire, the dilator is removed, and the sidearm of the sheath is flushed to remove any clot or air. An appropriate catheter is inserted over the wire through the sheath into the arterial system under fluoroscopic guidance throughout the procedure. The catheter is advanced retrograde through the arterial system to the ascending aorta. The wire is removed, and the catheter is attached to the pressure manifold. Pressure is measured in the aortic root. The catheter is then used to cross the aortic valve retrograde into the left ventricle. Left ventricular pressure is measured. The catheter is then attached to a power injector, with careful removal of any air from the tubing. Power injection is then performed to fill the ventricle, allowing examination of systolic function and the competence of the mitral valve in an appropriate angiographic view. The power injector is disconnected from the catheter, the catheter is reattached to the manifold, all air is removed, and a careful pullback is performed across the aortic valve to ensure no aortic valve gradient. The patient's arterial pressure, electrocardiogram, and oxygen saturation are constantly monitored throughout the procedure. All catheters are removed once angiography is completed. Images are reviewed to ensure no additional views are required before leaving the procedure suite. Angiography of the peripheral vessel is performed as needed to assess problems with retrograde passage of the sheath, wire, or catheters, and longer sheaths or stiffer wires are used when necessary.

Hypertension, hypotension, and oxygen desaturation are common and are treated appropriately with medications and/or oxygen as needed during the procedure. Angiography of the access site may be performed to assess for any complications and suitability for a percutaneous closure device. The catheters and sheaths are removed, and hemostasis is achieved by appropriate means by the physician or technician under the physician's supervision.

Description of Service for Code ⊙93454

Moderate sedation is administered, and adequate moderate sedation monitoring is verified. A thin-walled

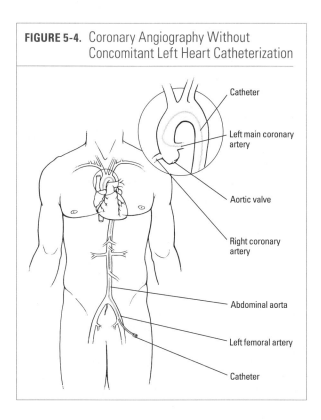

FIGURE 5-4. Coronary Angiography Without Concomitant Left Heart Catheterization

Catheter

Left main coronary artery

Aortic valve

Right coronary artery

Abdominal aorta

Left femoral artery

Catheter

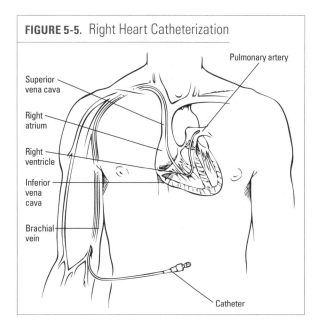

FIGURE 5-5. Right Heart Catheterization

Pulmonary artery

Superior vena cava

Right atrium

Right ventricle

Inferior vena cava

Brachial vein

Catheter

needle is inserted percutaneously into a peripheral artery, through which a flexible guidewire is inserted into the artery. The needle is removed over the wire, a sheath/dilator system is inserted over the guidewire, the dilator is removed, and the sidearm of the sheath is flushed to remove any clot or air. An appropriate catheter is inserted over the wire through the sheath into the arterial system under fluoroscopic guidance throughout the procedure. (See Figure 5-5.) The catheter is advanced retrograde through the arterial system to the ascending aorta. The wire is removed, and the catheter is attached to the injection manifold. Pressure is measured in the aortic root. The catheter is then manipulated using fluoroscopic guidance into the ostium of a coronary artery. The arterial pressure and waveform are checked to be sure there is no evidence of catheter malposition or impairment of coronary flow due to an ostial stenosis. Test contrast injections under fluoroscopy are performed to check catheter position. Multiple coronary injections are performed, each with the imaging system aligned in a different orientation, with simultaneous panning (moving the table) to assess for stenoses. The catheter is then removed over the wire. Additional catheters are introduced over the guidewire and manipulated into the ostia of other coronary arteries to inject them in multiple views while moving the table in similar fashion. Typically, a separate catheter is used for the left and right coronary arteries. The patient's arterial pressure, electrocardiogram, and oxygen saturation are constantly monitored throughout the procedure. All catheters are removed

once angiography is completed. Images are reviewed to ensure no additional views are required before leaving the procedure suite. Angiography of the access site may be performed to assess for any complications and suitability for a percutaneous closure device. Angiography of the peripheral vessel is performed as needed to assess problems with retrograde passage of the sheath, wire, or catheters, and longer sheaths or stiffer wires are used when necessary.

Hypertension, hypotension, and oxygen desaturation are common and are treated appropriately with medications and/or oxygen as needed during the procedure. The catheter and sheath are removed, and hemostasis is achieved by appropriate means by the physician or technician under the physician's supervision.

Description of Service for Code ⊙93455

Moderate sedation is administered, and adequate moderate sedation monitoring is verified. A thin-walled needle is inserted percutaneously into a peripheral artery, through which a flexible guidewire is inserted into the artery. The needle is removed over the wire, a sheath/dilator system is inserted over the guidewire, the dilator is removed, and the sidearm of the sheath is flushed to remove any clot or air. An appropriate catheter is inserted over the wire through the sheath into the arterial system under fluoroscopic guidance throughout the procedure. The catheter is advanced retrograde through the arterial system to the ascending aorta. The wire is removed, and the catheter is attached to the injection manifold. Pressure is measured in the aortic root. The catheter is then manipulated using fluoroscopic guidance into the ostium of a coronary artery. The arterial pressure and

CHAPTER 5

waveform are checked to be sure there is no evidence of catheter malposition or impairment of coronary flow due to an ostial stenosis. Test contrast injections under fluoroscopy are performed to check catheter position. Multiple coronary injections are performed, each with the imaging system aligned in a different orientation, with simultaneous panning (moving the table) to assess for stenoses. The catheter is then removed over the wire. Additional catheters are introduced over the guidewire and manipulated into the ostia of other coronary arteries to inject them in multiple views while moving the table in similar fashion. Typically, a separate catheter is used for the left and right coronary arteries. Additional catheters are used to engage the vein grafts (typically one catheter for the vein graft to the right coronary and one catheter for left-sided vein grafts). One or more catheters are typically needed to engage the left subclavian artery. Once the catheter is successfully positioned in the left subclavian artery, a wire is directed through it into the distal left subclavian artery, and the catheter is advanced over the wire to the level of the internal mammary artery origin. The wire is removed, and the catheter is reattached to the injection manifold and meticulously flushed to avoid thrombus or air embolus to the cerebral vessels. The catheter is then manipulated using fluoroscopic guidance to engage the ostium of the left internal mammary artery atraumatically. The arterial pressure and waveform are checked to be sure there is no evidence of catheter malposition or impairment of mammary flow due to an ostial stenosis. Typically, the catheter used to enter the left subclavian artery will not engage the internal mammary artery, and the original catheter must be exchanged over the wire for a catheter specially designed to cannulate the internal mammary artery. A similar procedure is performed on the right side if a right internal mammary artery graft has been placed previously. The patient's arterial pressure, electrocardiogram, and oxygen saturation are constantly monitored throughout the procedure. All catheters are removed once angiography is completed. Images are reviewed to ensure no additional views are required before leaving the procedure suite. Angiography of the peripheral vessel is performed as needed to assess problems with retrograde passage of the sheath, wire, or catheters, and longer sheaths or stiffer wires are used when necessary.

Hypertension, hypotension, and oxygen desaturation are common and are treated appropriately with medications and/or oxygen as needed during the procedure. Angiography of the access site may be performed to assess for any complications and suitability for a percutaneous closure device. The catheter and sheath are removed, and hemostasis is achieved by appropri-

ate means by the physician or technician under the physician's supervision.

Description of Service for Code ⊙⊘93456

Moderate sedation is administered, and adequate moderate sedation monitoring is verified. Percutaneous venous access is obtained, typically through the internal jugular, subclavian, or femoral vein. A thin-walled needle is inserted percutaneously into the vein, through which a flexible guidewire is inserted into the vein. The needle is removed over the wire, a sheath/dilator system is inserted over the guidewire, the dilator is removed, and the sidearm of the sheath is flushed to remove any clot or air. A pulmonary artery catheter is inserted through the sheath, a balloon on the tip of the catheter is inflated, and the catheter is passed through the right atrium and right ventricle and into the pulmonary artery. Fluoroscopic guidance is used throughout the procedure. As the catheter tip passes through the heart into the lungs, pressure measurements are obtained within the cardiac chambers and pulmonary artery. The catheter is advanced farther to a point that the balloon tip occludes the pulmonary artery. The pressure transduced from the tip of the catheter in this position represents a pulmonary wedge pressure, an indirect measurement of left atrial and left ventricular end diastolic pressure. Oxygen saturation measurements are obtained to assess for intracardiac shunts and to assess Fick cardiac output. Serial injections may be performed through the catheter to measure thermodilution cardiac output.

A thin-walled needle is inserted percutaneously into a peripheral artery, through which a flexible guidewire is inserted into the artery. The needle is removed over the wire, a sheath/dilator system is inserted over the guidewire, the dilator is removed, and the sidearm of the sheath is flushed to remove any clot or air. An appropriate catheter is inserted over the wire through the sheath into the arterial system under fluoroscopic guidance throughout the procedure. The catheter is advanced retrograde through the arterial system to the ascending aorta. The wire is removed, and the catheter is attached to the injection manifold. Pressure is measured in the aortic root. The catheter is then manipulated using fluoroscopic guidance into the ostium of a coronary artery. The arterial pressure and waveform are checked to be sure there is no evidence of catheter malposition or impairment of coronary flow due to an ostial stenosis. Test contrast injections under fluoroscopy are performed to check catheter position. Multiple coronary injections are performed, each with the imaging system aligned in a different orientation, with simultaneous panning (moving the table) to assess for stenoses. The catheter is then removed over the wire. Additional catheters are introduced over the guidewire and manipulated into the ostia of other coronary arteries to inject them in multiple views while moving the table in similar fashion. Typically, a separate catheter is used for the left and right coronary arteries. The patient's arterial pressure, electrocardiogram, and oxygen saturation are constantly monitored throughout the procedure. All catheters are removed once angiography is completed. Images are reviewed to ensure no additional views are required before leaving the procedure suite. Angiography of the peripheral vessel is performed as needed to assess problems with retrograde passage of the sheath, wire, or catheters, and longer sheaths or stiffer wires are used when necessary.

Hypertension, hypotension, and oxygen desaturation are common and are treated appropriately with medications and/or oxygen as needed during the procedure. Angiography of the access site may be performed to assess for any complications and suitability for a percutaneous closure device. The catheters and sheaths are removed, and hemostasis is achieved by appropriate means by the physician or technician under the physician's supervision.

Description of Service for Code ⊙93457

Moderate sedation is administered, and adequate moderate sedation monitoring is verified. Percutaneous venous access is obtained, typically through the internal jugular, subclavian, or femoral vein. A thin-walled needle is inserted percutaneously into the vein, through which a flexible guidewire is inserted into the vein. The needle is removed over the wire, a sheath/dilator system is inserted over the guidewire, the dilator is removed, and the sidearm of the sheath is flushed to remove any clot or air. A pulmonary artery catheter is inserted through the sheath, a balloon on the tip of the catheter is inflated, and the catheter is passed through the right atrium and right ventricle and into the pulmonary artery. Fluoroscopic guidance is used throughout the procedure. As the catheter tip passes through the heart into the lungs, pressure measurements are obtained within the cardiac chambers and pulmonary artery. The catheter is advanced farther to a point that the balloon tip occludes the pulmonary artery. The pressure transduced from the tip of the catheter in this position represents a pulmonary wedge pressure, an indirect measurement of left atrial and left ventricular end diastolic pressure. Oxygen saturation measurements are obtained to assess for intracardiac shunts and to assess Fick cardiac output. Serial injections may be performed through the catheter to measure thermodilution cardiac output.

A thin-walled needle is inserted percutaneously into a peripheral artery, through which a flexible guidewire is inserted into the artery. The needle is removed over the wire, a sheath/dilator system is inserted over the guidewire, the dilator is removed, and the sidearm of the sheath is flushed to remove any clot or air. An appropriate catheter is inserted over the wire through the sheath into the arterial system under fluoroscopic guidance throughout the procedure. The catheter is advanced retrograde through the arterial system to the ascending aorta. The wire is removed, and the catheter is attached to the injection manifold. Pressure is measured in the aortic root. The catheter is then manipulated using fluoroscopic guidance into the ostium of a coronary artery. The arterial pressure and waveform are checked to be sure there is no evidence of catheter malposition or impairment of coronary flow due to an ostial stenosis. Test contrast injections under fluoroscopy are performed to check catheter position. Multiple coronary injections are performed, each with the imaging system aligned in a different orientation, with simultaneous panning (moving the table) to assess for stenoses. The catheter is then removed over the wire. Additional catheters are introduced over the guidewire and manipulated into the ostia of other coronary arteries to inject them in multiple views while moving the table in similar fashion. Typically, a separate catheter is used for the left and right coronary arteries. Additional catheters are used to engage the vein grafts (typically one catheter for the vein graft to the right coronary and one catheter for left-sided vein grafts). One or more catheters are typically needed to engage the left subclavian artery. Once the catheter is successfully positioned in the left subclavian artery, a wire is directed through it into the distal left subclavian artery, and the catheter is advanced over the wire to the level of the internal mammary artery origin. The wire is removed, and the catheter is reattached to the injection manifold and meticulously flushed to avoid thrombus or air embolus to the cerebral vessels. The catheter is then manipulated using fluoroscopic guidance to engage the ostium of the left internal mammary artery atraumatically. Typically, the catheter used to enter the left subclavian artery will not engage the internal mammary artery, and the original catheter must be exchanged over the wire for a catheter specially designed to cannulate the internal mammary artery. The arterial pressure and waveform are checked to be sure there is no evidence of catheter malposition or impairment of mammary flow due to an ostial stenosis. A similar procedure is performed on the right side if a right internal mammary artery graft has been placed previously. The patient's arterial pressure, electrocardiogram, and oxygen saturation are constantly monitored throughout the procedure. Angiography of the peripheral vessel is performed as needed to assess problems with retrograde passage of the sheath, wire, or catheters, and longer sheaths or stiffer wires are used when necessary.

Hypertension, hypotension, and oxygen desaturation are common and are treated appropriately with medications and/or oxygen as needed during the procedure. All catheters are removed once angiography is completed. Images are reviewed to ensure no additional views are required before leaving the procedure suite. Angiography of the access site may be performed to assess for any complications and suitability for a percutaneous closure device. The catheters and sheaths are removed, and hemostasis is achieved.

Description of Service for Code ⊙93458

Moderate sedation is administered, and adequate moderate sedation monitoring is verified. A thin-walled needle is inserted percutaneously into a peripheral artery, through which a flexible guidewire is inserted into the artery. The needle is removed over the wire, a sheath/dilator system is inserted over the guidewire, the dilator is removed, and the sidearm of the sheath is flushed to remove any clot or air. An appropriate catheter is inserted over the wire through the sheath into the arterial system under fluoroscopic guidance throughout the procedure. The catheter is advanced retrograde through the arterial system to the ascending aorta. The wire is removed, and the catheter is attached to the injection manifold. Pressure is measured in the aortic root. The catheter is then manipulated using fluoroscopic guidance into the ostium of a coronary artery. The arterial pressure and waveform are checked to be sure there is no evidence of catheter malposition or impairment of coronary flow due to an ostial stenosis. Test contrast injections under fluoroscopy are performed to check catheter position. Multiple coronary injections are performed, each with the imaging system aligned in a different orientation, with simultaneous panning (moving the table) to assess for stenoses. The catheter is then removed over the wire. Additional catheters are introduced over the guidewire and manipulated into the ostia of other coronary arteries to inject them in multiple views while moving the table in similar fashion. Typically, a separate catheter is used for the left and right coronary arteries.

A separate catheter is used to cross the aortic valve retrograde into the left ventricle. Left ventricular pressure is measured. The catheter is then attached to a power injector with careful removal of any air from the tubing. Power injection is then performed to fill the ventricle, allowing examination of systolic function and the competence of the mitral valve in

an appropriate angiographic view. The power injector is disconnected from the catheter, the catheter is reattached to the manifold, all air is removed, and a careful pullback is performed across the aortic valve to ensure no aortic valve gradient. The patient's arterial pressure, electrocardiogram, and oxygen saturation are constantly monitored throughout the procedure. All catheters are removed once angiography is completed. Images are reviewed to ensure no additional views are required before leaving the procedure suite. Angiography of the peripheral vessel is performed as needed to assess problems with retrograde passage of the sheath, wire, or catheters, and longer sheaths or stiffer wires are used when necessary.

Hypertension, hypotension, and oxygen desaturation are common and are treated appropriately with medications and/or oxygen as needed during the procedure. Angiography of the access site may be performed to assess for any complications and suitability for a percutaneous closure device. The catheter and sheath are removed, and hemostasis is achieved by appropriate means by the physician or technician under the physician's supervision.

Description of Service for Code ⊙93459

Moderate sedation is administered, and adequate moderate sedation monitoring is verified. A thin-walled needle is inserted percutaneously into a peripheral artery, through which a flexible guidewire is inserted into the artery. The needle is removed over the wire, a sheath/dilator system is inserted over the guidewire, the dilator is removed, and the sidearm of the sheath is flushed to remove any clot or air. An appropriate catheter is inserted over the wire through the sheath into the arterial system under fluoroscopic guidance throughout the procedure. The catheter is advanced retrograde through the arterial system to the ascending aorta. The wire is removed, and the catheter is attached to the injection manifold. Pressure is measured in the aortic root. The catheter is then manipulated using fluoroscopic guidance into the ostium of a coronary artery. The arterial pressure and waveform are checked to be sure there is no evidence of catheter malposition or impairment of coronary flow due to an ostial stenosis. Test contrast injections under fluoroscopy are performed to check catheter position. Multiple coronary injections are performed, each with the imaging system aligned in a different orientation, with simultaneous panning (moving the table) to assess for stenoses. The catheter is then removed over the wire. Additional catheters are introduced over the guidewire and manipulated into the ostia of other coronary arteries to inject them in multiple views while moving the table in similar fashion. Typically, a separate catheter is used for the left and right coronary arteries.

Additional catheters are used to engage the vein grafts (typically one catheter for the vein graft to the right coronary and one catheter for left-sided vein grafts). One or more catheters are typically needed to engage the left subclavian artery. Once the catheter is successfully positioned in the left subclavian artery, a wire is directed through it into the distal left subclavian artery, and the catheter is advanced over the wire to the level of the internal mammary artery origin. The wire is removed, and the catheter is reattached to the injection manifold and meticulously flushed to avoid thrombus or air embolus to the cerebral vessels. The catheter is then manipulated using fluoroscopic guidance to engage the ostium of the left internal mammary artery atraumatically. Typically, the catheter used to enter the left subclavian artery will not engage the internal mammary artery, and the original catheter must be exchanged over the wire for a catheter specially designed to cannulate the internal mammary artery. The arterial pressure and waveform are checked to be sure there is no evidence of catheter malposition or impairment of mammary flow due to an ostial stenosis. A similar procedure is performed on the right side if a right internal mammary artery graft has been placed previously.

A separate catheter is used to cross the aortic valve retrograde into the left ventricle. Left ventricular pressure is measured. The catheter is then attached to a power injector with careful removal of any air from the tubing. Power injection is then performed to fill the ventricle, allowing examination of systolic function and the competence of the mitral valve in an appropriate angiographic view. The power injector is disconnected from the catheter, the catheter is reattached to the manifold, all air is removed, and a careful pullback is performed across the aortic valve to ensure no aortic valve gradient. The patient's arterial pressure, electrocardiogram, and oxygen saturation are constantly monitored throughout the procedure. All catheters are removed once angiography is completed. Images are reviewed to ensure no additional views are required before leaving the procedure suite. Angiography of the peripheral vessel is performed as needed to assess problems with retrograde passage of the sheath, wire, or catheters, and longer sheaths or stiffer wires are used when necessary.

Hypertension, hypotension, and oxygen desaturation are common and are treated appropriately with medications and/or oxygen as needed during the procedure. Angiography of the access site may be performed to assess for any complications and suitability for a

percutaneous closure device. The catheter and sheath are removed, and hemostasis is achieved by appropriate means by the physician or technician under the physician's supervision.

Description of Service for Code ⊙93460

Moderate sedation is administered, and adequate moderate sedation monitoring is verified. Percutaneous venous access is obtained, typically through the internal jugular, subclavian, or femoral vein. A thin-walled needle is inserted percutaneously into the vein, through which a flexible guidewire is inserted into the vein. The needle is removed over the wire, a sheath/dilator system is inserted over the guidewire, the dilator is removed, and the sidearm of the sheath is flushed to remove any clot or air. A pulmonary artery catheter is inserted through the sheath, a balloon on the tip of the catheter is inflated, and the catheter is passed through the right atrium and right ventricle and into the pulmonary artery. Fluoroscopic guidance is used throughout the procedure. As the catheter tip passes through the heart into the lungs, pressure measurements are obtained within the cardiac chambers and pulmonary artery. The catheter is advanced farther to a point that the balloon tip occludes the pulmonary artery. The pressure transduced from the tip of the catheter in this position represents a pulmonary wedge pressure, an indirect measurement of left atrial and left ventricular end diastolic pressure. Oxygen saturation measurements are obtained to assess for intracardiac shunts and to assess Fick cardiac output. Serial injections may be performed through the catheter to measure thermodilution cardiac output.

A thin-walled needle is inserted percutaneously into a peripheral artery, through which a flexible guidewire is inserted into the artery. The needle is removed over the wire, a sheath/dilator system is inserted over the guidewire, the dilator is removed, and the sidearm of the sheath is flushed to remove any clot or air. An appropriate catheter is inserted over the wire through the sheath into the arterial system under fluoroscopic guidance throughout the procedure. The catheter is advanced retrograde through the arterial system to the ascending aorta. The wire is removed, and the catheter is attached to the injection manifold. Pressure is measured in the aortic root. The catheter is then manipulated using fluoroscopic guidance into the ostium of a coronary artery. The arterial pressure and waveform are checked to be sure there is no evidence of catheter malposition or impairment of coronary flow due to an ostial stenosis. Test contrast injections under fluoroscopy are performed to check catheter position. Multiple coronary injections are performed, each with the imaging system aligned in a different orientation, with simultaneous panning (moving the table) to assess for stenoses. The catheter is then removed over the wire. Additional catheters are introduced over the guidewire and manipulated into the ostia of other coronary arteries to inject them in multiple views while moving the table in similar fashion. Typically, a separate catheter is used for the left and right coronary arteries.

A separate catheter is used to cross the aortic valve retrograde into the left ventricle. Left ventricular pressure is measured simultaneously with aortic pressure to assess the transaortic valve gradient. These data are combined with the right heart catheterization cardiac output data to calculate an aortic valve area. The catheter is then attached to a power injector with careful removal of any air from the tubing. Power injection is then performed to fill the ventricle, allowing examination of systolic function and the competence of the mitral valve in an appropriate angiographic view. The power injector is disconnected from the catheter, the catheter is reattached to the manifold, all air is removed, and a careful pullback is performed across the aortic valve to ensure no aortic valve gradient. The patient's arterial pressure, electrocardiogram, and oxygen saturation are constantly monitored throughout the procedure. All catheters are removed once angiography is completed. Images are reviewed to ensure no additional views are required before leaving the procedure suite. Angiography of the peripheral vessel is performed as needed to assess problems with retrograde passage of the sheath, wire, or catheters, and longer sheaths or stiffer wires are used when necessary.

Hypertension, hypotension, and oxygen desaturation are common and are treated appropriately with medications and/or oxygen as needed during the procedure. Angiography of the access site may be performed to assess for any complications and suitability for a percutaneous closure device. The catheters and sheaths are removed, and hemostasis is achieved by appropriate means by the physician or technician under the physician's supervision.

Description of Service for Code ⊙93461

Moderate sedation is administered, and adequate moderate sedation monitoring is verified. Percutaneous venous access is obtained, typically through the internal jugular, subclavian, or femoral vein. A thin-walled needle is inserted percutaneously into the vein, through which a flexible guidewire is inserted into the vein. The needle is removed over the wire, a sheath/dilator system is inserted over the guidewire, the dilator is removed, and the sidearm of the sheath is flushed to remove any clot or air. A pulmonary artery catheter

is inserted through the sheath, a balloon on the tip of the catheter is inflated, and the catheter is passed through the right atrium and right ventricle and into the pulmonary artery. Fluoroscopic guidance is used throughout the procedure. As the catheter tip passes through the heart into the lungs, pressure measurements are obtained within the cardiac chambers and pulmonary artery. The catheter is advanced farther to a point that the balloon tip occludes the pulmonary artery. The pressure transduced from the tip of the catheter in this position represents a pulmonary wedge pressure, an indirect measurement of left atrial and left ventricular end diastolic pressure. Oxygen saturation measurements are obtained to assess for intracardiac shunts and to assess Fick cardiac output. Serial injections may be performed through the catheter to measure thermodilution cardiac output.

A thin-walled needle is inserted percutaneously into a peripheral artery, through which a flexible guidewire is inserted into the artery. The needle is removed over the wire, a sheath/dilator system is inserted over the guidewire, the dilator is removed, and the sidearm of the sheath is flushed to remove any clot or air. An appropriate catheter is inserted over the wire through the sheath into the arterial system under fluoroscopic guidance throughout the procedure. The catheter is advanced retrograde through the arterial system to the ascending aorta. The wire is removed, and the catheter is attached to the injection manifold. Pressure is measured in the aortic root. The catheter is then manipulated using fluoroscopic guidance into the ostium of a coronary artery. The arterial pressure and waveform are checked to be sure there is no evidence of catheter malposition or impairment of coronary flow due to an ostial stenosis. Test contrast injections under fluoroscopy are performed to check catheter position. Multiple coronary injections are performed, each with the imaging system aligned in a different orientation, with simultaneous panning (moving the table) to assess for stenoses. The catheter is then removed over the wire. Additional catheters are introduced over the guidewire and manipulated into the ostia of other coronary arteries to inject them in multiple views while moving the table in similar fashion. Typically, a separate catheter is used for the left and right coronary arteries. Additional catheters are used to engage the vein grafts (typically one catheter for the vein graft to the right coronary and one catheter for left-sided vein grafts). One or more catheters are typically needed to engage the left subclavian artery. Once the catheter is successfully positioned in the left subclavian artery, a wire is directed through it, into the distal left subclavian artery, and the catheter is advanced over the wire to the level of the internal mammary artery origin. The wire is removed, and the catheter is reattached to the injection manifold and meticulously flushed to avoid thrombus or air embolus to the cerebral vessels. The catheter is then manipulated using fluoroscopic guidance to engage the ostium of the left internal mammary artery atraumatically. Typically, the catheter used to enter the left subclavian artery will not engage the internal mammary artery, and the original catheter must be exchanged over the wire for a catheter specially designed to cannulate the internal mammary artery. The arterial pressure and waveform are checked to be sure there is no evidence of catheter malposition or impairment of mammary flow due to an ostial stenosis. A similar procedure is performed on the right side if a right internal mammary artery graft has been placed previously.

A separate catheter is used to cross the aortic valve retrograde into the left ventricle. Left ventricular pressure is measured simultaneously with aortic pressure to assess the transaortic valve gradient. These data are combined with the right heart catheterization cardiac output data to calculate an aortic valve area. The catheter is then attached to a power injector with careful removal of any air from the tubing. Power injection is then performed to fill the ventricle, allowing examination of systolic function and the competence of the mitral valve in an appropriate angiographic view. The power injector is disconnected from the catheter, the catheter is reattached to the manifold, all air is removed, and a careful pullback is performed across the aortic valve to ensure no aortic valve gradient.

The patient's arterial pressure, electrocardiogram, and oxygen saturation are constantly monitored throughout the procedure. All catheters are removed once angiography is completed. Images are reviewed to ensure no additional views are required before leaving the procedure suite. Angiography of the peripheral vessel is performed as needed to assess problems with retrograde passage of the sheath, wire, or catheters, and longer sheaths or stiffer wires are used when necessary.

Hypertension, hypotension, and oxygen desaturation are common and are treated appropriately with medications and/or oxygen as needed during the procedure. Angiography of the access site may be performed to assess for any complications and suitability for a percutaneous closure device. The catheters and sheaths are removed, and hemostasis is achieved by appropriate means by the physician or technician under the physician's supervision.

CODING TIP When left heart catheterization is performed using either transapical puncture of the left ventricle or transseptal puncture of an intact septum, report code **93462** in conjunction with codes **93452**, **93453**, **93458-93461**, **93651**, and **93652**.

Description of Service for Code ⊙+93462

Prepare the interactive system of a needle, stylet, dilator, and catheter, which is used to puncture and then cross the atrial septum. Typically, separate venous access must be obtained as part of this procedure, typically through the femoral vein. A thin-walled needle is inserted percutaneously into the vein, through which a flexible guidewire is inserted into the vein. The needle is removed over the wire, a sheath/dilator system is inserted over the guidewire, the dilator is removed, and the sidearm of the sheath is flushed to remove any clot or air. Fluoroscopic guidance is used throughout the procedure. An appropriate catheter is inserted over a wire through the venous sheath into the venous system and advanced under fluoroscopic guidance up to the superior vena cava. The wire is removed. A rigid transseptal puncture needle is carefully advanced through the catheter, stopping just short of the end of the catheter. The needle-catheter unit is flushed and attached to a second pressure manifold and then withdrawn to the level of the fossa ovalis in the interatrial septum under fluoroscopic guidance. The imaging system is rotated in both the anterior and lateral positions to confirm proper positioning with respect to the arterial catheter, which has been positioned just above the aortic valve. Exquisite precision of the needle-catheter unit is imperative, as improper positioning can lead to puncture of the aorta or perforation through the atrial wall into the pericardium. Typically, the needle-catheter unit may not be positioned properly on the first attempt and one or more repositionings of the unit may be required. This typically requires removal of the needle, reinsertion of the guidewire, readvancement of the wire and catheter to the superior vena cava, removal of the wire, reinsertion of the needle, and then repeating the process of positioning the needle-catheter unit in the proper spot on the interatrial septum. Once successful positioning is achieved, the needle-catheter unit is then advanced several millimeters across the interatrial septum to the left atrium while observing the pressure waveform. The transseptal puncture is achieved. Left atrial position is confirmed by pressure waveform analysis, oxygen saturation measurement, and contrast injection through the system. If the needle-catheter unit has not traversed the septum properly, complications are first excluded and then the device is repositioned

CHAPTER 5

and repeat attempt(s) performed until successful. The transseptal needle is removed from the catheter, which is now in the left atrium. The catheter is flushed, and a wire is advanced through the catheter into the left atrium. (As part of the work reported separately as part of other codes **93451-93461**, an appropriate left heart catheter is advanced over the wire to the left atrium and/or the left ventricle.)

Description of Service for Code ⊙+**93463**

Inhaled nitric oxide (a selective pulmonary vasodilator) is administered for 10 minutes. Alternative pulmonary vasodilators may be used instead or in addition. The patient's arterial pressure, pulmonary arterial pressure, electrocardiogram, and oxygen saturation are constantly monitored throughout the procedure via a right heart catheter that was previously placed (coded separately). Repeat right heart measurements are then performed after administration of the pulmonary vasodilators to determine the responsiveness of the pulmonary circulation. Typically, this involves repositioning the right heart catheter into the pulmonary wedge positioning to obtain a wedge pressure, withdrawing it to the pulmonary artery position to obtain a pulmonary artery pressure, and re-measuring cardiac output with Fick or thermodilution techniques. The entire process may be repeated with additional vasodilators if a satisfactory hemodynamic response is not achieved with the first agent. Additional waveforms, pressure measurements, saturation data, and cardiac output calculations are reviewed when performed and are included in the report of the procedure.

> **CODING TIP** It is not appropriate to report code **93463** in conjunction with codes **92975**, **92977**, **92980**, **92982**, or **92995** for intracoronary administration of pharmacologic agents during percutaneous coronary interventional procedures, during intracoronary assessment of coronary pressure, flow, or resistance, or during intracoronary imaging procedures.

Description of Service for Code ⊙+**96464**

The patient is exercised or treated with agents to increase heart rate and/or contractility with catheters in place to measure appropriate pressures, oxygen saturations, and cardiac output when performed. The patient's arterial pressure, left ventricular end diastolic pressure, pulmonary arterial pressure, electrocardiogram, and oxygen saturation are constantly monitored throughout the procedure via a right heart catheter that was previously placed (coded separately).. The patient is coached to exercise vigorously using an

exercise bicycle to maximum capacity until limiting dyspnea is achieved. If a pharmacologic agent is used instead of exercise, the agent is administered over time, titrating it to a level that achieves the desired heart rate, hemodynamic response, or limiting symptoms. Repeat right and left heart measurements are then performed after the exercise/pharmacologic stress to determine the physiologic response. Typically, this involves repositioning the right heart catheter to the wedge position and adjusting the left ventricular catheter, which has often moved during the study. Typically, repeat cardiac output measurements and oxygen saturation measurements are obtained. Additional waveforms, pressure measurements, saturation data, and cardiac output calculations are reviewed when performed and added to the report of the procedure.

FLOW-DIRECTED MONITORING CATHETER INSERTION (⊘**93503**)

⊘**93503** Insertion and placement of flow directed catheter (eg, Swan-Ganz) for monitoring purposes
CPT Changes: An Insider's View 2011

Intent and Use of Code ⊘**93503**

Code **93503** is used only to describe the placement of a flow-directed catheter (Swan-Ganz) for the purpose of hemodynamic monitoring not in conjunction with other catheterizations services. Code **93503** includes vascular access, sedation and monitoring, insertion and positioning of the right heart catheter, and eventual removal of the catheter.

Code **93503** is distinguished from code **93451** (right heart catheterization) in that the service described by code **93503** is not typically performed in the cardiac catheterization laboratory. Placement of a flow-directed catheter for monitoring in an intensive care setting is done to monitor critically ill patients or preoperatively to allow monitoring of hemodynamics during surgery. The right heart catheterization described by code **93451** is diagnostic in nature and often performed in conjunction with other cardiac catheterization procedures.

Code **93503** represents the placement (in the pulmonary artery) of this multiple lumen, balloon-tipped flotation catheter (ie, Swan-Ganz) with a thermistor at the end of the catheter. A thermistor is a device that monitors the temperature. This balloon-tipped, flow-directed catheter provides intermittent occlusion of the pulmonary artery for the initial and serial assessment of right and left ventricle failure and allows monitoring of therapy associated with complications of acute myocardial infarction (eg, cardiogenic shock, pulmonary edema, fluid-related hypovolemia, hypotension, systolic murmur, unexplained sinus tachycardia, cardiac arrhythmias, fluid status due to serious burns, or renal disease). An indirect measurement of left atrial filling pressure is obtained when the catheter is "wedged." This type of catheter (having a thermistor) allows for measurement of cardiac output. Other hemodynamic parameters such as systemic vascular resistance, mixed venous oxygen saturation, and intrapulmonary shunt fraction(s) may also be measured. For serial determinations, it is not uncommon for this type of catheter to remain in place for 48 to 72 hours, or as long as the patient's needs require, for serial determinations.

> **CODING TIP** Do not report code **93503** in addition to the diagnostic cardiac catheterization codes, as recordings of intracardiac and intravascular pressures, blood sampling for measurement of oxygen saturation or blood gases, or cardiac output measurements are considered an integral component of cardiac catheterization diagnostic procedures.

Description of Service for Code ⊘**93503**

Before placement of the flow-directed catheter, the physician examines the patient, discusses the procedure with the patient or other legally responsible individual, and obtains informed consent for the procedure. Additional preprocedural functions include writing orders for adequate sedation and patient support and reviewing study arrangements and procedures with assisting personnel.

Flow-directed catheterization is generally performed via the subclavian, internal jugular, brachial, or femoral vein, utilizing sterile technique, local anesthetic, and appropriate sedation. Placement of a flow-directed catheter typically involves percutaneous insertion of a needle in the target vein, followed by placement of flexible guidewire, removal of the needle, insertion of a sheath/dilator system over the guidewire, removal of the dilator and guidewire, and subsequent insertion of the flow-directed catheter through the sheath. The catheter is connected to the pressure-measuring system for constant monitoring while the catheter is advanced to the desired site within the right heart, pulmonary artery, or pulmonary capillary wedge position. The patient's electrocardiogram is monitored during the insertion to detect and avoid significant arrhythmias. Baseline pressure measurements and blood sampling may be conducted in each of the desired sites, and

cardiac output may be measured. Measurements may be repeated following exercise or other interventions.

Following catheterization, the catheter may be secured in place for subsequent serial measurements, or the catheter and sheath may be removed and hemostasis achieved by the physician or technician (or nurse) under the physician's supervision.

ENDOMYOCARDIAL BIOPSY (⊙**93505**)

⊙**93505** Endomyocardial biopsy
CPT Assistant Apr 98:2, Apr 00:10; *CPT Changes: An Insider's View* 2008

Intent and Use of Code ⊙**93505**

An endomyocardial biopsy involves the percutaneous introduction of a venous sheath system into the internal jugular or femoral vein using sterile techniques, local anesthesia, and appropriate sedation. Using a procedure similar to that described for right heart catheterization (**93451**), a guiding sheath is directed into the internal jugular or femoral vein. Under fluoroscopic guidance, a bioptome is directed through the sheath to the right ventricular endocardium where a biopsy sample is excised from the myocardium, withdrawn with the bioptome, and placed in fixative. The bioptome insertion and biopsy are repeated until three to eight samples have been obtained. Following the endomyocardial biopsy, the catheter and sheath are removed, and hemostasis is achieved by appropriate actions of the physician or technician under his or her supervision. A report is prepared by the physician summarizing the procedure.

> **CODING TIP** When endomyocardial biopsy is performed in conjunction with a diagnostic cardiac catheterization, code **93505** should be reported in addition to the component cardiac catheterization codes. However, if the physician performs the cardiac catheterization only as a means of obtaining the endomyocardial biopsy and does not perform a separate diagnostic heart catheterization, then only the endomyocardial biopsy would be reported.

TABLE 5-1. Cardiac Catheterization Table

Effective 2012		CATHETER PLACEMENT TYPE				ADD-ON PROCEDURES (Can Be Reported Separately)					
CPT Code	Code Descriptor	RHC	LHC	Coronary Artery Placement	Bypass Graft(s)	With Transseptal or Transapical Puncture 93462	With Pharmacological Study 93463	With Exercise Study 93464	Injection Procedure for Selective Right Ventricular or Right Atrial Angiography 93566	Injection Procedure for Supravalvular Aortography 93567	Injection Procedure for Pulmonary Angiography 93568
93451	**Right heart catheterization including measurement(s) of oxygen saturation and cardiac output, when performed**	X					X	X	X		X
93452	**Left heart catheterization including intraprocedural injection(s) for left ventriculography, imaging supervision and interpretation, when performed**		X			X	X	X		X	
93453	**Combined right and left heart catheterization including intraprocedural injection(s) for left ventriculography, imaging supervision and interpretation, when performed**	X	X			X	X	X	X	X	X
93454	**Catheter placement in coronary artery(s) for coronary angiography, including intraprocedural injection(s) for coronary angiography, imaging supervision and interpretation;**			X						X	
93455	Catheter placement in coronary artery(s) for coronary angiography, including intraprocedural injection(s) for coronary angiography, imaging supervision and interpretation; **with catheter placement(s) in bypass graft(s) (internal mammary, free arterial venous grafts) including intraprocedural injection(s) for bypass graft angiography**			X	X					X	
93456	Catheter placement in coronary artery(s) for coronary angiography, including intraprocedural injection(s) for coronary angiography, imaging supervision and interpretation; **with right heart catheterization**	X		X			X	X	X	X	X
93457	Catheter placement in coronary artery(s) for coronary angiography, including intraprocedural injection(s) for coronary angiography, imaging supervision and interpretation; **with catheter placement(s) in bypass graft(s) (internal mammary, free arterial, venous grafts) including intraprocedural injection(s) for bypass graft angiography and right heart catheterization**	X		X	X	X	X	X	X	X	X
93458	Catheter placement in coronary artery(s) for coronary angiography, including intraprocedural injection(s) for coronary angiography, imaging supervision and interpretation; **with left heart catheterization including intraprocedural injection(s) for left ventriculography, when performed**		X	X		X	X	X		X	

continued

TABLE 5-1. Cardiac Catheterization Table, *continued*

Effective 2012		CATHETER PLACEMENT TYPE				ADD-ON PROCEDURES (Can Be Reported Separately)					
CPT Code	Code Descriptor	RHC	LHC	Coronary Artery Placement	Bypass Graft(s)	With Transseptal or Transapical Puncture	With Pharmacological Study	With Exercise Study	Injection Procedure for Selective Right Ventricular or Right Atrial Angiography	Injection Procedure for Supravalvular Aortography	Injection Procedure for Pulmonary Angiography
						93462	93463	93464	93566	93567	93568
93459	Catheter placement in coronary artery(s) for coronary angiography, including intraprocedural injection(s) for coronary angiography, imaging supervision and interpretation; **with left heart catheterization including intraprocedural injection(s) for left ventriculography, when performed, catheter placement(s) in bypass graft(s) (internal mammary, free arterial, venous grafts) with bypass graft angiography**		X	X	X	X	X	X		X	X
93460	Catheter placement in coronary artery(s) for coronary angiography, including intraprocedural injection(s) for coronary angiography, imaging supervision and interpretation; **with right and left heart catheterization including intraprocedural injection(s) for left ventriculography, when performed**	X	X	X		X	X	X	X	X	
93461	Catheter placement in coronary artery(s) for coronary angiography, including intraprocedural injection(s) for coronary angiography, imaging supervision and interpretation; **with right and left heart catheterization including intraprocedural injection(s) for left ventriculography, when performed, catheter placement(s) in bypass graft(s) (internal mammary, free arterial, venous grafts) with bypass graft angiography**	X	X	X	X	X	X	X	X	X	

PAYMENT POLICY ALERT Code **93505** was removed from the list of **modifier 51** (Multiple Procedure [multiple surgery reduction]) exempt codes and appears in the CPT code set without the **modifier 51** exempt symbol because it does not meet the **modifier 51** Exemption—Inclusion/Exclusion Criteria approved by the CPT Editorial Panel. (See the rationales in Appendix E of the CPT 2012 codebook.) Because **modifier 51** exempt codes are typically reported with more extensive procedures or services, there should be minimal pre- and postservice time (compared to the intraservice time) and minimal postoperative visits associated with the valuation of these procedures. (Refer to the AMA publication, *Medicare RBRVS: The Physicians Guide 2012*, which is available in March 2012) for definitions of service time and work relative values.) The data obtained from the AMA's RVS Update Committee (RUC) indicated that code **93505** involves significant pre- and postservice time (compared to intraservice time). In addition, code **93505** is currently subjected to the Medicare payment rule for multiple surgery reduction; therefore, **modifier 51** exemption was removed because payment reductions already apply under this rule.

CARDIAC CATHETERIZATION FOR THE PATIENT WITH CONGENITAL HEART DISEASE (⊙**93530-93533**)

The CPT codes most often used by pediatric cardiologists include some that are commonly used by adult cardiologists as well as some that are unique to pediatric cardiology. In the last 16 years, a number of cardiology services codes designed to be used in reporting on the diagnosis and management of patients with congenital heart disease have been created. The code descriptions and related relative value unit (RVU) assignments are primarily based on the care of pediatric patients, but they may be applied to adults whose primary cardiovascular disease is related to congenital heart disease. Many insurance programs, both public (eg, Medicaid) and private, have adopted the relative value scale used by Medicare, necessitating re-evaluation of the RVU assignment for services provided to children as well as adults.

The work relative values in the Resource-Based Relative Value Scale (RBRVS) are intended to reflect the typical patient treated by the typical doctor, based on the premise that while any specific patient may not be typical, such inequities are corrected by the broad experience of an individual physician's practice. Such an assumption creates obvious problems for the physician whose practice does not consist of typical

adults. Therefore, appropriate valuation of the physician work effort involved in providing services for the typical pediatric patient requires different norms. In fact, physician work relative values for many pediatric cardiology services have been demonstrated to be different from corresponding adult values.

⊙**93530** Right heart catheterization, for congenital cardiac anomalies
CPT Assistant Nov 97:45, Jan 98:11, Mar 98:11, Apr 98:3, 6-7; *CPT Changes: An Insider's View* 2008

93531 Combined right heart catheterization and retrograde left heart catheterization, for congenital cardiac anomalies
CPT Assistant Nov 97:45, Jan 98:11, Mar 98:11, Apr 98:8, 10-11; *CPT Changes: An Insider's View* 2008

93532 Combined right heart catheterization and transseptal left heart catheterization through intact septum with or without retrograde left heart catheterization, for congenital cardiac anomalies
CPT Assistant Nov 97:45, Jan 98:11, Mar 98:11, Apr 98:10-11; *CPT Changes: An Insider's View* 2008

93533 Combined right heart catheterization and transseptal left heart catheterization through existing septal opening, with or without retrograde left heart catheterization, for congenital cardiac anomalies
CPT Assistant Nov 97:45, Jan 98:11, Mar 98:11, Apr 98:12-13; *CPT Changes: An Insider's View* 2008

Intent and Use of Codes ⊙93530-93533

Congenital heart diseases are diverse, and their variety and complexity set them apart from acquired heart disease. More young adults with congenital heart disease are surviving into adolescence and young adulthood. However, the vast majority of patients undergoing congenital heart disease catheterization procedures (**93530-93533**) are children, frequently newborns or infants younger than 2 years. The risks and technical skills required are greater in this group due to:

- complexity of the anomalies;

- small patient and vessel size; and

- high frequency of severe hypoxemia, congestive heart failure, and cardiogenic shock.

Congenital heart disease presents a much broader range of anatomic abnormalities than does acquired heart disease. The catheter maneuvers required for the complete range of diagnostic and therapeutic studies are correspondingly more difficult with vessel and valvular misalignment, especially in the small heart. There is, therefore, no "standard" way to catheterize patients with congenital heart disease. For each technique employed, the congenital cardiac catheterization codes may or may not include all of the required maneuvers and selective catheterizations.

Codes **93530-93533** describe cardiac catheterization for congenital cardiac anomalies. While these codes may be used for reporting catheterization of adults with congenital heart disease, the majority of patients undergoing these procedures are within the pediatric age range.

- Code **93530** is used to report right heart catheterization.

- Code **93531** is used to report combined right heart catheterization and retrograde left heart catheterization.

- Code **93532** is used to report combined right heart catheterization and transseptal left heart catheterization through an intact atrial septum, with or without retrograde left heart catheterization.

- Code **93533** is used to report combined right heart catheterization through an existing septal opening, with or without retrograde left heart catheterization.

- Codes **93530-93533** also require additional reporting when injection procedures and radiological supervision and interpretation services are performed.

Injection procedures (**93563-93568**) represent separate identifiable services and may be coded in conjunction with one another when appropriate. The technical details of angiography, supervision of filming and processing, interpretation, and report are included. Therefore, it is not appropriate to report radiology codes **75605, 75625, 75741,** or **75743** to represent the radiological supervision and interpretation and report when performing the services described by add-on codes **93563-93568**. Add-on code **93568** is reported in addition to **93530-93533** and **93451, 93453, 93456, 93460,** and **93461.**

When contrast injection(s) are performed in conjunction with cardiac catheterization for congenital cardiac anomalies (**93530-93533**), see codes **93563-93568.**

When injection procedures are performed in conjunction with cardiac catheterization, these services do not include introduction of catheters but do include repositioning of catheters, when necessary, and use

of automatic power injectors. Injection procedures (**93563-93568**) represent separate identifiable services and may be coded in conjunction with one another when appropriate.

Coding for cardiac catheterizations to evaluate congenital heart disease can be quite complex. If the physician must selectively catheterize other vessels (both venous and/or arterial), in addition to the common catheter insertion routes performed in conjunction with diagnostic cardiac catheterization, these additional selective procedures should be reported in addition to the multiple cardiac catheterization codes required to accurately identify the overall intervention.

Because the cardiac catheterization codes for congenital anomalies may require additional access to other vessels not normally required in normal cardiac anatomy (eg, pulmonary vein, azygous vein), it is appropriate to additionally report selective catheterization codes from the **36000-36248** series and/or their respective radiologic supervision and interpretation codes. (For further information pertaining to the reporting of noncoronary selective/nonselective catheterization reporting at the time of congenital cardiac catheterization, refer to the coding examples provided in this chapter.)

CODING TIP It is not appropriate to report code **37202**, *Transcatheter therapy, infusion for other than thrombolysis,* for intracoronary infusions during cardiac catheterization procedures. Intracoronary administration of pharmacologic agents during percutaneous coronary interventional procedures is considered a routine and integral part of both the diagnostic cardiac catheterization codes **93530-93533, 93451-93453,** and **93456-93461** and the coronary intervention codes **92980-92996.** Code **37202** is intended to be reported for prolonged infusions into peripheral arteries.

Description of Service for Code ⊙93530

The majority of catheter introductions are performed percutaneously into the internal jugular, subclavian, brachial, or femoral venous systems under local anesthesia. Frequently, multiple attempts much be made because of very small vessels and/or venous thrombosis from previous studies. Typically, a venous sheath is placed in a large peripheral vein and the catheter passed through this sheath under fluoroscopic guidance. The catheter is then directed from the venous system into the superior vena cava, right atrium, right ventricle, right and left pulmonary arteries, and pulmonary capillary wedge position. Baseline measurements and blood sampling may be conducted in each of these chambers. Cardiac output is measured using thermodilution or using measured oxygen consumption via the Fick method if intracardiac shunting is suspected. Positioning for angiography may occur in any of the right heart chambers, usually after exchanging a catheter used for physiologic data for an angiographic catheter. After measurement of baseline values, pharmacologic intervention may be performed and the measurements repeated. Supplementary sedation is frequently necessary, especially in younger children. After the conduct of the catheterization proper, the catheter is extracted, and compression hemostasis is achieved, usually by the physician.

After catheterization, a report that includes interpretation of the hemodynamic information and response to intervention is generated, with pulmonary and systemic blood flow, left-to-right and right-to-left shunts, and pulmonary vascular resistances generated. After the patient has left the catheterization laboratory, there usually is at least one physician visit to ascertain clinical stability and satisfactory hemostasis. Typical patients who undergo isolated right heart catheterization are those with simple congenital heart lesions being evaluated preoperatively or postoperative patients in whom significant residual defects may be diagnosed and quantified from a single right heart catheterization. Examples include patients with atrial septal and ventricular septal defects and postoperative tetralogy of Fallot, patients with primary pulmonary hypertension for measurement of pulmonary pressure and resistance to characterize the disease and monitor the prognosis, and patients with end-stage congenital heart disease who are being evaluated for cardiac transplantation.

Description of Service for Code 93531

A venous catheterizaton is performed similar to the described for code **93530**. In addition, an arterial catheter is inserted into the brachial, axillary, or femoral artery. Frequently, multiple attempts will be necessary because of the reduced size of the artery in children and thrombosis from previous catheterization. A separate local anesthetic is often required because the artery may not be near the vein used for venous access. The catheter is directed from the arterial system into the ascending aorta and left ventricle, frequently across stenosis in the vessels or valve. Occasionally, the catheter must be passed across an aortopulmonary shunt (Blalock-Taussig) to gain access to the pulmonary artery. With catheters in both arterial and venous systems, the physiologic measurements including blood sampling for oxygen saturation and pressure recordings in pulmonary wedge, pulmonary artery, right ventricle,

right atrium, and superior vena cava from the venous side and left ventricle ascending aorta and descending aorta from the arterial side are obtained in close proximity, for measurement of left-to-right and right-to-left shunts, cardiac output, gradient across valves, and valve area. Positioning for angiography is performed, sometimes involving several injections and different angles. For many patients, if baseline values are abnormal (eg, showing increased pulmonary vascular resistance), pharmacologic intervention with oxygen, nitric oxide, isoproterenol (Isuprel), or dopamine may be performed with measurements repeated with each of the pharmacologic interventions. Following the conduct of the catheterization, the catheter is extracted and compression hemostasis achieved, either conducted or supervised by the physician.

Description of Service for Code 93532

After completing the right heart catheterization, the catheter is removed and replaced with a venous sheath that is placed in the right atrium against the wall of the left atrium. A long needle is placed through the sheath against the atrial septum and advanced sharply, puncturing the septum. After confirmation of position within the left atrium, the sheath is advanced through the hole and the needle replaced with a physiologic and later an angiographic catheter. After the catheterization is completed, the interpretation of the data and total postprocedure time are similar to code **93531**. The typical person who needs this procedure is someone with complex cyanotic heart disease, with mitral stenosis or atresia, for access to the left ventricle in a child a prosthetic aortic valve in whom retrograde left heart catheterization cannot be performed, for tetralogy of Fallot with pulmonary atresia, for pulmonary venous wedge angiography to outline the hypoplastic pulmonary arteries, or for a child with severe aortic stenosis in whom the valve cannot be crossed in retrograde fashion.

Description of Service for Code 93533

After passing the catheter through the right heart chambers, it is withdrawn to the right atrium, passed posterior into the left atrium and pulmonary veins, and then anterior through the mitral valve into the left ventricle. Occasionally, the catheter is then passed into the aorta. Pressures are measured at each location and blood samples obtained for oxygen level and shunt calculations. The catheter is frequently exchanged for an angiographic catheter and, after positioning the child, one or more angiograms obtained in the different chambers. (See Figure 5-6.)

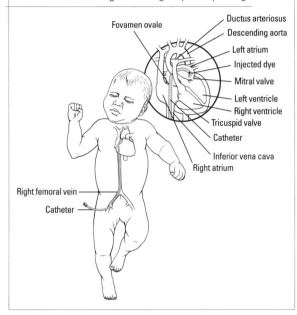

FIGURE 5-6. Right Heart Catheterization and Transseptal Left Heart Catheterization Through Existing Septal Openings

THERMODILUTION STUDY OTHER THAN CARDIAC CATHETERIZATION (⊙▲93561, ⊙▲93562)

⊙▲**93561** Indicator dilution studies such as dye or thermodilution, including arterial and/or venous catheterization; with cardiac output measurement (separate procedure)

CPT Assistant Winter 91:25, Summer 95:2, Aug 00:2, Feb 07:10, Jul 07:1; CPT Changes: An Insider's View 2012

⊙▲**93562** subsequent measurement of cardiac output

CPT Assistant Winter 91:25, Summer 95:2, Aug 00:2, Feb 07:10, Jul 07:1; CPT Changes: An Insider's View 2012

Intent and Use of Codes ⊙▲93561 and ⊙▲93562

Codes **93561** and **93562** are used to report measurement of cardiac output using indicator dilution studies that are performed at any time other than the time of cardiac catheterization. These two codes cannot be used with cardiac catheterization codes because the measurement of cardiac output by dye dilution curves, the Fick method, or any other method, is included in cardiac catheterization codes **93451-93461**. The interpretation, final evaluation, and report are also included in those codes. In addition, codes **93561** and **93562** are not used to report bedside measurements of cardiac output obtained in the intensive care unit.

Code **93561** is the arterial and/or venous catheterization code for cardiac output.

Code **93562** is to be used once code **93561** has been performed and subsequent measurements of cardiac output are performed using indicator dilution studies.

> **CODING TIP** Do not report codes **93561**, **93562** in conjunction with cardiac catheterization codes **93451-93462**.

CARDIAC CATHETERIZATION (NONCONGENITAL AND CONGENITAL) INJECTION PROCEDURES (⊙+93563-⊙+93568)

⊙+**93563** Injection procedure during cardiac catheterization including imaging supervision, interpretation, and report; for selective coronary angiography during congenital heart catheterization (List separately in addition to code for primary procedure)

CPT Changes: An Insider's View 2011

⊙+**93564** for selective opacification of aortocoronary venous or arterial bypass graft(s) (eg, aortocoronary saphenous vein, free radial artery, or free mammary artery graft) to one or more coronary arteries and in situ arterial conduits (eg, internal mammary), whether native or used for bypass to one or more coronary arteries during congenital heart catheterization, when performed (List separately in addition to code for primary procedure)

CPT Changes: An Insider's View 2011

⊙+**93565** for selective left ventricular or left atrial angiography (List separately in addition to code for primary procedure)

CPT Changes: An Insider's View 2011

⊙+**93566** for selective right ventricular or right atrial angiography (List separately in addition to code for primary procedure)

CPT Changes: An Insider's View 2011

⊙+**93567** for supravalvular aortography (List separately in addition to code for primary procedure)

CPT Changes: An Insider's View 2011

⊙+**93568** for pulmonary angiography (List separately in addition to code for primary procedure)

CPT Changes: An Insider's View 2011

Intent and Use of Codes ⊙+93563-⊙+93568

When injection procedures are performed in conjunction with congenital cardiac catheterization, these services do not include introduction of catheters but do include repositioning of catheters, when necessary, and use of automatic power injectors. Injection procedures (93563-93568) represent separate identifiable services and may be coded in conjunction with one another when appropriate.

All injection codes (93563-93568) include radiological supervision and interpretation and report. Therefore, it is not appropriate to report radiology codes 75605, 75625, 75741, or 75743 to represent the radiological supervision and interpretation and report when performing the services described by add-on codes 93563-93568.

Cardiac catheterization codes (93452-93461), other than those for congenital heart disease, include contrast injection(s) for imaging typically performed during these procedures (see Cardiac Catheterization above). Do not report codes 93563-93565 in conjunction with codes 93452-93461.

Coding for cardiac catheterizations to evaluate congenital heart disease can be quite complex. If the physician must selectively catheterize other vessels (both venous and/or arterial), in addition to the common catheter insertion routes performed in conjunction with diagnostic cardiac catheterization, these additional selective procedures should be reported in addition to the multiple cardiac catheterization codes required to accurately identify the overall intervention.

When contrast injection(s) are performed in conjunction with cardiac catheterization for congenital cardiac anomalies (93530-93533), see codes 93563-93568. Injection procedure codes 93563-93568 include imaging supervision, interpretation, and report.

Injection procedures (93563-93568) represent separate identifiable services and may be coded in conjunction with one another when appropriate. The technical details of angiography, supervision of filming and processing, interpretation, and report are included.

> **CODING TIP** It is not appropriate to report code **37202**, *Transcatheter therapy, infusion for other than thrombolysis,* for intracoronary infusions during cardiac catheterization procedures. Intracoronary administration of pharmacologic agents during percutaneous coronary interventional procedures is considered a routine and integral part of both the diagnostic cardiac catheterization codes (**93530-93533, 93451-93453, and 93456-93461**) and the coronary intervention codes (**92980-92996**). Code **37202** is intended to be reported for prolonged infusions into peripheral arteries.

Description of Service for Code ⊙+93563

Codes 93530-93533 include the work of passing a catheter into the aortic root. The work of add-on code 93563 begins when the catheter is manipulated into the ostium of a coronary artery using fluoroscopic guidance. The arterial pressure and waveform are checked to be sure there is no evidence of catheter malposition or impairment of coronary flow due to an ostial stenosis. Test contrast injections under fluoroscopy are performed to check catheter position. Multiple coronary injections are performed, each with the imaging system aligned in a different orientation, with simultaneous panning (moving the table) to assess for stenoses. The catheter is then removed over the wire. Additional catheters are introduced over the guidewire and manipulated into the ostia of other coronary arteries to inject them in multiple views while moving the table in similar fashion. Typically, a separate catheter is used for the left and right coronary arteries. The patient's arterial pressure, electrocardiogram, and oxygen saturation are constantly monitored throughout the procedure. Additional images obtained by coronary angiography are reviewed and are described in the report of the procedure.

Description of Service for Code ⊙+93564

Additional review of original operative report from the previous bypass surgery to identify the exact number, location, and nature of bypass grafts. Codes 93530-93533 include the work of passing a catheter into the aortic root. The work of 93564 begins when the catheter is manipulated, using fluoroscopic guidance, into the ostium of a bypass graft. The arterial pressure and waveform are checked to ensure there is no evidence of catheter malposition or impairment of graft flow because of an ostial stenosis. Test-contrast injections under fluoroscopy are performed to check catheter position. Multiple graft injections are performed, each with the imaging system aligned in a different orientation, with simultaneous panning (moving the table) to assess for stenoses. Engagement of different bypass grafts typically requires differently shaped catheters. Additional catheters are introduced over the guidewire and manipulated into the ostium(a) of other graft(s) to inject them in multiple views, while moving the table in similar fashion. Typically, two or more different catheters are used to engage the aorto-coronary bypass grafts. Catheters are repositioned to engage the in situ arterial conduits. One or more catheters are typically needed to engage the left subclavian artery. Once the catheter is successfully positioned in the left subclavian artery, a wire is directed through it into the distal left subclavian artery and the catheter is advanced over the wire to the level of the internal mammary artery origin. The wire is removed and the catheter is reattached to the injection manifold and meticulously flushed to avoid thrombus or air embolus to the cerebral vessels. The catheter is then manipulated using fluoroscopic guidance to engage the ostium of the left internal mammary artery atraumatically. Typically, the catheter used to enter the left subclavian artery will not engage the internal mammary artery, and the original catheter must be exchanged over the wire for a catheter specially designed to cannulate the internal mammary artery. The arterial pressure and waveform are checked to ensure there is no evidence of catheter malposition or impairment of mammary flow due to an ostial stenosis. Multiple mammary artery injections are performed, each with the imaging system aligned in a different orientation, with simultaneous panning (moving the table) to assess for stenoses. A similar procedure is performed on the right side if a right internal mammary artery graft has been previously placed. The patient's arterial pressure, electrocardiogram, and oxygen saturation are constantly monitored throughout the procedure. Fluoroscopic guidance is used throughout the procedure. Additional images obtained by coronary angiography are reviewed and are described in the report of the procedure.

Additional monitoring related to contrast injection is necessary to detect and treat heart failure symptoms and/or contrast-induced nephropathy.

Description of Service for Code ⊙+93565

Codes **93530-93533** include the work of passing a catheter into the left ventricle. The work of add-on code **93565** begins when the catheter is then attached to a power injector with careful removal of any air from the tubing. Fluoroscopic guidance is used to ensure proper positioning of the catheter. Power injection is then performed to fill the ventricle, allowing examination of systolic function and the competence of the mitral valve in an appropriate angiographic view. The power injector is disconnected from the catheter, the

catheter is reattached to the manifold, and all air is removed. The patient's arterial pressure, electrocardiogram, and oxygen saturation are constantly monitored throughout the procedure. Additional images obtained by coronary angiography are reviewed and are described in the report of the procedure.

Additional monitoring related to contrast injection is necessary to detect and treat heart failure symptoms and/or contrast-induced nephropathy.

Description of Service for Code ⊙+93566

Codes **93530-93533** or codes **93451-93461** include the work of passing a catheter into the right ventricle. The work of add-on code **93566** begins when the catheter is then attached to a power injector with careful removal of any air from the tubing. Fluoroscopic guidance is used to ensure proper positioning of the catheter. Power injection is then performed to fill the ventricle, allowing examination of systolic function and the competence of the tricuspid valve in an appropriate angiographic view. The power injector is disconnected from the catheter, the catheter is reattached to the manifold, and all air is removed. The patient's arterial pressure, electrocardiogram, and oxygen saturation are constantly monitored throughout the procedure. Additional images obtained by coronary angiography are reviewed and are described in the report of the procedure. Additional monitoring related to contrast injection is necessary to detect and treat heart failure symptoms and/or contrast-induced nephropathy.

Description of Service for Code ⊙+93567

Codes **93530-93533** or codes **93451-93461** include the work of passing a catheter into the aorta. The work of add-on code **93567** begins with repositioning of catheter for aortogram. The catheter is then attached to a power injector, with careful removal of any air from the tubing. The catheter is positioned to inject the area of interest. Fluoroscopic guidance is used to ensure proper positioning of the catheter. Power injection is then performed to fill the aorta. The power injector is disconnected from the catheter, and the catheter is reattached to the manifold. The patient's arterial pressure, electrocardiogram, and oxygen saturation are constantly monitored throughout the procedure. Additional images obtained by coronary angiography are reviewed and are described in the report of the procedure.

Additional monitoring related to contrast injection is necessary to detect and treat heart failure symptoms and/or contrast-induced nephropathy.

Description of Service for Code ⊙+93568

Codes **93530-93533** or codes **93451-93461** include the work of passing a catheter into the main pulmonary artery. The work of add-on code **93568** begins when the catheter is then attached to a power injector, with careful removal of any air from the tubing. The catheter is positioned to inject the area of interest. Fluoroscopic guidance is used to ensure proper positioning of the catheter. Power injection is then performed to fill the pulmonary artery. Repositioning of the catheter into the left and right pulmonary arteries is frequently performed with additional power injections at each site. The power injector is disconnected from the catheter, and the catheter is reattached to the manifold. The patient's arterial pressure, electrocardiogram, and oxygen saturation are constantly monitored throughout the procedure. Additional images obtained by coronary angiography are reviewed and are described in the report of the procedure.

Additional monitoring related to contrast injection is necessary to detect and treat heart failure symptoms and/or contrast-induced nephropathy.

PAYMENT POLICY ALERT CMS has recognized that, at times, nonselective study of one or both renal arteries or one or both iliac arteries may be medically indicated at time of cardiac catheterization and/or coronary angiography. The following two codes have been generated by CMS for proper coding of these procedures:

- **Code G0275** is used to report renal artery angiography, nonselective, one or both kidneys, performed at the time of cardiac catheterization and/or coronary angiography. This procedure includes positioning or placement of any catheter in the abdominal aorta at or near the origins (ostia) of the renal arteries, injection of dye, flush aortography, production of permanent images, and radiologic supervision and interpretation. (List each separately in addition to the primary procedure.)

- Code **G0278** is used to report iliac and/or femoral artery angiography, nonselective, bilateral or ipsilateral to catheter insertion. This procedure is performed at the same time as cardiac catheterization and/or coronary angiography, includes positioning or placement of the catheter in the distal aorta or ipsilateral femoral or iliac artery, injection of dye, production of permanent images, and radiologic supervision and interpretation. (List each separately in addition to primary procedure.)

CPT codes should be utilized if a selective study is performed. In this case, documentation of the complete findings in a formal report is required. For example, if bilateral selective renal angiography is performed at the time of cardiac catheterization, codes **36252 LT** and **36252 RT** should be reported.

In addition, concern has been expressed by CMS about inappropriate utilization of renal angiography at the time of cardiac catheterization procedures. It is essential to document the indication for performing the procedure as well as the findings in the medical record. Practitioners who perform renal angiography in a substantial proportion of catheterization patients without documentation of medical necessity may be subject to medical review audits.

CODING EXAMPLES: PERIPHERAL ARTERIAL PROCEDURES AND CARDIAC CATHETERIZATION PROCEDURES

EXAMPLE 1: The right femoral artery is entered, and a catheter is advanced to the left ventricle. An injection of contrast is made in the left ventricle. The ventricular catheter is withdrawn and exchanged for a coronary catheter, and selective angiograms are made of the right coronary artery and the left coronary arteries. The coronary catheter is withdrawn and exchanged for a catheter that is positioned in the left renal artery for injection of contrast; this catheter is then repositioned in the right renal artery, and a contrast injection is made for the right renal angiogram. The catheter is removed, and hemostasis is achieved.

Coding Solution (Non-Medicare Patient): Use the following codes to report the procedures performed:

⊙**93458** Catheter placement in coronary artery(s) for coronary angiography, including intraprocedural injection(s) for coronary angiography, imaging supervision and interpretation; with left heart catheterization including intraprocedural injection(s) for left entriculography, when performed

⊙●**36252** Selective catheter placement (first-order), main renal artery and any accessory renal artery(s) for renal angiography, including arterial puncture and catheter placement(s), fluoroscopy, contrast injection(s), image postprocessing, permanent recording of images, and radiologic supervision and interpretation, including pressure gradient measurements when performed, and flush aortogram when performed; bilateral

Coding Solution (Medicare Patient): Use the following codes to report the procedures performed:

⊙**93458** Catheter placement in coronary artery(s) for coronary angiography, including intraprocedural injection(s) for coronary angiography, imaging supervision and interpretation; with left heart catheterization including intraprocedural injection(s) for left entriculography, when performed

⊙●**36252** Selective catheter placement (first-order), main renal artery and any accessory renal artery(s) for renal angiography, including arterial puncture and catheter placement(s), fluoroscopy, contrast injection(s), image postprocessing, permanent recording of images, and radiologic supervision and interpretation, including pressure gradient measurements when performed, and flush aortogram when performed; bilateral

Rationale: Per CMS, CPT codes should be utilized if a selective study is performed. In Example 1, HCPCS Level II code **G0275** is not reported because a "selective" catheterization of the right renal artery was performed.

PAYMENT POLICY ALERT CMS required the use of G codes for iliac angiograms and renal angiograms performed at the time of cardiac catheterization for Medicare patients.

Initially, these codes were mandated for both selective and nonselective injection of bilateral renal arteries at the time of catheterization; however, this has been modified and clarified to include only nonselective catheter placement with aortography at the level of the renal and iliac arteries. Selective renal angiography performed at the time of cardiac catheterization should be recorded in the standard way (see Example 1). If selective renal angiography is performed at the time of diagnostic catheterization, the indications for it should be carefully documented.

For nonselective catheter placement and aortography with nonselective renal artery angiography at the time of cardiac catheterization, code **G0275** should be used. Code **G0275** should be used as an add-on code to report nonselective renal angiography performed at the time of cardiac catheterization. This includes the catheter placement at the level of the renal artery, injection of dye, aortogram, radiologic supervision and interpretation, and production of images.

For iliac angiography performed at the time of cardiac catheterization to assess for hemostatic closure devices, code **G0278** should be used as an add-on code. This reports the iliac artery angiography performed at the time of cardiac catheterization, including the catheter placement in the iliac artery, injection of dye, radiologic supervision and interpretation, and production of images.

EXAMPLE 2: The right brachial artery is entered, and a coronary catheter is advanced to the aortic root. Selective angiograms are made of the right coronary artery and the left coronary arteries. The coronary catheter is withdrawn and exchanged for a catheter that is then positioned in the infrarenal aorta for injection of contrast for aortography and bilateral iliofemoral angiograms with runoff films. The catheter is removed, and hemostasis is achieved.

Coding Solution (Non-Medicare Patient): Use the following codes to report the procedures performed:

⊙**93454** Catheter placement in coronary artery(s) for coronary angiography, including intraprocedural injection(s) for coronary angiography, imaging supervision and interpretation;

75630 Aortography, abdominal plus bilateral lower extremity, catheter, by serialography, radiological supervision and interpretation

Coding Solution (Medicare Patient): Use the following codes to report the procedures performed:

⊙**93454** Catheter placement in coronary artery(s) for coronary angiography, including intraprocedural injection(s) for coronary angiography, imaging supervision and interpretation;

G0278 Iliac and/or femoral artery angiography, non-selective, bilateral or ipsilateral to catheter insertion, performed at the same time as cardiac catheterization and/or coronary angiography, includes positioning or placement of the catheter in the distal aorta or ipsilateral femoral or iliac artery, injection of dye, production of permanent images, and radiologic supervision and interpretation (List separately in addition to primary procedure)

Rationale: HCPCS Level II code **G0278** is not reported, since a "nonselective" catheterization was performed for the bilateral iliofemoral angiography with runoff. **G0278** is reported for iliac artery angiography performed at the time of cardiac catheterization, including the catheter placement in the iliac artery, injection of dye, radiologic supervision and interpretation, and production of images.

EXAMPLE 3: A 45-year-old male is seen in the emergency department with severe substernal chest pain. The ECG confirms acute inferior wall myocardial infarction (MI). Emergency cardiac catheterization is performed to define left heart hemodynamics; left ventriculography and coronary angiography are performed. The results of the study reveal total occlusion of the right coronary artery and severe occlusion of the LMCA. The patient is sent for emergency aortocoronary bypass. Prior to surgery, a Swan-Ganz catheter is inserted via the left subclavian vein, and an intra-aortic balloon catheter is inserted into the descending aorta.

Coding Solution (Medicare or Non-Medicare Patient): Use the following codes to report the procedures performed:

⊙**93458**	Catheter placement in coronary artery(s) for coronary angiography, including intraprocedural injection(s) for coronary angiography, imaging supervision and interpretation; with left heart catheterization including intraprocedural injection(s) for left ventriculography, when performed

93503 59	Insertion and placement of flow directed catheter (eg, Swan-Ganz) for monitoring purposes

33967 59	Insertion of intra-aortic balloon assist device, percutaneous

The patient has successful surgery—a quadruple bypass, performed using the left internal mammary artery and three saphenous vein grafts—and leaves the hospital. Two years later, the patient presents with chest pain, pulmonary edema, and acute anterior myocardial infarction. After initial stabilization, right and left heart catheterization is performed. Angiograms include left ventriculography, supravalvular aortography, coronary angiography, and opacification of all bypass conduits. The additional services are reported as follows:

Coding Solution (Medicare or Non-Medicare Patient): Use the following codes to report the procedures performed:

⊙**93461**	Catheter placement in coronary artery(s) for coronary angiography, including intraprocedural injection(s) for coronary angiography, imaging supervision and interpretation; with right and left heart catheterization including intraprocedural injection(s) for left ventriculography,when performed, catheter placement(s) in bypass graft(s) (internal mammary, free arterial, venous grafts) with bypass graft angiography

⊙+**93567**	Injection procedure during cardiac catheterization includeing imaging supervision, interpretation, and report; for supravalvular aortography (List separately in addition to code for primary procedure)

> **PAYMENT POLICY ALERT** CPT codes **01920, 01924, 01925,** and **01926** are used to describe anesthesia services for catheterization and therapeutic interventional radiologic procedures. However, Medicare payment rules state that these codes are reimbursable only when a different physician (eg, an anesthesiologist or another cardiologist) is present and actively managing the patient's anesthesia care. CMS payment policy specifically excludes separate payment for anesthesia care during routine coronary interventions. (Refer to Appendix G for discussion of coding for moderate sedation.)

EXAMPLE 4: Left heart catheterization from femoral artery; coronary angiography; descending aorta arteriography to visualize renal arteries.

Coding Solution (Non-Medicare Patient): Use the following codes to report the procedures performed:

⊙**93458**	Catheter placement in coronary artery(s) for coronary angiography, including intraprocedural injection (s) for coronary angiography, imaging supervision and interpretation; with left heart catheterization including intraprocedural injection(s) for left ventriculography, when performed

75625	Aortography, abdominal, radiological supervision and interpretation

Coding Solution (Medicare Patient): Use the following codes to report the procedures performed:

⊙**93458**	Catheter placement in coronary artery(s) for coronary angiography, including intraprocedural injection (s) for coronary angiography, imaging supervision and interpretation; with left heart catheterization including intraprocedural injection(s) for left ventriculography, when performed

G0275	Renal angiography, non-selective, one or both kidneys, performed at the same time as cardiac catheterization and/or coronary angiography, includes positioning or placement of any catheter in the abdominal aorta at or near the origins (ostia) of the renal arteries, injection of dye, flush aortogram, production of permanent images, and radiologic supervision and interpretation (list separately in addition to primary procedure)

Rationale: Code **G0275** should be used as an add-on code to report nonselective renal angiography performed at the time of cardiac catheterization. This includes the catheter placement at the level of the renal artery, injection of dye, aortogram, radiologic supervision and interpretation, and production of images.

PAYMENT POLICY ALERT When peripheral angiography is reported together with cardiac angiography, Medicare carriers will invoke the "multiple surgical procedures" rule, in which the highest valued surgical procedure code is reimbursed at 100%, while each additional surgical code is reimbursed at 50%. Imaging codes are not affected by the "multiple surgical procedures" rule.

EXAMPLE 5: The right femoral artery is entered, and a catheter is advanced to the left ventricle. An injection of contrast is made in the left ventricle. The ventricular catheter is withdrawn and exchanged for a coronary catheter, and selective angiograms are made of the right coronary artery and the left coronary arteries. The coronary catheter is withdrawn and exchanged for a catheter that is positioned in the left iliac artery. This catheter is then exchanged for a balloon catheter for angioplasty of the iliac artery. After angiographic evaluation of the angioplasty result, a stent is placed in the dilated segment of the iliac artery. The catheter is removed, and hemostasis is achieved.

Coding Solution (Medicare and Non-Medicare Patients): Use the following codes to report the procedures performed:

⊙**93458** Catheter placement in coronary artery(s) for coronary angiography, including intraprocedural injection(s) for coronary angiography, imaging supervision and interpretation; with left heart catheterization including intraprocedural injection(s) for left ventriculography, when performed

⊙**37221** Revascularization, endovascular, open or percutaneous, iliac artery, unilateral, initial vessel; with transluminal stent placement(s), includees angioplasty within same vessel, when performed

Rationale: The work of accessing and selectively catheterizing the left iliac artery and traversing the lesion is considered an inclusive service of code **37221**. Therefore, code **36245** should not be reported in addition to code **37221**. The radiological supervision and interpretation directly related

to the intervention(s) performed and imaging performed to document completion of the intervention in addition to the intervention(s), are also inclusive services.

PAYMENT POLICY ALERT Modifier application may vary by payer. For Medicare, **modifier 26** is used for codes with a technical component–professional component (TC/PC) split, if the service is performed in the facility setting. (Refer to Chapter 6 and Appendix B for further information regarding the use of the HCPCS Level II **TC modifier** and CPT **modifier 26**.)

CODING TIP More information on coding for peripheral vascular procedures can be obtained by ordering the Interventional Radiology Coding Users' Guide from the Society of Interventional Radiology at (888) 695-9733 or online at www.sirweb.org.

CODING EXAMPLES: CONGENITAL CARDIAC CATHETERIZATION PROCEDURES

EXAMPLE 1: A 23-year-old female with a history of cyanotic congenital heart disease; postoperative modified Fontan operation for repair of double outlet right ventricle or single ventricle with severe valvular pulmonary stenosis; single atria-ventricular valve with prolapse and minimal insufficiency; anomalous systemic venous drainage with absent hepatic segment of left inferior vena cava with drainage through an azygous to left superior vena cava; right-sided aortic arch; mesoversion, probable polysplenia syndrome; postoperative cardiac arrest; postoperative systemic venous hypertension with peripheral hypoxia; arrhythmias. The following procedures were performed:

- right heart catheterization;
- percutaneous catheterization of the left jugular vein;
- selective biplane cineangiocardiograms to the inferior vena cava, azygous vein, right pulmonary artery, left superior vena cava, right femoral vein; and
- intra-arterial line placement for monitoring.

This adult patient had anomalous left and right inferior vena cavi and left and right superior vena cavi, thus requiring separate catheter accesses to these structures and other venous routes (ie, jugular and azygous veins to reach the right pulmonary artery, which is ordinarily reached through the right ventricle). The left inferior vena cava did not reach to the thorax. The left superior vena cava was previously anastomosed to the left pulmonary artery. This patient also had prior repair for a single ventricle. (The patient had only one ventricle.) Therefore, access route coding ordinarily considered part of attaining the final destination, required selective catheterization, and warranted additional reporting of certain **36000** and **70000** series codes.

Coding Solution: Use the following codes to report the procedure performed:

⊙**93530 26** Right heart catheterization, for congenital cardiac anomalies

36010 26 Introduction of catheter, superior or inferior vena cava

Rationale: This is reported for the selective catheterization of the left inferior vena cava.

36010 26 59 Introduction of catheter, superior or inferior vena cava

Rationale: This is reported for the selective catheterization of the left superior vena cava.

36011 26 Selective catheter placement, venous system; first order branch (eg, renal vein, jugular vein)

Rationale: This is reported for the selective catheterization of the azygous vein.

36014 26 Selective catheter placement, left or right pulmonary artery

Rationale: The left and right pulmonary arteries were not accessible from the ventricle (ie, right heart catheter).

36620 26 Arterial catheterization or cannulation for sampling, monitoring or transfusion (separate procedure); percutaneous

Rationale: A right radial artery line was established during this intervention and was not used as an access route. Therefore, additional reporting of this procedure is warranted.

75743 26 Angiography, pulmonary, bilateral, selective, radiological supervision and interpretation

Rationale: This should be reported in addition, provided the interventionalist performed the supervision of filming, interpretation of all necessary filming, and written report.

75825 26 Venography, caval inferior, with serialography, radiological supervision and interpretation

Rationale: This should be reported in addition, provided the interventionalist performed the

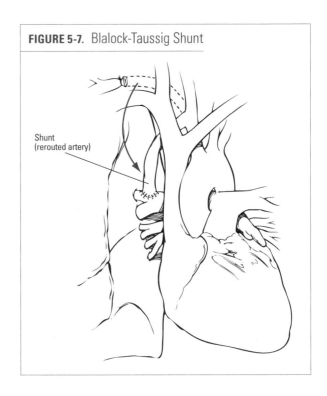

FIGURE 5-7. Blalock-Taussig Shunt

Shunt (rerouted artery)

supervision of filming, interpretation of all necessary filming, and written report.

75827 26 Venography, caval, superior, with serialography, radiological supervision and interpretation

Rationale: This should be reported in addition, provided the interventionalist performed the supervision of filming, interpretation of all necessary filming, and written report.

EXAMPLE 2: A 14-month-old male with cyanotic congenital heart disease; double inlet single ventricle; infundibular, valvular, supravalvular pulmonary stenosis; postoperative modified right Blalock-Taussig shunt functioning. (See Figure 5-7.) The following procedures were performed:

- right heart catheterization;
- left heart catheterization; and
- selective biplane cineangiocardiograms to the innominate artery and ventricle and pulmonary artery (via the Blalock-Taussig shunt).

In this procedure, the left atrium could not be entered from the right atrium. The pulmonary artery could not be entered from the right ventricle) and pulmonary artery (via the Blalock-Taussig shunt).

Coding Solution: Use the following codes to report the procedure performed:

FIGURE 5-8. Types of Ventricular Septal Defects

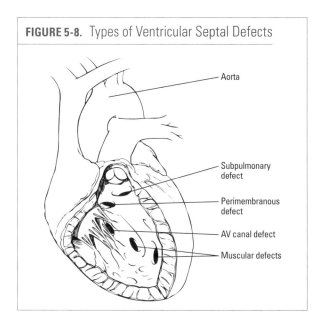

Aorta

Subpulmonary defect

Perimembranous defect

AV canal defect

Muscular defects

FIGURE 5-9. Shunting of Blood With a Ventricular Septal Defect

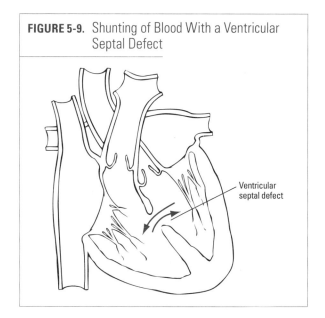

Ventricular septal defect

93531 Combined right heart catheterization and retrograde left heart catheterization, for congenital cardiac anomalies

⊙**+93565** Injection procedure during cardiac catheterization including imaging supervision, interpretation, and report; for selective left ventricular or left atrial angiography (List separately in addition to code for primary procedure)

Rationale: This is reported for left ventriculography.

⊙**+93568** Injection procedure during cardiac catheterization including imaging supervision, interpretation, and report; for pulmonary angiography (List separately in addition to code for primary procedure)

Rationale: This is reported for the injection procedures related to the Blalock-Taussig shunt and the right and left pulmonary arteries.

36215 26 Selective catheter placement, arterial system; each first order thoracic or brachiocephalic branch, within a vascular family

Rationale: This is reported for the selective catheterization of the innominate artery and the injection procedure. This is not an inclusive component of the common approach to the right and left heart, as identified by code **93453**. An additional selective catheterization procedure was performed in addition to the diagnostic cardiac catheterization procedure and should be individually reported.

75650 26 Angiography, cervicocerebral, catheter, including vessel origin, radiological supervision and interpretation

Rationale: The documentation indicated that the radiological supervision and interpretation was also performed, therefore code **75650** should be reported in addition to code **36215 26**.

EXAMPLE 3: A 10-year-old male with multiple left-sided obstructive lesions (Shone's syndrome) including mitral stenosis, coarctation of the aorta, a bicuspid aortic valve, and a ventricular septal defect with repair of his coarctation of the aorta. At 2 years old, due to the appearance of pulmonary edema, he underwent resection of a supra valvar mitral ring and closure of a membranous ventricular septal defect. Because of a recurrence of congestive heart failure and failure to thrive with suggestive evidence of pulmonary artery hypertension, he underwent this cardiac catheterization to evaluate the success of repair of ventricular septal defect and severity of residual mitral stenosis and coarctation. The following procedures were performed:

- right heart catheterization;
- left heart catheterization; and
- selective biplane cineangiocardiograms to the left and right atria, left ventricle, root of aorta, and pulmonary artery.

Coding Solution: Use the following codes to report the procedure performed:

93532 Combined right heart catheterization and transseptal left heart catheterization through intact septum with or without retrograde left heart catheterization, for congenital cardiac anomalies

FIGURE 5-10. Patent Ductus Arteriosus

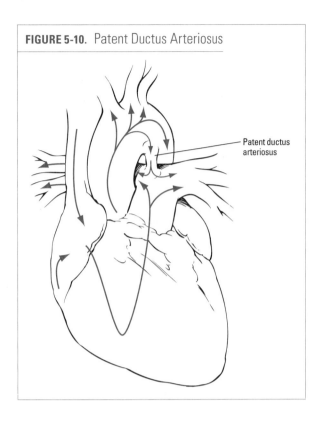

Patent ductus
arteriosus

FIGURE 5-11. Types of Atrial Septal Defects

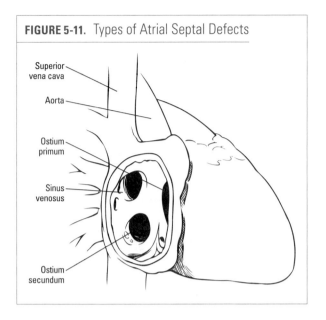

Superior
vena cava

Aorta

Ostium
primum

Sinus
venosus

Ostium
secundum

⊙**+93568** Injection procedure during cardiac
catheterization including imaging supervision,
interpretation, and report; for pulmonary
angiography (List separately in addition to code
for primary procedure)

⊙**+93565** Injection procedure during cardiac
catheterization including imaging supervision,
interpretation, and report; for selective
left ventricular or left atrial angiography
(List separately in addition to code for
primary procedure)

Rationale: This is reported for left atrial
angiography.

⊙**+93565** Injection procedure during cardiac
catheterization including imaging supervision,
interpretation, and report; for selective
left ventricular or left atrial angiography
(List separately in addition to code for
primary procedure)

Rationale: This is reported for left ventriculography.

⊙**93566** Injection procedure during cardiac
catheterization including imaging supervision,
interpretation, and report; for selective
right ventricular or right atrial angiography
(List separately in addition to code for
primary procedure)

Rationale: This is reported for right atrial
angiography.

⊙**+93567** Injection procedure during cardiac
catheterization including imaging supervision,
interpretation, and report; for supravalvular
aortography (List separately in addition to code
for primary procedure)

EXAMPLE 4: A 3-day-old female with cyanotic congenital heart disease; tricuspid atresia; atrial septal
defect; ventricular septal defect; and patent ductus
arteriosus. The following procedures were performed:

- right heart catheterization;

- left heart catheterization; and

- selective biplane cineangiocardiograms to the
main pulmonary artery, left ventricle, superior
vena cava, and umbilical artery catheter.

Coding Solution: Use the following codes to report
the procedure performed:

93533 26 Combined right heart catheterization and
transseptal left heart catheterization through
existing septal opening, with or without
retrograde left heart catheterization, for
congenital cardiac anomalies

36010 26 Introduction of catheter, superior or inferior
vena cava

Rationale: This is reported as this patient had
an anomalous left superior vena cava in addition
to the superior vena cava. Therefore, this represents an additional selective catheterization and
injection procedure, not included in the cardiac
catheterization procedure.

FIGURE 5-12. Shunting of Blood with an Atrial Septal Defect

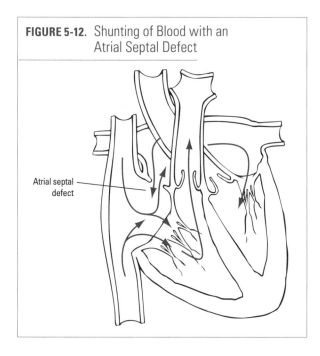

FIGURE 5-13. Intravascular Distal Blood Flow Velocity

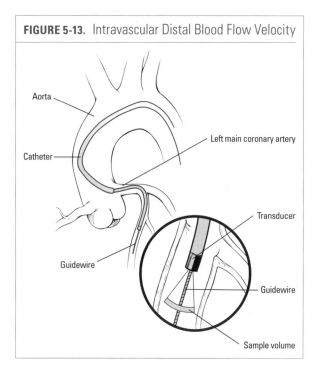

75827 26 Venography, caval, superior, with serialography, radiological supervision and interpretation

Rationale: This code should be reported in addition to code **36010 26**, provided the interventionalist performed the supervision of filming, interpretation of all necessary filming, and written report.

⊙**+93567** Injection procedure during cardiac catheterization including imaging supervision, interpretation, and report; for supravalvular aortography (List separately in addition to code for primary procedure)

Rationale: This is reported for the injection procedure for aortography, which was additionally performed demonstrating this patient had a normal-size aorta taking off from the left ventricle with a left-sided aortic arch and left descending aorta.

Right atrial or ventricular angiography was not reported due to the inability to access the right atrium/right ventricle. The catheter could not be advanced to the right atrium and the right ventricle en route to the pulmonary artery. Instead, the catheter was advanced through the left atrium through an intra-atrial communication to the left ventricle; and, in an antegrade manner, through a ventricular septal defect into the main pulmonary artery.

⊙**+93565** Injection procedure during cardiac catheterization including imaging supervision, interpretation, and report; for selective left ventricular or left atrial angiography (List separately in addition to code for primary procedure)

Rationale: The previously placed umbilical artery catheter was replaced with an angiographic catheter and used for injection of contrast and visualization of the ascending aorta and pulmonary arteries. No additional reporting is warranted. The ascending aorta filming is not reported individually. The aortography is reported with code **93567**. The pulmonary arteriography is reported with code **93568**.

⊙**+93568** Injection procedure during cardiac catheterization including imaging supervision, interpretation, and report; for pulmonary angiography (List separately in addition to code for primary procedure)

INTRAVASCULAR DOPPLER VELOCITY AND/OR PRESSURE-DERIVED CORONARY FLOW RESERVE MEASUREMENT (**+93571**, **+93572**)

⊙**+93571** Intravascular Doppler velocity and/or pressure derived coronary flow reserve measurement (coronary vessel or graft) during coronary angiography including pharmacologically induced stress; initial vessel (List separately in addition to code for primary procedure)
CPT Assistant Nov 98:33, Apr 00:2, Mar 08:4

⊙**+93572** each additional vessel (List separately in addition to code for primary procedure)
CPT Assistant Nov 98:34, Apr 00:2

Intent and Use of Codes ⊙+93571 and ⊙+93572

Codes **93571** and **93572** are add-on codes used to report intravascular Doppler velocity and/or pressure-derived coronary flow reserve measurement during coronary angiography for coronary vessels or grafts. These codes include pharmacologically induced stress. All Doppler transducer manipulations and repositioning within the specific vessel being examined during coronary angiography or therapeutic intervention are included as well. Velocity measurement of additional vessels in the same session is reported using the "each additional vessel" code **93572**.

CPT guidelines instruct that intravascular distal coronary blood flow velocity measurements include all Doppler transducer manipulations and repositioning within the specific vessel being examined during coronary angiography or therapeutic intervention (eg, angioplasty).

Description of Service for Code ⊙+93571

Intravascular Doppler velocity and/or pressure-derived coronary flow reserve measurement are performed during coronary angiography or intervention. A specialized guidewire with a miniaturized Doppler or pressure transducer mounted in the distal tip is advanced through the diagnostic or guiding catheter and positioned 2 to 3 cm distal to the coronary lesion in question. The wire is manipulated until a stable signal is obtained (as seen on the console to which the Doppler guide is attached). Baseline blood flow velocity or pressure is recorded. A pharmacological stress agent such as adenosine is given by intracoronary bolus to induce hyperemia. Over the hyperemic period, coronary pressure will decrease and then return to normal, and the velocity of the blood in the coronary arteries will increase and then return to baseline. Comparison of the hyperemic and baseline measurements indicates the extent to which the lesion is limiting blood flow. The Doppler guidewire is then withdrawn.

CATHETER CLOSURE OF ATRIAL SEPTAL DEFECT/VENTRICULAR SEPTAL DEFECT (**93580, 93581**)

93580   Percutaneous transcatheter closure of congenital interatrial communication (ie, Fontan fenestration, atrial septal defect) with implant
CPT Assistant Mar 03:23; *CPT Changes: An Insider's View* 2003

93581   Percutaneous transcatheter closure of a congenital ventricular septal defect with implant
CPT Assistant Mar 03:23, Mar 08:4; *CPT Changes: An Insider's View* 2003

Intent and Use of Codes 93580 and 93581

Code **93580** describes percutaneous transcatheter closure of a congenital interatrial communication (ie, Fontan fenestration, atrial septal defect). This may describe closure of a patent foramen ovale. Code **93581** describes percutaneous transcatheter closure of congenital ventricular septal defects. These codes are not intended for postmyocardial infarction septal defects but are intended for reporting the repair of congenital defects. Patients range from infants to adults. The physician work is comparable whether the patient is an infant or an adult.

As indicated in the CPT guidelines, percutaneous transcatheter closure of atrial septal defect includes a right heart catheterization procedure. Code **93580** includes injection of contrast for atrial and ventricular angiograms. Codes **93451-93453, 93455-93461, 93530-93533,** and **93564-93566** should not be reported separately in addition to code **93580**.

If transthoracic echocardiography (TTE), transesophageal echocardiography (TEE), or intracardiac echocardiography (ICE) is used as part of the procedure, codes **93303-93317** and code **93662** should be reported separately.

Description of Service for Code 93580

TEE or ICE may be required (separately reported). General anesthesia (separately reported) is commonly used when TEE is required; otherwise conscious sedation is usually employed. The patient is heparinized, and the activated clotting time (ACT) is maintained throughout the case. Prophylactic antibiotics are given. A combined right heart catheterization and left heart catheterization through existing septal opening including angiography is performed to delineate the anatomy and physiology.

Using an end-hole catheter, wedge, or preformed catheter such as a multipurpose catheter, the atrial defect is crossed from the right to left atrium. The catheter is then advanced into the left upper pulmonary vein. This catheter is exchanged for a sizing balloon over a guidewire. The balloon is positioned across the defect and inflated at low pressure to measure the "stretched" diameter. The device size is based on this measurement. In patients with fenestrated Fontans, and in some with right-to-left shunts through the atrial defect, right-sided pressures and saturations are re-measured while temporarily balloon occluding the defect to ensure that device closure will be hemodynamically tolerated.

A long sheath and dilator are then advanced over the wire and positioned in the left atrium. The device is then deployed across the atrial opening. The position of the device must be evaluated by echocardiography and fluoroscopy prior to release. If the device is in good position, the release mechanism is activated and the device position checked again. Abnormal placement or an inappropriate-sized device may have to be removed if there is a large leak, potential encroachment on cardiac structures, or risk of embolization, and a second device is placed.

After device position is confirmed using TEE or angiography, the catheters and sheaths are removed, and hemostasis is achieved.

Description of Service for Code 93581

The ventricular septal defect (VSD) closure is performed using general anesthesia (separately reported). TEE or ICE may be performed. The patient is prepared and draped.

Percutaneous access is obtained in the femoral vein and artery, and sheaths are placed. The patient is heparinized, and the activated clotting time (ACT) is maintained throughout the case. Prophylactic antibiotics are given.

Depending on the location of the VSD, additional venous access will be required in the other femoral vein or the internal jugular vein. A right and left heart catheterization, including angiography, is performed to define the anatomy and physiology of the defect(s).

Device closure of VSDs involves crossing the VSD, sizing the defect, and then delivering the device. Multiple options to cross the defect are available and depend on the anatomy and location of the defect. Usually the VSD is crossed from left to right ventricle rather than right to left from the trabeculated right ventricle. From the left ventricle, the VSD can be crossed using a retrograde approach from the femoral artery or antegrade using the catheter in the femoral vein. The latter is accomplished by performing a transseptal (atrial septum) puncture (Brockenbrough) to enter the left atrium. The catheter is then passed from the left atrium to the left ventricle. The VSD can be crossed using a flow-directed, balloon-tipped wedge catheter or, more commonly, preformed catheters are used to aim a guidewire, which is then advanced through the defect into the right ventricle and then into a pulmonary artery or retrograde through the tricuspid valve in the right atrium. This wire is then snared from the venous side. The venous site from which the wire is snared will depend on how one intends to deliver the device.

Devices are occasionally delivered retrograde from an artery. Mid- and apical-muscular defects are most easily closed using the internal jugular vein. Anterior muscular defects and residual membranous and cono-ventricular defects are most easily closed from the femoral vein. At the completion of this stage, there is an exchange-length guidewire entering the body at one site, passing through the VSD, and exiting the body at another site.

An angiographic catheter is passed over the wire for selective contrast injections in the defect to define the commonly complex anatomy. Following this, a balloon-tipped catheter (over the wire) is pulled through or inflated in the defect to determine the "stretched" diameter. With this information, the appropriate device can be chosen. A long sheath and dilator are advanced over the guidewire and positioned across the VSD. The guidewire and dilator are removed, and the device is delivered. Angiography, using a retrograde left ventricular catheter, is performed during delivery to ensure correct positioning of the device. Following delivery, angiography is performed to confirm device position, and hemodynamics are repeated to determine residual shunting.

If there is a large leak, potential encroachment on cardiac structures, or risk of embolization, the device may have to be removed and a second device placed. Occasionally (10- to 15% of the time), multiple devices must be placed to close separate muscular defects that cannot be covered with a single device.

Intracardiac Electrophysiological Procedures/Studies

In an intracardiac electrophysiology study, several electrode catheters are positioned in various areas of the heart.

The heart's normal conduction pattern can be disrupted by different causes. In both pediatric and adult patients, abnormal electrical activity can occur at single or multiple sites along the cardiac conduction system. Depending upon the location(s) of the abnormality, certain rhythm disorders may place the patient at risk for future cardiac events, even sudden cardiac death. The diagnosis, treatment, and continued assessment of cardiac rhythm disorders can be very complex. New therapeutic approaches and specific noninvasive and invasive procedures assist in the diagnosis and management of cardiovascular disease.

Because there are many types of rhythm abnormalities that can occur singly or in combination along the cardiac conduction system, rhythm patterns may be chaotic, episodic, and/or have very different electrical tracings. At times it is difficult to detect and document the event(s) during other diagnostic studies (eg, ECG, ambulatory electrocardiography monitoring, cardiovascular stress testing [**93015-93018, 93303-93308, 93320-93325, 93350-93352**]).

Electrophysiological studies are viewed as supplements to the analysis of standard ECG studies, which, in most patients, are adequate for diagnosis and clinical decisions. (For additional information pertaining to ECG recordings, refer to the discussions about codes **93000-93010** and **93040-93052** earlier in this chapter.) Because the intracardiacelectrophysiology catheter is placed closer to the cardiac conduction system than external or esophageal electrodes, electrophysiology studies may provide important insights into many other conduction disturbances, especially those related to significant symptoms.

Codes **93600-93652** reflect electrophysiologic procedures performed for diagnostic and/or therapeutic purposes. Intracardiac electrophysiology study(s) include systematic intracardiac assessment of the heart's electrical event timing in various locations during rest and after a stimulated (induced) state. Recorded responses reveal the type, site, origin, and activity path of various cardiac conduction and rhythm disturbances. In addition to the induction of arrhythmias and their response to pharmacotherapy or device therapy, electrophysiologic studies are used in the diagnosis and treatment of life-threatening and non–life-threatening cardiac arrhythmias. Therefore, electrophysiology studies offer a wealth of information about the heart's electrical activity to:

- investigate the patient's sinus node, AV conduction, and tachyarrhythmias;

- locate the origin of dangerous arrhythmias;

- evaluate the effect of antiarrhythmic drugs;

- assess supraventricular tachycardia, ventricular tachycardia, and AV conduction disorders (heart block);

- evaluate the effectiveness of drug therapy or an automatic implantable cardioverter-defibrillator; and

- perform a radio frequency ablation to destroy accessory conduction pathways or other sites of abnormal electrical activity that cause tachycardias.

According to CPT guidelines, intracardiac electrophysiologic studies are an invasive diagnostic medical procedure that include the insertion and repositioning of electrode catheters, recording of electrograms before and during pacing or programmed stimulation of multiple locations in the heart, analysis of recorded information, and report of the procedure.

Electrophysiologic studies are most often performed with two or more electrode catheters. In many circumstances, patients with arrhythmias are evaluated and treated at the same encounter. In this situation, a diagnostic electrophysiologic study is performed, induced tachycardia(s) are mapped, and on the basis of the diagnostic and mapping information, the tissue is ablated. Electrophysiologic study(ies), mapping, and ablation represent distinctly different procedures, requiring individual reporting whether performed on the same or subsequent dates. CPT guidelines provide the following definitions and usage.

Arrhythmia induction: In most electrophysiologic studies, an attempt is made to induce arrhythmia(s) from single or multiple sites within the heart. Arrhythmia induction is achieved by performing pacing at different rates, programmed stimulation (introduction of critically timed electrical impulses), and other techniques. Because arrhythmia induction occurs via the same catheter(s) inserted for the electrophysiologic study(ies), catheter insertion and temporary pacemaker codes are not additionally reported.

Code **93619** describes only evaluation of the sinus node, AV node, and His-Purkinje conduction system, without arrhythmia induction.

Codes **93620-93624** and **93640-93642** all include recording, pacing, and attempted arrhythmia induction from one or more site(s) in the heart.

Mapping: Mapping is a distinct procedure performed in addition to a diagnostic electrophysiologic procedure and should be separately reported using code **93609** or **93613**. Do not report standard mapping (**93609**) in addition to three-dimensional mapping (**93613**). When a tachycardia is induced, the site of tachycardia origination or its electrical path through the heart is often defined by mapping. Mapping creates a multidimensional depiction of a tachycardia by recording multiple electrograms obtained sequentially or simultaneously from multiple catheter sites in the heart. Depending upon the technique, certain types of mapping catheters may be repositioned from point-to-point within the heart, allowing sequential recording from the various sites to construct maps. Other types of mapping catheters allow mapping without a point-to-point technique

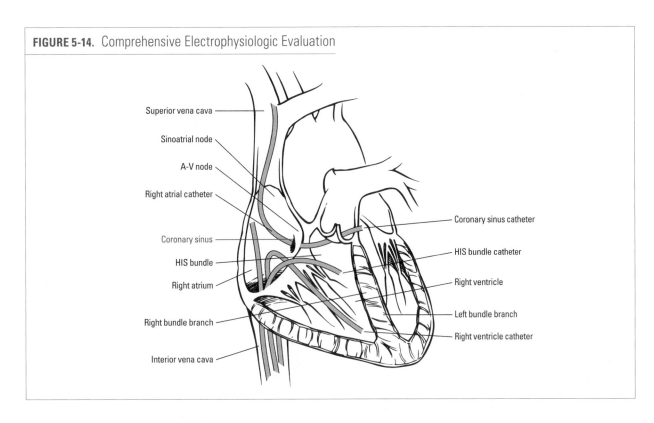

FIGURE 5-14. Comprehensive Electrophysiologic Evaluation

by allowing simultaneous recording from many electrodes on the same catheter and computer-assisted three-dimensional reconstruction of the tachycardia activation sequence.

Ablation: Once the part of the heart involved in the tachycardia is localized, the tachycardia may be treated by ablation (the delivery of a radiofrequency energy to the area to selectively destroy cardiac tissue). Ablation procedures (**93651-93652**) may be performed independently on a date subsequent to a diagnostic electrophysiologic study and mapping; or at the time a diagnostic electrophysiologic study, tachycardia(s) induction, and mapping are performed. When an electrophysiologic study, mapping, and ablation are performed on the same date, each procedure should be separately reported. In reporting catheter ablation, code **93651** and/or code **93652** should be reported once to describe ablation of cardiac arrhythmias, regardless of the number of arrhythmias ablated.

EDITOR'S NOTE To provide instructional continuity, the diagnostic intracardiac electrophysiology study(ies) and therapeutic procedure codes are not listed in strict chronological order. The intent and use of this series of codes is presented according to the respective procedural elements: (1) recording and pacing; (2) mapping; and (3) ablation.

RECORDING AND PACING (⊘**93600**-⊘**93612**)

⊘**93600** Bundle of His recording
CPT Assistant Summer 94:12, Aug 97:9, Apr 04:9, Jul 04:13, Aug 05:13, Dec 07:16, Mar 08:4

⊘**93602** Intra-atrial recording
CPT Assistant Summer 94:12, Aug 97:9, Apr 04:9, Jul 04:13, Aug 05:13

⊘**93603** Right ventricular recording
CPT Assistant Summer 94:12, Aug 97:9, Apr 04:9, Jul 04:13, Aug 05:13

⊘**93610** Intra-atrial pacing
CPT Assistant Summer 94:12, Aug 97:9, Apr 04:9, Jul 04:13

⊘**93612** Intraventricular pacing
CPT Assistant Summer 94:12, Aug 97:9, Apr 04:9, Jul 04:13

Intent and Use of Codes ⊘93600-93603 and ⊘93610-93612

As previously stated, an electrophysiology study requires the placement of electrode catheter(s) for pacing and recording in single or multiple cardiac chambers. The designs of the catheters and the sites appropriate for their placement are determined according to the nature of the arrhythmia under investigation. Typically, each catheter will have multiple electrode poles for both recording and local stimulation. The intracardiac signals are acquired, amplified, filtered, displayed, stored, and analyzed, either in real time or for subsequent offline review.

The commonality among the single-catheter electrophysiology procedures is that each procedure requires the placement and repositioning of a single arterial or venous catheter under fluoroscopic guidance to derive the diagnostic information. Although it is extremely unusual to record and pace from only one or two sites within the heart, there are still occasional circumstances for which single catheter studies for either recording and/or pacing might be undertaken. Nonetheless, single catheter studies for either recording and/or pacing are useful in a variety of circumstances.

Codes **93600**, **93602**, **93603**, **93610**, and **93612** describe separately distinct procedures performed independently or in combination to obtain specific diagnostic information from a specific intracardiac site. Single catheter studies for either recording and/or pacing are performed, for example, to help identify the site of a heart block in a patient having second- or third degree block symptoms. A combination of a single catheter recording and pacing studies of a specific intracardiac site is commonly performed in arrhythmia termination (eg, to assess the electrical activity in the atria associated with a wide-complex tachycardia of uncertain mechanism).

If recording electrograms alone are performed, codes **93600-93603** would be chosen either singly or in combination. Pacing alone would be coded with either code **93610** or code **93612**. Codes **93600**, **93602**, **93603**, **93610**, and **93612** are performed under ECG, blood pressure, and pulse oximetry monitoring. Conscious sedation and local anesthetic is administered. For codes **93600**, **93602**, **93603**, and **93610**, the physician inserts a single electrical catheter (with electrodes on the tip) from a groin vein (usually femoral) into the right heart using fluoroscopic guidance. For code **93612**, the catheter is placed into the right ventricle. (Refer to Appendix G for further information regarding the use of conscious sedation codes.)

Codes **93600-93603** and **93610-93612** specify recording or pacing from particular intracardiac sites. While historically the use of individual site codes was useful for diagnostic purposes (eg, using code **93602** to report evaluation of atrial activity during a wide-complex tachycardia of uncertain mechanism), most electrophysiology studies today are comprehensive and performed using multiple catheters to record electrical activity and pace from two or more sites within the heart. These comprehensive electrophysiologic

procedures are reported with code **93619** or 93620, depending on whether attempts to induce arrhythmia were undertaken.

> **CODING TIP** Temporary pacemaker insertion codes (**33210-33213**) are not reported in conjunction with electrophysiologic study(ies) codes **93600-93624**, **93640-93642**, or **93650-93652**. However, permanent pacemaker insertion performed at the time of ablation (**93650-93652**) should be separately reported.

> **CODING TIP** Currently there is no code to delineate the placement of a single coronary sinus catheter without comprehensive study. Codes for intra-atrial recording and pacing (**93602**, **93610**) are the most appropriate. Left atrial recording achieved from the transseptal catheterization should be separately coded (eg, with code **93462**).

Description of Service for Code ⊘**93600**

To obtain intracardiac electrograms, the physician uses a catheter with electrodes on the tip, attaches the catheter to an electrical recording device, and positions the catheter at the bundle of His. If necessary, left ventricular outflow tract recordings of the bundle of His can be obtained via the aorta.

Description of Service for Code ⊘**93602**

To obtain intracardiac electrograms, the physician uses a catheter with electrodes on the tip, attaches the catheter to an electrical recording device, and positions the catheter in the right atrium. If necessary, left atrial recordings can be obtained using a retrograde technique involving placement of an arterial catheter into the aorta, across the aortic and mitral valves.

Description of Service for Code ⊘**93603**

To obtain intracardiac electrograms, the physician uses a catheter with electrodes on the tip, attaches the catheter to an electrical recording device, and positions the catheter in the right ventricle.

Description of Service for Code ⊘**93610**

To perform atrial pacing, the physician uses a catheter with electrodes on the tip and attaches the catheter to an electrical pacing device to transmit pacing impulses to the right atrium. Left atrial pacing requires additional positioning of the catheter in the coronary sinus.

(It should be noted that transseptal catheterization is not needed for placement of a coronary sinus catheter.)

Description of Service for Code ⊘93612

To perform ventricular pacing, the physician uses a catheter with electrodes on the tip and attaches the catheter to an electrical pacing device to transmit pacing impulses to the right ventricle. Left ventricular pacing requires additional positioning of the catheter in the right atrium using a transseptal technique across the interatrial septum and mitral valve. Alternatively, using an arterial route, the physician may access the left ventricle via the aorta, across the aortic valve.

INTRACARDIAC MAPPING (⊙+93609, ⊙+93613)

⊙+93609 Intraventricular and/or intra-atrial mapping of tachycardia site(s) with catheter manipulation to record from multiple sites to identify origin of tachycardia (List separately in addition to code for primary procedure)

CPT Assistant Summer 94:12, Aug 97:9, Apr 04:8, Apr 04:9, Aug 05:13; *CPT Changes: An Insider's View* 2002

⊙+93613 Intracardiac electrophysiologic 3-dimensional mapping (List separately in addition to code for primary procedure)

CPT Assistant Apr 04:8, Aug 05:13; *CPT Changes: An Insider's View* 2002

Intent and Use of Codes ⊙+93609 and ⊙+93613

Not included in the comprehensive electrophysiology evaluation codes (93619-93622) is the localization of the site of an accessory pathway or origin of a tachycardia by intracardiac mapping. Therefore, code 93609 should be reported in addition to the appropriate comprehensive electrophysiology evaluation codes 93619-93622.

If intracardiac mapping of tachycardia site(s) is performed in order to localize the site of an accessory pathway or the site of origin of a tachycardia, then code 93609 or 93613 should be reported in combination with the appropriate comprehensive codes described earlier. Thus, for a complex supraventricular tachycardia study in a patient with Wolff-Parkinson-White syndrome, code 93609 or 93613 would be used in combination with codes 93620 and 93621, denoting localization of the bypass tract(s). In a patient with mappable monomorphic ventricular tachycardia undergoing assessment for possible radiofrequency catheterization, code 93620, plus codes 93622 and

93609, would describe procedures used in the electrophysiologic laboratory to localize the site of origin of the ventricular tachycardia.

> **CODING TIP** CPT add-on codes are not reported for intraventricular and/or intra-atrial mapping (**93609**) and intracardiac electrophysiologic three-dimensional mapping (**93613**) in addition to codes **93600-93603**, **93610-93612**, and **93615-93618**. Code **93613** is not reported in addition to code **93609**.

Intent and Use of Code ⊙+93613

Code 93613 describes the use of three-dimensional mapping systems. It is to be used in addition to a primary code for comprehensive electrophysiologic study (93620) or catheter ablation procedures (93651 or 93652).

ESOPHAGEAL ELECTROCARDIOGRAPHY (⊙⊘93615, ⊙⊘93616)

⊙⊘93615 Esophageal recording of atrial electrogram with or without ventricular electrogram(s);

CPT Assistant Summer 94:12, Aug 97:9, Apr 04:9, Aug 05:13

⊙⊘93616 with pacing

CPT Assistant Summer 94:12, Aug 97:9, Apr 04:9, Aug 05:13

Intent and Use of Codes ⊙⊘93615 and ⊙⊘93616

Esophageal electrocardiography has been employed both in the diagnosis and therapy of supraventricular arrhythmias. Codes 93615 and 93616 describe insertion of a catheter to a specific esophageal site. The electrodes on the tip of the catheter detect the optimal location to receive the signal to obtain esophageal electrograms of the atria (with or without ventricular recording/pacing). Because the esophagus passes close to the posterior surface of the left atrium, a swallowed exploring electrode attached to a fine piece of wire can be used to detect atrial activity during arrhythmias.

Code 93615 describes esophageal recordings alone for the purpose of identifying the atrial mechanism.

Code 93616 includes both esophageal recording and pacing, for example, for termination of atrial flutter using esophageal pacing.

Description of Service for Code ⊙⊗93615

To obtain esophageal electrograms, the physician uses either an oropharyngeal or nasopharyngeal route to place a catheter at a specific site in the esophagus. The recording electrodes on the tip of the catheter provide atrial and/or ventricular recordings of the heart's electrical activity.

Description of Service for Code ⊙⊗93616

To obtain esophageal pacing, the physician uses either an oropharyngeal or nasopharyngeal route to place a catheter at a specific site in the esophagus. The recording electrodes on the tip of the catheter perform atrial pacing, with or without recording ventricular activity.

ARRHYTHMIA INDUCTION (⊙⊗**93618**)

⊙⊗**93618**   Induction of arrhythmia by electrical pacing

> *CPT Assistant* Summer 94:12, Aug 97:9, Oct 97:10, Apr 99:10, Jun 00:5, Nov 00:9, Apr 04:9, Jul 04:13, Aug 05:13, Dec 07:16

Intent and Use of Code ⊙⊗93618

The combination of recording and pacing codes for a specific intracardiac site is common in situations requiring termination of an arrhythmia. Note, however, that a specific code (**93618**) is used for induction of arrhythmia. This code is rarely used alone because there are few clinical circumstances that warrant only induction of an arrhythmia without further diagnostic study or mapping procedures.

Code **93618** is used to report insertion of a catheter for the purpose of inducing an arrhythmia. This procedure is rarely performed in and of itself, as in most instances further evaluative studies and mapping of the arrhythmia would also be performed.

Description of Service for Code ⊙⊗93618

To perform programmed electrical stimulation or pacing to induce or attempt induction of an arrhythmia, under fluoroscopic guidance, the physician uses an arterial or venous access to place the catheter at a specific site in the heart. A pacing device is attached to the catheter to transmit intracardiac pacing impulses.

COMPREHENSIVE ELECTROPHYSIOLOGIC EVALUATION (⊙**93619**-⊙**+93622**)

⊙**93619**   Comprehensive electrophysiologic evaluation with right atrial pacing and recording, right ventricular pacing and recording, His bundle recording, including insertion and repositioning of multiple electrode catheters, without induction or attempted induction of arrhythmia

> *CPT Assistant* Aug 97:9, Oct 97:10, Nov 00:9, Apr 04:9, Jul 04:13, Aug 05:13, Dec 07:16; *CPT Changes: An Insider's View* 2002, 2008

⊙**93620**   Comprehensive electrophysiologic evaluation including insertion and repositioning of multiple electrode catheters with induction or attempted induction of arrhythmia; with right atrial pacing and recording, right ventricular pacing and recording, His bundle recording

> *CPT Assistant* Summer 94:12, Aug 97:9, Oct 97:10, Jul 98:10, Aug 98:7, Nov 00:9, Apr 04:9, Jul 04:13, Aug 05:13, Dec 07:16, Oct 08:10; *CPT Changes: An Insider's View* 2002, 2003, 2008

⊙**+93621**   with left atrial pacing and recording from coronary sinus or left atrium (List separately in addition to code for primary procedure)

> *CPT Assistant* Summer 94:12, Aug 97:9, Oct 97:10, Jul 98:10, Aug 98:7, Nov 98:34, Nov 00:9, Apr 04:9, Jul 04:13, Aug 05:13, Dec 07:16, Oct 08:10; *CPT Changes: An Insider's View* 2002

⊙**+93622**   with left ventricular pacing and recording (List separately in addition to code for primary procedure)

> *CPT Assistant* Summer 94:14, Aug 97:9, Oct 97:10, Jul 98:10, Aug 98:7, Nov 98:34, Nov 00:9, Apr 04:9, Jul 04:13, Aug 05:13, Dec 07:16, Mar 08:4; *CPT Changes: An Insider's View* 2002

Intent and Use of Codes ⊙93619-⊙+93622

Codes **93619-93622** reflect recording and/or pacing from a combination of sites. Codes **93619-93622** describe diagnostic electrophysiologic studies as they are most commonly performed. Typically, three or more diagnostic catheters are employed. Such studies are undertaken to evaluate syncope of uncertain origin, to evaluate known or suspected supraventricular tachycardias (particularly when the mechanism is uncertain), to assess properties of AV conduction, and to evaluate known or suspected ventricular tachycardias, as in a patient resuscitated from out-of-hospital cardiac arrest.

Depending on the type of arrhythmia suspected, the electrophysiology study includes placement of varying numbers of intracardiac catheters (three or more) in one or more of the heart chambers for the attempted induction of an arrhythmia. Therefore, it is possible to report code **93621** and/or code **93622**, in addition to electrophysiology study(s) of the right atrium and ventricle (**93620**), in order to more accurately describe the following procedures:

- placement of additional catheter(s) in appropriate cardiac chamber(s);

- further electrophysiology study(s) of the left atrium and/or ventricle;

- successful or unsuccessful arrhythmia induction; and

- recording (with or without pacing).

To use the comprehensive electrophysiology add-on codes **93621** and **93622**, a base code must first be reported. If all the elements are not done, it is appropriate to append **modifier 52** to the base code. It is not appropriate to append either **modifier 22** or **modifier 52** to add-on codes **93621-93622** to describe successful or unsuccessful arrhythmia induction.

However, it is usually proper to perform a complete study once a sinus rhythm is obtained after cardioversion or ablation for atrial flutter and fibrillation. This is to ensure that there is not a hidden accessory pathway or another problem. If atrial and ventricular pacing is done before or after the ablation, the code for a complete electrophysiologic study can be reported. Whether the induction of arrhythmia is successful is irrelevant, because the code describes the attempt at induction, not the success of the procedure, and supports the use of code **93620**. The number of catheters used is determined by the technician and the specific clinical condition addressed.

Intent and Use of Code ⊙93619

Code **93619** is reported if a combination of catheters is used to record and/or pace from the right atrium, His bundle, and right ventricle without attempted induction of arrhythmia. This procedure may be required, for example, to localize the site of block in a patient with Mobitz II heart block and syncope.

Code **93619** includes the services represented by codes **93600**, **93602**, **93603**, **93610**, and **93612**. Also included are vascular access, sedation, and monitoring; insertion and repositioning of multiple catheters; pacing of different heart chambers; and removal of the catheters.

Do not report code **93619** in conjunction with codes **93600**, **93602**, **93610**, **93612**, **93618**, or **93620-93622**.

Description of Service for Code ⊙93619

The risks and benefits of, and alternatives to, a comprehensive electrophysiologic procedure without induction of arrhythmia are discussed with the patient, and informed consent is obtained. The procedure is performed under ECG, blood pressure, and pulse oximetry monitoring. The patient is prepared and given conscious sedation and local anesthesia. Multiple transvenous electrode catheters are inserted and positioned in the high right atrium, His bundle region, and right ventricle. Right atrial pacing and recording, His bundle recording, and right ventricular pacing and recording are performed, and conduction intervals are measured. At the conclusion of the procedure, the catheters are withdrawn, and hemostasis is attained. The physician documents these services, generates a report, and communicates with the referring physician.

Intent and Use of Code ⊙93620

Code **93620** is used if induction of arrhythmia is attempted (or is successful). Code **93620** includes the services described by code **93618** and code **93619**.

Description of Service for Code ⊙93620

The risks and benefits of, and alternatives to, comprehensive electrophysiologic evaluation with induction of arrhythmia are discussed with the patient, and informed consent is obtained. The procedure is performed under ECG, blood pressure, and pulse oximetry monitoring. The patient is prepared and given conscious sedation and local anesthesia. Multiple transvenous electrode catheters are inserted and positioned in the high right atrium, His bundle region, and right ventricle. Right atrial pacing and recording, His bundle recording, and right ventricular pacing and recording are performed. Programmed stimulation is undertaken in an effort to induce arrhythmias and diagnose their mechanism. Arrhythmias are terminated by pacing methods or direct countershock. At the conclusion of the procedure, the catheters are withdrawn, and hemostasis is attained. The physician documents these services, generates a report, and communicates with the referring physician.

> **CODING TIP** If intracardiac mapping of tachycardia site(s) is performed to localize the site of an accessory pathway or the site of origin of a tachycardia, code **93609** or **93613** should be reported in combination with the appropriate comprehensive codes (**93619-93622**).

Intent and Use of Code ⊙+93621

Add-on code **93621** is used if a coronary sinus or left atrial recording is also performed as part of an electrophysiologic study. Use add-on code **93621** in addition to code **93620**.

In patients with supraventricular tachycardias, and in some patients with atrial fibrillation, recording from the coronary sinus or left atrium is necessary to make an accurate diagnosis of the mechanism of an arrhythmia.

Description of Service for Code ⊙+93621

The patient is undergoing an electrophysiology procedure (code **93620**, reported separately), and it is necessary to place a catheter in the coronary sinus to record left atrial activity. The venous access site is prepared and draped (this work is in addition to the work of code **93620**), and a sheath is placed either in the internal jugular vein or subclavian vein using standard percutaneous techniques. The catheter is then introduced into the sheath and advanced into the right atrium where the ostium of the coronary sinus is engaged and the catheter advanced into the coronary sinus. The multi-electrode catheter is used to record electrical activity from the left atrium and, at times, pace the left atrium to attempt arrhythmia induction. Catheter repositioning may occur throughout the course of the electrophysiology study (**93620**) to optimize recordings and pacing thresholds. At the conclusion of the procedure, the catheter is removed, hemostasis obtained, and a description of the catheter use and associated findings are entered into the procedure report.

> **CODING TIP** Neither **modifier 22** nor **modifier 52** should be appended to codes **93621-93622** to describe successful or unsuccessful arrhythmia induction.

Intent and Use of Code ⊙+93622

Code **93622** is reported in addition to code **93620** when left ventricular recording and pacing are performed. Some patients with complex arrhythmias may require a left ventricular catheter insertion as part of a comprehensive electrophysiologic study.

Description of Service for Code ⊙+93622

The patient is undergoing an electrophysiology procedure (code **93620**, reported separately), and it is necessary to place a catheter in the left ventricle to record left ventricular activity. A sheath is placed in the femoral artery using standard percutaneous techniques. The preparation and draping of the site is included as part of the baseline procedure work (**93620**). A catheter is placed through the sheath and advanced retrograde through the aorta, across the aortic valve, and into the left ventricle. The multi-electrode catheter is used for recording electrical activity from the left ventricle and, at times, pace the left ventricle to attempt arrhythmia induction. Catheter repositioning may occur throughout the course of the electrophysiology study (**93620**) to optimize recordings and pacing thresholds. The catheter is removed at the conclusion of the study, hemostasis obtained, and a description of the catheter use and associated findings are entered into the procedure report.

ACUTE DRUG TESTING (**+93623**)

+93623 Programmed stimulation and pacing after intravenous drug infusion (List separately in addition to code for primary procedure)
CPT Assistant Summer 94:14, Aug 97:9, Nov 00:9, Aug 05:13, Dec 07:16, Oct 08:10

Intent and Use of Code +93623

Add-on code **93623** is often used in combination with one of the comprehensive codes described earlier when intravenous agents are used either diagnostically or therapeutically at the time of baseline electrophysiologic assessment.

The procedure of serial drug testing is often employed to evaluate patients with tachycardia. In some cases, an intravenous drug is infused as a diagnostic measure to induce the arrhythmia whether or not arrhythmia induction was performed as a component of the intracardiac catheter-based electrophysiologic evaluation. Therefore, add-on code **93623** is used to describe this procedure and should be used in combination with the appropriate CPT code describing the actual electrophysiologic evaluation being performed (**93619** or **93620**).

When catheters are used for recording only, without attempted induction of arrhythmia, code **93619** should be used. This approach may be undertaken for example to identify the site of block in a patient with high-grade second degree heart block and syncope. Because code **93619** describes only evaluation of the sinus node, AV node, and His-Purkinje conduction system (without arrhythmia induction), if intravenous programmed drug stimulation is performed, add-on code **93623** is additionally reported. Some typical types of drugs infused for programmed stimulation include isoproterenol (Isuprel), procainamide, epinephrine, and atropine.

Add-on code 93623 may also represent an additional therapeutic assessment wherein intravenous drug infusion is performed to suppress an inducible arrhythmia during comprehensive electrophysiology evaluation (93620).

When an agent is infused for intravenous programmed stimulation performed immediately postablation to test the effectiveness of the ablation procedure, add-on code 93623 may be reported, but only if a comprehensive diagnostic electrophysiologic study was also performed during the same session (93619, 93620).

Isoproterenol infusion, for example, is often employed in the assessment of supraventricular tachycardias and would be reported as a combination of codes 93623, 93620, and add-on code 93621, if left atrial recording is used. If therapeutic assessment of an intravenous agent is undertaken to evaluate for suppression of inducible tachycardia (as in the use of intravenous procainamide for patients with inducible ventricular tachycardia), code 93623 should always be used as an add-on in combination with the appropriate comprehensive code (93619, 93620).

In the event the isoproterenol study is performed postablation following a single catheter electrophysiologic study with induction of arrhythymia, ablation of supraventricular tachycardia, and postablation injection of isoproterenol, code 93624 would be reported to describe follow-up electrophysiologic study of the efficacy of any therapy undertaken, including any therapy initiated, whether pharmacologic, surgical or catheter ablation, or device therapy. This procedure is rarely performed in and of itself because, in most instances, further evaluative studies and mapping of the arrhythmia would also be performed. Therefore, also reportable for the postablation isoproterenol study is code 93618, which is used to represent the insertion of a single catheter for the purpose of inducing an arrhythmia. Code 93561 is reported to describe the catheter ablation procedure.

> **CODING TIP** Modifier 51 should not be appended to codes **93600**, **93618**, **93621-93623**, or **93631**.

FOLLOW-UP ELECTROPHYSIOLOGIC STUDY (⊙93624)

⊙**93624** Electrophysiologic follow-up study with pacing and recording to test effectiveness of therapy, including induction or attempted induction of arrhythmia
CPT Assistant Summer 94:14, Aug 97:9, Nov 00:9, Aug 05:13, Dec 07:16; *CPT Changes: An Insider's View* 2008

Intent and Use of Code ⊙93624

Code 93624 is employed to describe a follow-up electrophysiologic study of the efficacy of any therapy undertaken after the baseline comprehensive intracardiac electrophysiologic study. This applies to any therapy initiated, whether pharmacologic, surgical or catheter ablation, or device therapy. This code should not be used to report intravenous drug testing employed at the time of the electrophysiologic study (93623). Code 93623 could, however, be used in conjunction with code 93624 if, in addition to testing chronic therapy, other intravenous agents are used for further evaluation. In general, whenever a repeat electrophysiologic study is performed to evaluate the efficacy of chronic therapy, code 93624 is reported, whereas code 93623 should be used when the effectiveness of intravenous therapy is being evaluated.

Code 93624 is not used for reporting a generator evaluation of a cardioverter-defibrillator in an office setting during which an electrophysiologic study is not performed; codes 93741 and 93744 refer to the appropriate procedures for electronic analysis of a defibrillator with and without reprogramming, respectively. Code 93624 has been previously used to describe follow-up electrophysiologic studies in which arrhythmias are induced and previously implanted defibrillators are employed as therapies to be assessed. Code 93642 is better used to describe such a procedure, particularly if defibrillation thresholds are being assessed in the laboratory. This code should be differentiated, however, from code 93640, which describes the electrophysiologic evaluation required for the implantation or replacement of a defibrillator.

> **CODING TIP** For physician reporting, it is appropriate to append **modifier 26** to the code range **93600-93642**. However, codes **93650-93652** for intracardiac catheter ablation procedures are valued to include the physician component service only. Therefore, it is not necessary to append **modifier 26** with respect to the **93650-93652** code range.

INTRAOPERATIVE CARDIAC PACING AND MAPPING (⊘**93631**)

⊘**93631**   Intra-operative epicardial and endocardial pacing and mapping to localize the site of tachycardia or zone of slow conduction for surgical correction

CPT Assistant Summer 94:14, Aug 97:9, Nov 00:9, Aug 05:13, Dec 07:16

Intent and Use of Code ⊘93631

Code **93631** refers to intraoperative epicardial and endocardial pacing and mapping used to localize the site(s) of tachycardia or zone(s) of slow conduction for surgical ablation (cardiac electrosurgery). It specifically refers to the electrophysiologist's role in this procedure. This code should not be used to describe mapping during catheter ablation procedures; codes **93609** and **93613** are used for mapping associated with electrophysiologic studies or catheter ablation procedures. Cardiac electrosurgery may be performed alone or with other surgical procedures such as aneurysmectomy or coronary revascularization.

Code **93631** is reported when epicardial and endocardial pacing and mapping are performed via an open incision with the heart exposed. The cardiothoracic surgeon exposes the heart; then the electrophysiologist performs the mapping. Once the arrhythmogenic focus is determined, the cardiothoracic surgeon ablates the specific focus. (Refer to Chapter 3 for more information pertaining to ablation of arrhythomogenic foci codes **33250, 33251, 33260,** and **33261**.)

ELECTROPHYSIOLOGIC EVALUATION OF INTERNAL CARDIOVERTER-DEFIBRILLATORS (⊙**93640**-⊙**93642**)

⊙**93640**   Electrophysiologic evaluation of single or dual chamber pacing cardioverter-defibrillator leads including defibrillation threshold evaluation (induction of arrhythmia, evaluation of sensing and pacing for arrhythmia termination) at time of initial implantation or replacement;

CPT Assistant Summer 94:14, Aug 97:9, Apr 99:10, Nov 99:50, Nov 00:9, Aug 05:13; *CPT Changes: An Insider's View* 2000, 2008

⊙**93641**   with testing of single or dual chamber pacing cardioverter-defibrillator pulse generator

CPT Assistant Summer 94:14, Aug 97:9, Apr 99:10, Nov 99:50, Jun 00:5, Jul 00:5, Nov 00:9, Aug 05:13; *CPT Changes: An Insider's View* 2000, 2008

⊙**93642**   Electrophysiologic evaluation of single or dual chamber pacing cardioverter-defibrillator (includes defibrillation threshold evaluation, induction of arrhythmia, evaluation of sensing and pacing for arrhythmia termination, and programming or reprogramming of sensing or therapeutic parameters)

CPT Assistant Summer 94:14, Aug 97:9, Nov 99:50, Jun 00:5, Nov 00:9, Aug 05:13; *CPT Changes: An Insider's View* 2000, 2008

Intent and Use of Codes ⊙93640 and ⊙93641

Codes **93640** and **93642** refer to procedures undertaken by the electrophysiologist for the evaluation of newly implanted or replaced cardioverter-defibrillators, during which arrhythmias are induced and defibrillation thresholds and sensing thresholds are determined. (The actual implanting of the device is coded separately [eg, **33249**], even if this is also performed by the electrophysiologist.)

Intent and Use of Code ⊙93640

Code **93640** is used for electrophysiology evaluation of implantable cardioverter-defibrillator (ICD) leads. Use this code to report evaluation at the time of initial implantation, generator replacement, or system electrophysiologic evaluation, including arrhythmia induction, sensing function, and defibrillation threshold testing of lead configurations. This code is particularly appropriate where defibrillator leads are implanted but not connected to a generator.

Description of Service for Code ⊙93640

Code **93640** is used to report electrophysiologic evaluation of ICD leads at the time of placement. Increasingly, ICD systems are equipped with self-testing capabilities, which may eliminate the need for testing with an external device. Patient preparation is described in the ICD lead implantation or repair procedure description (**33218**). The pacing and sensing leads are tested to determine the pacing threshold, ventricular electrogram amplitude, and lead impedance. Ventricular fibrillation is induced multiple times and terminated with the implantable defibrillator using decrementing energy levels to determine the defibrillation threshold. The defibrillation lead impedance is assessed. Ventricular tachycardia may be induced to assess for pace-termination capabilities of the lead system and to assess cardioversion thresholds. If inadequate sensing/pacing or defibrillation thresholds are obtained, lead repositioning followed by repeat threshold testing is performed. The physician documents these services, generates a report, and communicates with the referring physician.

Intent and Use of Code ⊙93641

Code **93641** is used for electrophysiologic evaluation of the ICD pulse generator, during which, typically, the lead configuration is tested and the connected generator is tested in vivo.

Description of Service for Code ⊙93641

Code **93641** is used to report electrophysiologic evaluation of ICD leads and the pulse generator at the time of implantation or replacement. Patient preparation is described in the ICD system implantation or pulse generator replacement procedure description (codes 33212, 33240, or 33249). The pacing and sensing leads are tested to determine the pacing threshold, ventricular electrogram amplitude, and lead impedance. Ventricular fibrillation is induced multiple times and terminated with the ICD or an external defibrillator, using decrementing energy levels to determine the defibrillation threshold. The defibrillation lead impedance is assessed. When satisfactory lead function is confirmed, the ICD pulse generator is attached. If possible, the pacing threshold, ventricular electrogram amplitude, and pacing lead impedance are reassessed through the device. If possible, ventricular tachycardia is induced to confirm adequate arrhythmia sensing and termination. Ventricular fibrillation is induced to confirm adequate arrhythmia sensing and termination. Defibrillation lead impedance is reassessed through the device. If possible, stored event markers and electrograms are assessed. Pacing, sensing and arrhythmia detection, and therapy parameters are programmed. The physician documents these services, generates a report, and communicates with the referring physician.

> **PAYMENT POLICY ALERT** The National Correct Coding Initiative has identified code **93640** or **93641** and the diagnostic electrophysiologic codes **93620-93624** as mutually exclusive activities if performed on the same day. Because electrophysiologists may legitimately perform a diagnostic electrophysiologic study to confirm the diagnosis of a ventricular tachyarrhythmia, followed by implantation of an ICD with appropriate device testing, these mutually exclusive codes will be accepted with the addition of **modifier 59**.

Intent and Use of Code ⊙93642

Code **93642** is used if the purpose of the procedure is to evaluate a previously implanted device, induce

an arrhythmia, and evaluate thresholds (including possible reprogramming).

Description of Service for Code ⊙93642

The risks and benefits of, and the alternatives to, electrophysiologic evaluation of an ICD are discussed with the patient, and informed consent is obtained. The procedure is performed under ECG, blood pressure, and pulse oximetry monitoring. The ICD device is interrogated, and programmed parameters and stored information, including information about stored episodes, are reviewed and analyzed. If possible, fluoroscopic visualization of the lead system is undertaken. If possible, the pacing threshold, ventricular electrogram amplitude, and pacing lead impedance are evaluated. Sedation is given, and ventricular tachycardia is induced with programmed stimulation through the device, if possible, or by using a transvenous pacing catheter, if necessary. Several inductions are performed to confirm proper arrhythmia sensing and therapy programming. Reprogramming and retesting are performed, if necessary. Ventricular fibrillation is induced to confirm proper arrhythmia sensing and termination. Reprogramming and retesting are performed, if necessary. The physician documents these services, generates a report, and communicates with the referring physician.

INTRACARDIAC ABLATION (⊙**93650**-⊙**93652**)

⊙**93650** Intracardiac catheter ablation of atrioventricular node function, atrioventricular conduction for creation of complete heart block, with or without temporary pacemaker placement
CPT Assistant Summer 94:15, Aug 97:9, Aug 05:13; *CPT Changes: An Insider's View* 2008

⊙**93651** for treatment of ventricular tachycardia
CPT Assistant Summer 94:15, Aug 97:9, Aug 05:13, Mar 08:4; *CPT Changes: An Insider's View* 2008

⊙**93652** for treatment of ventricular tachycardia
CPT Assistant Summer 94:15, Aug 97:9, Aug 05:13, Mar 08:4; *CPT Changes: An Insider's View* 2008

Intent and Use of Codes ⊙93650-⊙93652

Catheter ablation of cardiac arrhythmias has made it possible to cure many heart rhythm abnormalities without surgery and without the need for long-term medication. This is especially the case for patients with supraventricular arrhythmias. Supraventricular arrhythmias may arise within the AV node; they may utilize accessory pathways, or they may arise in other areas in the atrium. In all these circumstances, it is possible to cure the arrhythmia by undertaking a procedure called mapping to localize the part of the heart involved in the tachycardia and then deliver radiofrequency ablation energy to the area to selectively destroy cardiac tissue. This procedure is complex because of the requirements of careful attention to detail in the construction of a map.

In some patients with atrial fibrillation in which it has been impossible to control ventricular rate with medication, ablation of the AV node to cause complete heart block, followed by insertion of a permanent pacemaker, is an effective treatment. In this procedure, complex mapping is not required, and the delivery of ablation energy to the AV node can be accomplished with a minimum of catheter manipulation. Therefore, this is usually a very short procedure.

Catheter ablation of ventricular arrhythmias is effective in those patients for whom the electrophysiologist can map the arrhythmia to a specific focus. The treatment of ventricular tachycardia by catheter ablation is tedious and requires several hours of intracardiac mapping followed by ablation. The differences in the techniques involved for ablation of supraventricular arrhythmias, AV node, and ventricular arrhythmias requires the use of two codes to describe catheter ablation for different rhythm abnormalities (**93561** and **93652**). In catheter ablation coding, a single code is used to describe ablation of cardiac arrhythmias, regardless of the number of arrhythmias ablated.

If ablation is undertaken to cause complete heart block, code **93650** is used. Because a temporary pacemaker is required, code **93650** includes the placement of a temporary backup pacemaker, but an additional and separate code is then used to describe insertion of the permanent pacemaker.

Catheter ablation undertaken for treatment of supraventricular tachycardia caused by dual AV nodal pathways or accessory AV connections or other atrial foci is reported with code **93651**.

Code **93652** describes catheter ablation undertaken for treatment of ventricular tachycardia.

Detailed electrophysiologic evaluation is often performed with catheter ablation as an initial diagnostic study before catheter ablation, all at the same session. In these cases, the electrophysiologic evaluation should be reported in addition to the therapeutic procedure. Catheter ablation of atrial fibrillation may be attempted in select patients who are thought to have a focal origin of the arrhythmia. Focal atrial fibrillation

often originates in or near the orifice of the pulmonary veins in the left atrium. Successful ablation of this arrhythmia requires placement of a catheter in the left atrium. Although it may be possible to maneuver a catheter into the left atrium through a patent foramen ovale, it is more often necessary to perform transseptal catheterization of the left atrium. The additional work involved in this left atrial catheterization can be coded with code **93527**. If mapping is included in the ablation procedure, code **93609** or **93613** should also be reported.

Codes **93650-93652** refer to intracardiac catheter ablation as a therapeutic modality. This represents an expansion from the previous single code **93650**. These codes define the target site of the ablation.

Intent and Use of Code ⊙**93650**

Code **93650** is used if ablation is undertaken at the level of the AV node with the intent of creating complete heart block. Typically this requires concomitant pacer therapy; this code includes the placement of a temporary backup pacer (not reported separately).

A permanent pacemaker inserted at the same time or subsequently is reported separately.

Description of Service for Code ⊙**93650**

The risks and benefits of, and alternatives to, ablation of the AV node are discussed with the patient, and informed consent is obtained. The procedure is performed under ECG, blood pressure, and pulse oximetry monitoring. The patient is prepared and given conscious sedation and local anesthesia. A temporary pacing catheter is positioned in the right ventricle transvenously. An ablation catheter is advanced via the femoral vein across the tricuspid annulus and positioned proximal to the His bundle. Radiofrequency or other energy applications are delivered to this region until persistent, complete heart block develops. On occasion, this region must be ablated from the left heart via a transaortic approach. Temporary ventricular pacing is performed until a permanent pacemaker is implanted. The physician documents these services, generates a report, and communicates with the referring physician.

Intent and Use of Code ⊙**93651**

Code **93651** refers to catheter ablation undertaken for treatment of supraventricular tachycardia due to dual AV nodal pathways, accessory AV connections, or other atrial foci. At present, the single code **93651** is used regardless of whether the ablation effort is undertaken for one or more than one supraventricular target(s). (The code is valued to compensate for the occasional case with more than one pathway.) Thus, if a patient has both AV nodal re-entrant tachycardia and a concealed bypass tract, and ablation is undertaken simultaneously for both, a single code **93651** describes the procedure. There is no separate code for ablation of atrial tachycardia, pulmonary vein focus, or atrial flutter; these should be reported with code **93651** as well.

Intent and Use of Code ⊙93652

Code **93652** refers to catheter ablation undertaken for ventricular tachycardia, again independent of the number of ventricular sites ablated.

> **PAYMENT POLICY ALERT** Often the catheter ablation procedure requires the presence and skill of two electrophysiologists. When reporting codes **93650**, **93651**, and **93652** for procedures performed by two electrophysiologists, use the assistant surgeon **modifier 80** (if the procedure is performed in a nonacademic hospital) or **modifier 82** (if the procedure is performed in a teaching hospital), in addition to the base ablation code. The report documenting the need for an assistant physician should be sent directly to the medical director of the carrier.

> **CODING TIP** Internal cardioversion code **92961** should not be reported with codes **93282-93284**, **93287**, **93289**, **93295**, **93296**, **93618-93624**, **93631**, **93640-93642**, **93650-93652**, and **93662**.

CARDIOVASCULAR FUNCTION TILT TABLE EVALUATION (**93660**)

93660 Evaluation of cardiovascular function with tilt table evaluation, with continuous ECG monitoring and intermittent blood pressure monitoring, with or without pharmacological intervention
CPT Changes: An Insider's View 2008

Intent and Use of Code 93660

Patients with symptoms of recurrent near-syncope or syncope may have abnormalities of the sinus node, AV node, or His-Purkinje system function that lead to significant slowing of their heart rate. Many patients with such symptoms will suffer from neurocardiogenic or

vasodepressor syncope in which autonomically mediated hypotension and/or bradycardia causes reduced circulation to the brain and symptoms of near-syncope or syncope. These symptoms are frequently evaluated with tilt table testing done either alone or in conjunction with a comprehensive electrophysiologic study.

Code **93660** refers to cardiovascular evaluation using tilt-table testing, including pharmacological intervention such as isoproterenol infusion, when necessary.

Because tilt-table testing is a separate and distinctive service from a comprehensive electrophysiologic study, code **93660** is listed in addition to the code for the comprehensive electrophysiologic study when both are performed on the same date.

In some circumstances, during tilt-table testing, administration of isoproterenol or mechanical manipulation of peripheral blood flow using a variety of compression devices may be used to try to provoke symptoms of near-syncope or syncope.

Codes **95921-95923** should be reported for testing of autonomic nervous system function.

Description of Service for Code 93660

Informed consent is obtained, and the patient is placed on the tilt table. Surface electrodes are placed, and intravenous access established. Noninvasive blood pressure cuffs are also applied. Baseline hemodynamic and rhythm determinations are made for 15 minutes. Following this, head-up tilt is advanced to 70 to 80 degrees. During this time, the patient is observed for any symptoms or changes in heart rhythm, pulse rate, or blood pressure. The duration of the head-up tilt may range from 20 to 60 minutes. If no abnormalities are identified during baseline tilt testing, an isoproterenol infusion is often undertaken as an adjunct to induce a potential response. The infusion rate is variable depending on the resting heart rate but is usually undertaken to bring about an increase in the heart rate of at least 25%. If the patient still has a negative test after 45 minutes, sublingual nitrates are often applied as an additional adjunct. If a positive response is encountered, the patient is placed in the supine position, sometimes with fluids and/or atropine administered to reverse any bradycardia.

INTRACARDIAC ECHOCARDIOGRAPHY (+93662)

+93662 Intracardiac echocardiography during therapeutic/
diagnostic intervention, including imaging
supervision and interpretation (List separately in
addition to code for primary procedure)
*CPT Assistant Mar 03:23; CPT Changes: An Insider's
View 2001*

Intent and Use of Code +93662

Add-on code **93662** is used to report intracardiac
echocardiography during therapeutic or diagnostic
interventions. The description for the code includes
imaging supervision and interpretation. This is an add-
on code and should be listed separately, in addition to a
code for a primary procedure. CPT guidelines indicate
that add-on code **93662** should be used in conjunction with codes **92987, 93527, 93532, 93620, 93621,
93622, 93651,** or **93652,** as appropriate.

Add-on code **93662** should not be used with code
92961 but may be reported with codes **93580**
and **93581.**

> **CODING TIP** It is appropriate to report add-on code
> **93662** in conjunction with code **93580,** *Percutaneous
> transcatheter closure of congenital interatrial communi-
> cation (ie, Fontan fenestration, atrial septal defect) with
> implant,* and code **93581,** *Percutaneous transcatheter
> closure of a congenital ventricular septal defect with
> implant,* when performed at the same operative session.

Description of Service for Code +93662

The patient is brought to the electrophysiologic lab
for a diagnostic electrophysiologic study with possible
catheter ablation. After the initial assessment, the
accessory pathway is localized to the left lateral mitral
annulus. The ICE catheter is introduced into the right
atrium. Evidence of a pericardial effusion is ruled out,
and the fossa ovalis is imaged, as well as the left atrium.
Using ICE, the transseptal apparatus is positioned to
the mid-portion of the fossa ovalis and transseptal
puncture is performed. The ablation catheter is then
advanced to the left atrium, and the accessory pathway
is mapped and ablated. Imaging continues throughout
the procedure to watch for the development of a pericardial effusion and to assess electrode/tissue contact
during ablation.

Noninvasive Cardiovascular/ Peripheral Vascular Services/Studies

PERIPHERAL ARTERIAL DISEASE REHABILITATION (93668)

93668 Peripheral arterial disease (PAD) rehabilitation,
per session
CPT Changes: An Insider's View 2001

Intent and Use of Code 93668

According to CPT guidelines, peripheral arterial
disease (PAD) rehabilitative physical exercise consists
of a series of sessions, lasting 45 to 60 minutes per session, involving the use of either a motorized treadmill
or a track to permit each patient to achieve symptom-
limited claudication. Each session is supervised by an
exercise physiologist or nurse. The supervising provider
monitors the individual patient's claudication threshold
and other cardiovascular limitations for adjustment of
workload. During this supervised rehabilitation program, the development of new arrhythmias, symptoms
that might suggest angina, or the continued inability of
the patient to progress to an adequate level of exercise
may require physician review and examination of the
patient. These physician services would be separately
reported with an appropriate level E/M service code.

Code **93668** delineates the services performed by nonphysician health care providers in the provision of PAD
rehabilitation to a group of patients and is intended
to be reported one time per session. This therapy is
intended to treat patients with intermittent claudication and patients recovering from peripheral vascular
surgeries or from peripheral angioplasty/stenting/
stent-grafting.

Description of Service for Code 93668

The treating physician is responsible for both the direct
care of the patient who receives PAD rehabilitation, as
well as programmatic responsibility for the efficacy of
the rehabilitation program. The work of the treating
physician includes his or her immediate availability
to the exercise provider and patient for direct supervision as is deemed clinically necessary. Physician work
also includes the global and ongoing supervision of
the rehabilitation program; supervision of the ongoing
training and efficacy of PAD rehabilitation personnel; supervision of clinical safety standards during

rehabilitation; and supervision of use of calibrated motorized treadmill and monitoring equipment.

The patient enters a series of rehabilitative physical exercise sessions that use either a motorized treadmill or a track to permit each patient to achieve his or her symptom-limited claudication threshold within 10 to 15 minutes of dynamic exercise. These sessions are usually supervised by an exercise physiologist or a nurse and may include the work of a vascular technologist. The supervising provider monitors the patient's claudication threshold and other cardiovascular limitations to adjust the workload accordingly. The patient rests and then repeats the exercise protocol so that exercise is continued until 30 to 45 minutes of exercise have been accrued. This program of exercise should occur at least three times per week for at least 12 weeks (ie, 36 visits). Whether patients require ECG monitoring should be determined on a case-by-case basis. The patient will also attend educational sessions that will include discussion of: (1) the causes of PAD; (2) the role of exercise in maintaining functional status; (3) management and normalization of atherosclerosis risk factors; (4) the importance of antiplatelet therapies to prevent heart attack, stroke, and death; and (5) other coronary and/or cerebral ischemic warning symptoms (eg, angina, MI, TIA, stroke). During this supervised rehabilitation program, the development of new arrhythmias, symptoms that might suggest angina, or the continued inability of the patient to progress to an adequate level of exercise may require physician review and examination of the patient.

NONINVASIVE PHYSIOLOGIC STUDIES AND PROCEDURES (**93701**)

___

93701   Bioimpedance-derived physiologic
             cardiovascular analysis
             CPT Assistant March 02:3, Mar 08:4; *CPT Changes: An Insider's View* 2002, 2010

___

Intent and Use of Code 93701

Code **93701** describes diagnostic (as opposed to continuous) monitoring of thoracic electrical bioimpedance, a noninvasive hemodynamic assessment of multiple cardiac parameters used to augment clinical assessment by providing data to assist in the choice and response to therapy.

Description of Service for Code 93701

The patient is greeted in the office, placed in an examination room, and instructed to put on an exam gown and lie down on the exam table. Vital signs are obtained, and the patient's neck and thorax are prepared with alcohol wipes for attachment of the four sets of dual sensors. Sensors are applied, the cardiac output monitor is turned on, and key data are entered into the monitor by the staff before the procedure/monitoring session can commence. The nurse assists the physician during the monitoring session by ensuring proper sensor placement and assisting the patient through positional changes.

By utilizing the diagnostic monitoring results obtained from thoracic electrical bioimpedance plethysmography (TEBP) to demonstrate a high systemic vascular resistance (SVR) and low volume (eg, low thoracic fluid content and low stroke volume), the physician concludes that the patient is actually vasoconstricted and hypovolemic. The physician decides to uptitrate the angiotensin-converting enzyme inhibitor and decrease the diuretic dose.

The patient is re-evaluated in two weeks to determine response to therapy. Upon reevaluation, the SVR, stroke volume, and thoracic fluid level are found to be in optimal ranges, so the patient is maintained on the current ACE inhibitor and diuretic dosages. TEBP allows the noninvasive evaluation of hemodynamic status previously obtainable only by invasive means.

PACEMAKER AND DEFIBRILLATOR MONITORING (**93724, 93745, 93750**)

___

93724   Electronic analysis of antitachycardia pacemaker
             system (includes electrocardiographic recording,
             programming of device, induction and termination
             of tachycardia via implanted pacemaker, and
             interpretation of recordings)
             CPT Assistant Summer 94:23

93745   Initial set-up and programming by a physician of
             wearable cardioverter-defibrillator includes initial
             programming of system, establishing baseline
             electronic ECG, transmission of data to data
             repository, patient instruction in wearing system
             and patient reporting of problems or events
             CPT Changes: An Insider's View 2005

93750   Interrogation of ventricular assist device (VAD),
             in person, with physician analysis of device
             parameters (eg, drivelines, alarms, power
             surges), review of device function (eg, flow and
             volume status, septum status, recovery), with
             programming, if performed, and report
             CPT Changes: An Insider's View 2010

___

CHAPTER 5

Intent and Use of Code 93724

Code **93724** is used to report the electronic analysis of antitachycardia pacemaker systems, usually prescribed for the treatment of supraventricular tachycardia. The analysis includes ECG recording, programming of the device, induction and termination of tachycardia by the device using noninvasive programmed stimulation, and interpretation of the corresponding recordings.

The evaluation of an antitachycardia pacemaker system is performed noninvasively utilizing a radiofrequency link between a programming device and the implanted pulse generator. Antitachycardia pacemaker systems are not commonly utilized in electrophysiologic practice today because of the ability to effectively cure tachycardia utilizing ablation techniques. However, when used, antitachycardia pacemakers are chosen for treatment of supraventricular arrhythmias rather than ventricular arrhythmias.

Description of Service for Code 93724

Electronic analysis of antitachycardia pacemaker system is performed under continuous ECG monitoring. An external defibrillator is available during ventricular arrhythmia induction in the event of arrhythmia acceleration during antitachycardia pacing. A standard 12-lead ECG with and without magnet application is performed and analyzed. The device is interrogated, and stored information (including programmed parameters, battery status, lead impedance, and summary of antitachycardia events) is retrieved and analyzed. The capture and sensing threshold are determined. Multiple episodes of tachycardia are induced using noninvasive programmed stimulation in order to assess the efficacy of antitachycardia pacing therapy. Reprogramming is performed as necessary to optimize battery life and to detect and terminate tachycardia. The physician documents these services, generates a report, and communicates with the referring physician.

Intent and Use of Code 93750

Code **93750** describes the in-person interrogation of a ventricular assist device (VAD). Code **93750** includes analysis of the device parameters by a physician and review of device function and programming, if performed. A report is also included in this service.

VAD programming and interrogation on a regular basis is necessary in longer-term VAD patients. Initially, these patients' conditions may not be stable, and the function of the VAD can be affected by minor changes in either exercise or activities of daily living. However, around the second month after the VAD insertion, patients typically tend to stabilize with less frequent interrogations. Code **93750** is used to report the work of the interrogation and programming of the device, which is similar, regardless of the condition of the patient.

The evaluation of the patient is not considered an inclusive component of code **93750**. Therefore, the level of E/M service provided depends on the status of the patient and may vary throughout the course of the patient visits.

> **CODING TIP** Because interrogation and programming are considered inclusive in the initial insertion or replacement, it is not appropriate to report code **93750** in conjunction with codes **33975**, **33976**, **33979**, and **33981-33983**.

Description of Service for Code 93750

The physician disconnects the patient from the battery and attaches the outflow conduit to a cable, which in turn is connected to a nonportable VAD systems monitor that downloads information from the patient's VAD and performs a series of diagnostic checks (ie, VAD stroke rate, flow volume, pump rate, alarm history) to ensure the VAD is functioning within specified parameters. This real-time data are compared to recorded data to determine functioning as well as patient compliance with VAD operating instructions when the patient is engaged in activities of daily living. (Refer to Chapter 3 for further information related to the insertion, removal, and replacement of ventricular assist devices.)

Noninvasive Vascular Diagnostic Studies

EXTREMITY ARTERIAL STUDIES (INCLUDING DIGITS) (**93922-93924**)

93922   Limited bilateral noninvasive physiologic studies of upper or lower extremity arteries, (eg, for lower extremity: ankle/brachial indices at distal posterior tibial and anterior tibial/dorsalis pedis arteries plus bidirectional, Doppler waveform recording and analysis at 1-2 levels, or ankle/brachial indices at distal posterior tibial and anterior tibial/dorsalis pedis arteries plus volume plethysmography at 1-2 levels, or ankle/brachial indices at distal posterior tibial and anterior tibial/dorsalis pedis arteries with transcutaneous oxygen tension measurements at 1-2 levels)

CPT Assistant Jun 96:9, Dec 05:3, Aug 09:3; *CPT Changes: An Insider's View* 2011

93923 Complete bilateral noninvasive physiologic studies of upper or lower extremity arteries, 3 or more levels (eg, for lower extremity: ankle/brachial indices at distal posterior tibial and anterior tibial/ dorsalis pedis arteries plus segmental blood pressure measurements with bidirectional Doppler waveform recording and analysis, at 3 or more levels, or ankle/brachial indices at distal posterior tibial and anterior tibial/dorsalis pedis arteries plus segmental volume plethysmography at 3 or more levels, or ankle/brachial indices at distal posterior tibial and anterior tibial/dorsalis pedis arteries plus segmental transcutaneous oxygen tension measurements at 3 or more level(s), or single level study with provocative functional maneuvers (eg, measurements with postural provocative tests, or measurements with reactive hyperemia)

CPT Assistant Jun 96:9, Jun 01:10, Dec 05:3, Aug 09:3; *CPT Changes: An Insider's View* 2011

93924 Noninvasive physiologic studies of lower extremity arteries, at rest and following treadmill stress testing, (ie, bidirectional Doppler waveform or volume plethysmography recording and analysis at rest with ankle/brachial indices immediately after and at timed intervals following performance of a standardized protocol on a motorized treadmill plus recording of time of onset of claudication or other symptoms, maximal walking time, and time to recovery) complete bilateral study

CPT Assistant Jun 96:9, Dec 05:3, Aug 09:3; *CPT Changes: An Insider's View* 2011

Intent and Use of Codes 93922-93924

Noninvasive physiologic peripheral arterial examinations are performed when significant signs and/or symptoms of either upper or lower limb ischemia are present. They assist in the decision whether to perform an invasive therapeutic procedure.

Indications for peripheral arterial evaluation may include, but are not limited to, the following:

- claudication that interferes significantly with the patient's occupation or lifestyle;

- rest pain (typically in the front part of the foot), usually associated with absent pulses;

- tissue loss of the extremity (eg, gangrene or pre- gangreneous changes, ischemic ulceration occurring in the absence of pulses);

- previously diagnosed peripheral vascular conditions or previous arterial interventions (eg, angioplasty, intravascular stent, intravascular stent-graft, or surgical bypass) that need to be monitored;

- aneurysmal disease;

- suspected arterial embolization and/or evidence of thromboembolic events;

- blunt or penetrating trauma (including complications of diagnostic and/or therapeutic procedures); and/or

- certain preoperative evaluations (eg, dialysis access, examination of the upper extremity arterial system prior to anticipated Cimino fistula or forearm fistula, evaluation of the radial artery prior to myocardial revascularization).

According to CPT guidelines, vascular studies include patient care required to perform the studies, supervision of the studies, and interpretation of study results with copies for patient records of hard copy output with analysis of all data, including bidirectional vascular flow or imaging when provided.

The use of a simple hand-held or other Doppler device that does not produce hard copy output, or that produces a record that does not permit analysis of bidirectional vascular flow, is considered to be part of the physical examination of the vascular system and is not separately reported. The Ankle-Brachial Index (ABI) is reported with code **93922** or **93923** as long as simultaneous Doppler recording and analysis of bidirectional blood flow, volume plethysmography, or transcutaneous oxygen tension measurements are also performed.

Noninvasive physiologic studies are performed using equipment separate and distinct from the duplex ultrasound imager. Codes **93875**, **93965**, **93922**, **93923**, and **93924** describe the evaluation of nonimaging physiologic recordings of pressures with Doppler analysis of bidirectional blood flow, plethysmography, and/or oxygen tension measurements appropriate for the anatomic area studied.

Limited studies for lower extremity require either: (1) ankle/brachial indices at distal posterior tibial and anterior tibial/dorsalis pedis arteries plus bidirectional Doppler waveform recording and analysis at one to two levels; or (2) ankle/brachial indices at distal posterior tibial and anterior tibial/dorsalis pedis arteries plus volume plethysmography at one to two levels; or (3) ankle/brachial indices at distal posterior tibial and anterior tibial/dorsalis pedis arteries with transcutaneous oxygen tension measurements at one to two levels. Potential levels include high thigh, low thigh, calf, ankle, metatarsal, and toes.

Limited studies for upper extremity require either: (1) Doppler-determined systolic pressures and bidirectional Doppler waveform recording and analysis at one to two levels; or (2) Doppler-determined systolic pressures and volume plethysmography at one to two levels; or (3) Doppler-determined systolic pressures and transcutaneous oxygen tension measurements at one to two levels. Potential levels include arm, forearm, wrist, and digits.

Complete studies for lower extremity require either: (1) ankle/brachial indices at distal posterior tibial and anterior tibial/dorsalis pedis arteries plus bidirectional Doppler waveform recording and analysis at three or more levels; or (2) ankle/brachial indices at distal posterior tibial and anterior tibial/dorsalis pedis arteries plus volume plethysmography at three or more levels; or (3) ankle/brachial indices at distal posterior tibial and anterior tibial/dorsalis pedis arteries with transcutaneous oxygen tension measurements at three or more levels.

Alternatively, a complete study may be reported with measurements at a single level if provocative functional maneuvers (eg, measurements with postural provocative tests or measurements with reactive hyperemia) are performed.

Complete studies for upper extremity requireeither: (1) Doppler-determined systolic pressures and bidirectional Doppler waveform recording and analysis at three or more levels; or (2) Doppler-determined systolic pressures and volume plethysmography at three or more levels; or (3) Doppler-determined systolic pressures and transcutaneous oxygen tension measurements at three or more levels. Potential levels include arm, forearm, wrist, and digits. Alternatively, a complete study may be reported with measurements at a single level if provocative functional maneuvers (eg, measurements with postural provocative tests or measurements with cold stress) are performed.

> **CODING TIP** The use of a simple hand-held or other Doppler device that does not produce hard copy output, or that does not permit analysis of bidirectional vascular flow, is considered to be part of the E/M service (physical examination) and is not separately reportable.

Intent and Use of Code 93922

Code **93922** represents a noninvasive physiologic arterial study of either both upper extremities or both lower extremities. An example of a single level study is an evaluation of nonimaging physiologic recordings of pressures, Doppler analysis of bidirectional blood flow, plethysmography, and/or oxygen tension measurements at each ankle. Again, if this evaluation does not produce hard copy output or, for Doppler testing produces a record that does not permit analysis of bidirectional blood flow direction, the evaluation is considered to be part of the part of the E/M service and is not separately reportable. When only one arm or leg is available for study, report code **93922** with **modifier 52** for a unilateral study when recording one to two levels. Report code **93922** when recording three or more levels or performing provocative functional maneuvers. Report code **93922** only once in the upper extremity(s) and/or once in the lower extremity(s). When both the upper and lower extremities are evaluated in the same setting, code **93923** may be reported twice adding **modifier 59** to the second procedure.

Description of Service for Code 93922

For an upper extremity evaluation, at least two of the following three possible elements must be performed to qualify to report code **93922**:

- bidirectional Doppler waveform recordings from one or two levels are analyzed;

- volume plethysmography from one or two levels is analyzed; and/or

- transcutaneous oxygen tension measurements obtained at one or two levels are analyzed.

In addition, the Doppler-derived upper arm systolic blood pressure in both extremities is evaluated, and any side-to-side gradient is noted, as this would represent an axillosubclavian arterial inflow obstruction. Doppler-derived systolic pressures of segments of the radial and ulnar arteries are noted. The ratios between the highest upper arm extremity blood pressure and the blood pressure at the wrist in each arm are compared, and the ratio is noted. Clinical disease severity is assessed and reported based on an integrated interpretation of all data that have been collected.

For a lower extremity evaluation, at least two of the following three possible elements must be performed to qualify to report code **93922**:

- bidirectional Doppler waveform recordings from one or two levels are analyzed;

- volume plethysmography from one or two levels is analyzed; and/or

- transcutaneous oxygen tension measurements obtained at one or two levels are analyzed.

In addition, the Doppler-derived systolic pressures of segments of the anterior tibial, posterior tibial, and/or peroneal arteries are noted. The ratios between the highest upper arm extremity blood pressure and the highest tibial artery blood pressure in each extremity are compared, and the ratio (ankle brachial index) is calculated and noted. Tibial artery incompressibility, if present, is identified. Clinical disease severity is assessed and reported based on an integrated interpretation of all data that has been collected.

Interpretation is rendered indicating the severity, chronicity, and laterality of the arterial occlusive disease in the involved extremity. Comparison to previous studies is included when prior results are available. An etiology of the patient's arterial occlusive disease may be identified.

> **CODING TIP** It is not appropriate to append **modifier 50**, *Bilateral procedure*, to codes **93922**, **93923**, and **93924**, as these codes inherently describe bilateral procedures. **Modifier 52**, *Reduced services*, may be used to indicate when a unilateral procedure was performed (eg, a lower extremity arterial study performed on a patient who previously had an above-the-knee amputation).

Intent and Use of Code 93923

Code **93923** represents a noninvasive physiologic arterial study of both upper extremities or both lower extremities performed at multiple levels of the involved extremities. An example of a multiple-level study is the evaluation of multiple levels of nonimaging physiologic recordings of pressures, Doppler analysis of bidirectional blood flow, plethysmography, and/or oxygen tension measurements of the two lower extremities or two upper extremities.

The reference to "provocative functional maneuvers" as described in code **93923** references "provocative functional maneuvers" that are designed to assess for a decrease or an increase in extremity arterial perfusion after an intervention. Pulse volume recordings (PVRs) are an attempt to give an objective assessment of a limb's or a digit's arterial perfusion. Perfusion in a resting state while the patient lies on a table or sits in a chair is self-explanatory. However, some patients may have adequate perfusion at rest and still have

underlying arterial issues that require provocative maneuvers in order to elicit them.

For example, a patient may have vasospasticity in which the arteries of the finger constrict when exposed to cold temperatures as seen in Raynaud's disease. PVRs may be taken before and after a provocative maneuver, known as "cold immersion of the digits" to assess the digit's arterial perfusion. A decreased waveform may be apparent to assist in the diagnosis of, in this case, Raynaud's disease.

Another example is when a PVR is performed in an extremity when an AV access graft is patent in that limb without concern for "steal syndrome." The PVRs are repeated distally after pressure is held to occlude the AV fistula or graft proximally. The technician puts pressure on the arm or leg to temporarily block the venous return and potentially augment the distal arterial flow.

When only one arm or leg is available for study, report code **93922** for a unilateral study; when recording three or more levels or when performing provocative functional maneuvers, report code **93923** only once in the upper extremity(s) and/or once in the lower extremity(s). When both the upper and lower extremities are evaluated in the same setting, code **93923** may be reported twice, adding **modifier 59** to the second procedure.

Description of Service for Code 93923

For an upper extremity evaluation, at least two of the following three possible elements must be performed to qualify to report code **93923**:

- bidirectional Doppler waveform recordings from three or more levels are analyzed;

- volume plethysmography from three or more levels is analyzed; and/or

- transcutaneous oxygen tension measurements obtained at three or more levels are analyzed.

In addition, the Doppler-derived upper arm systolic blood pressure in both extremities is evaluated, and any side-to-side gradient is noted, as this would represent an axillosubclavian arterial inflow obstruction. Doppler-derived systolic pressures of segments of the radial and ulnar arteries are noted. The ratio between the highest upper arm extremity blood pressure and the blood pressure at the wrist in each arm are compared, and the ratio is noted. Clinical disease severity is assessed and reported based on an integrated interpretation of all data that have been collected.

For a lower extremity evaluation, at least two of the following three possible elements must be performed to qualify to report code **93923**:

- bidirectional Doppler waveform recordings from three or more levels are analyzed;

- volume plethysmography from three or more levels is analyzed; and/or

- transcutaneous oxygen tension measurements obtained at three or more levels are analyzed.

In addition, the Doppler-derived systolic pressures of segments of the anterior tibial, posterior tibial, and/or peroneal arteries are noted. The ratios between the highest upper arm extremity blood pressure and the highest tibial artery blood pressure in each extremity are compared, and the ratio (ankle brachial index) is calculated and noted. Tibial artery incompressibility, if present, is identified. Clinical disease severity is assessed and reported based on an integrated interpretation of all data that have been collected.

Change in arterial pressure is noted following postural provocative maneuvers, reactive hyperemia, or cold stress.

Interpretation is rendered indicating the severity, chronicity, and laterality of the arterial occlusive disease in the involved extremity. Comparison to previous studies is included when prior results are available. An etiology of the patient's arterial occlusive disease may be identified.

Intent and Use of Code 93924

Code **93924** is used to report noninvasive physiologic studies of lower extremity arteries, at rest and following treadmill stress testing, and should not be reported in conjunction with either code **93922** or **93923**.

As stated in the descriptor of code **93924**, treadmill stress testing must be performed in order to report the code. Code **93922** or **93923** represent noninvasive, nontreadmill studies performed with or without other adjunctive maneuvers. Therefore, it would be inappropriate to report code **93924** for noninvasive physiologic studies of lower extremity arteries without treadmill stress testing.

When patients cannot execute a treadmill exercise, either code **93922** or **93923** can be reported when another type of adjunctive maneuver(s) (ie, rocking forward on the toes [toe raises]) is performed.

CODING TIP Report code **0286T** when performing near-infrared spectroscopy transcutaneous oxyhemoglobin measurement in a lower extremity wound.

Description of Service for Code 93924

Following a period of rest, Doppler-derived systolic pressures and Doppler-derived flow interrogation of segments of the anterior tibial, posterior tibial, and peroneal arteries are noted. The ratios between the highest upper arm extremity Doppler-derived systolic pressure and the highest tibial artery Doppler-derived systolic pressure in each extremity are compared, and the ratio (ankle brachial index) is noted.

A treadmill exercise regimen completed by the patient, including speed, grade, and distance, is noted. Doppler-derived systolic pressures and Doppler-derived flow interrogation of segments of the anterior tibial, posterior tibial, and/or peroneal arteries immediately and at subsequent timed intervals following the exercise regimen are noted, and the calculated ankle brachial index at each interval is noted. The time interval for ankle pressures to return to baseline prior to exercise is recorded.

Bidirectional Doppler waveform or volume plethysmography recordings from the tibial vessels are analyzed.

Interpretation is rendered indicating the severity, chronicity, and laterality of the arterial occlusive disease in the involved extremity. Comparison to previous studies is included when prior results are available. The effects of exercise on the patient's blood flow is interpreted and recorded. An etiology of the patient's arterial occlusive disease may be identified.

CAROTID SINUS BAROREFLEX ACTIVATION (0266T-0273T)

●**0266T** Implantation or replacement of carotid sinus baroreflex activation device; total system (includes generator placement, unilateral or bilateral lead placement, intra-operative interrogation, programming, and repositioning, when performed)
CPT Changes: An Insider's View 2012

●**0267T** lead only, unilateral (includes intra-operative interrogation, programming, and repositioning, when performed)
CPT Changes: An Insider's View 2012

●**0268T**   pulse generator only (includes intra-operative interrogation, programming, and repositioning, when performed)
CPT Changes: An Insider's View 2012

●**0269T**   Revision or removal of carotid sinus baroreflex activation device; total system (includes generator placement, unilateral or bilateral lead placement, intra-operative interrogation, programming, and repositioning, when performed)
CPT Changes: An Insider's View 2012

●**0270T**   lead only, unilateral (includes intra-operative interrogation, programming, and repositioning, when performed)
CPT Changes: An Insider's View 2012

●**0271T**   pulse generator only (includes intra-operative interrogation, programming, and repositioning, when performed)
CPT Changes: An Insider's View 2012

●**0272T**   Interrogation device evaluation (in person), carotid sinus baroreflex activation system, including telemetric iterative communication with the implantable device to monitor device diagnostics and programmed therapy values, with interpretation and report (eg, battery status, lead impedance, pulse amplitude, pulse width, therapy frequency, pathway mode, burst mode, therapy start/stop times each day)
CPT Changes: An Insider's View 2012

●**0273T**   with programming
CPT Changes: An Insider's View 2012

Intent and Use of Codes ●0266T-●0273T

Category III codes 0266T-0268T describe implantation, replacement, revision, removal, and interrogation of a carotid sinus baroreflex activation device. This device is used to treat cardiac conditions such as hypertension and heart failure. Implantation of this device involves placing the electrodes directly around the carotid arteries. The codes are structured based on whether the services are provided for the total system, lead only, or pulse generator only.

Codes 0266T-0268T describe implantation or replacement of the carotid sinus baroreflex activation device. Code 0266T describes implantation of the total system. Code 0267T is reported for implantation or placement of the lead only. **Modifier 50** should be appended to code 0267T when bilateral lead implantation or replacement is performed. Code 0268T describes implantation or replacement of the pulse generator only. Codes 0266T-0271T describe revision

or removal of the carotid sinus baroreflex activation device. Code 0270T is reported for revision or removal of the lead only. **Modifier 50** should be appended to code 0270T when bilateral lead revision or removal is performed. Code 0271T describes revision or removal of the pulse generator only.

Since Category III codes include descriptor language that specifies the components of a particular service, it may be appropriate to append a CPT modifier to accurately describe the Category III procedure or service. Modifiers are used to indicate that a service or procedure performed was altered by some specific circumstance, but not changed in its definition or code.

> **CODING TIP** Because Category III codes include descriptor language that specifies the components of a particular service, it may be appropriate to append a CPT modifier to accurately describe the Category III procedure and/or service.

It is not appropriate to report codes 0267T, 0268T in conjunction with codes 0266T, 0269T-0273T. For removal and replacement, see 0264T, 0265T, and 0268T. It is also not appropriate to report 0270T in conjunction with 0266T-0269T, 0271T-0273T.

When removal and replacement are performed, the appropriate code from the 0266T-0268T series should be reported. When the device is removed but not replaced, the appropriate code from the 0269T-0271T series should be reported.

Codes 0272T and 0273T describe an in-person interrogation device evaluation. Code 0273T includes programming. It is important to note that codes 0272T and 0273T should not be reported in conjunction with codes 0266T-0271T, as these codes include interrogation and programming. Codes 0272T and 0273T should not be reported together.

Clinical Example for Code ●0266T

A 53-year-old female presents with a long history of resistant hypertension. The patient is currently on medical therapy including maximal doses of a diuretic and two other classes of antihypertensive agents. Despite medications, the patient's blood pressure is still 178/103 and the patient is at a high risk for stroke, myocardial infarction, renal damage, and other sequellae of uncontrolled hypertension. The physician managing her hypertension prescribes treatment with baroreflex activation therapy.

Description of Service for Code ●0266T

Please note that every surgeon has his or her preferred method to perform an open surgical operation. In addition, each patient's anatomy and pathology require individualization. Thus, the following is a generic description. Individual procedures will vary.

On both sides of neck: incise skin from ear lobe to clavicle. On both sides: dissect through soft tissues until common carotid artery is located. On both sides: Circumferentially dissect artery and pass two soft rubber loops around. On both sides: dissect to expose carotid bifurcation, including distal common carotid, proximal external and internal carotid arteries. Pass loops around each artery for control. Incise the chest wall and create subcutaneous pocket in the pectoral region for placement of the implantable pulse generator. Create tunnel from each neck incision to the pulse generator pocket.

Tunnel each lead subcutaneously to the pulse generator pocket. Attach leads to the pulse generator. The optimal location for attaching each lead to the carotid sinus is determined by placing the lead on the carotid sinus, electrically activating it and monitoring the blood pressure response of the patient. Several different lead positions are evaluated by rotating the lead slightly and moving it upward and downward on the carotid sinus. The location associated with the optimal blood pressure response is selected for permanent attachment of the lead. The lead is secured in place by first suturing to the carotid artery wall, wrapping the lead around the sinus and suturing the lead back onto itself. This procedure is repeated for the contralateral carotid artery. The pulse generator is inserted into the pocket.

Irrigate incisions copiously with sterile saline. Use electrocautery or suture ligation to achieve final hemostasis. Close incisions in multiple layers with special attention. Close skin.

Clinical Example for Code ●0267T

A 58-year-old adult is being treated for hypertension with a carotid sinus baroreflex activation device. The patient received the total device system five years previously and has responded favorably to the therapy. One or both of the leads have lost function. Possible reasons for this include trauma or damage during surgery in proximity to the device for an unrelated medical problem. Based on the patient's positive response to therapy, the healthcare provider made the decision to replace the lead(s).

Description of Service for Code ●0267T

Please note that every surgeon has his or her preferred method to perform an open surgical operation. In addition, each patient's anatomy and pathology require individualization. Thus, the following is a generic description. Individual procedures will vary. The side of the neck with a malfunctioning lead is incised skin from ear lobe to clavicle. The soft tissue and scar are dissected until the common carotid artery is located avoiding the adherent neurovascular structures in the redo field. Circumferentially dissect artery and pass two soft rubber loops around. Dissect to expose carotid bifurcation, including distal common carotid, proximal external and internal carotid arteries. Pass loops around each artery for control. Incise the chest wall and open the subcutaneous pocket in the pectoral region for isolation of the implantable pulse generator. Free malfunctioning lead from tunnel from neck incision to the pulse generator pocket

Tunnel new lead subcutaneously to the pulse generator pocket. Attach lead to the pulse generator. The optimal location for attaching each lead to the carotid sinus is determined by placing the lead on the carotid sinus, electrically activating it and monitoring the blood pressure response of the patient. Several different lead positions are evaluated by rotating the lead slightly and moving it upward and downward on the carotid sinus. The location associated with the optimal blood pressure response is selected for permanent attachment of the lead. The lead is secured in place by first suturing to the carotid artery wall, wrapping the lead around the sinus and suturing the lead back onto itself. This procedure is repeated for the contralateral carotid artery.

Irrigate incisions copiously with sterile saline. Use electrocautery or suture ligation to achieve final hemostasis. Close incisions in multiple layers with special attention. Close skin.

Clinical Example for Code ●0268T

A 58-year-old adult is being treated for hypertension with a carotid sinus baroreflex activation device. The patient was previously implanted with a total carotid sinus baroreflex activation system and has responded favorably to the therapy. The pulse generator has reached the end of its battery life and needs to be replaced in order for the patient to continue to receive therapy.

Description of Service for Code ●0268T

Please note that every surgeon has his or her preferred method to perform an open surgical operation. In addition, each patient's anatomy and pathology require individualization. Thus, the following is a generic description. Individual procedures will vary. Incise the chest wall and subcutaneous pocket in the pectoral region for isolation of the implantable pulse generator. Remove malfunctioning device from pocket and disconnect leads.

Insert new device. Attach leads to the pulse generator. The pulse generator is inserted into the pocket.

Irrigate incisions copiously with sterile saline. Use electrocautery or suture ligation to achieve final hemostasis. Close incisions in multiple layers with special attention. Close skin.

Clinical Example for Code ●0269T

A 58-year-old adult is being treated for hypertension with a carotid sinus baroreflex activation device. The patient was previously implanted with a total carotid sinus baroreflex activation system. The patient has developed an infection that has localized to the area of the implant. Based on medical necessity in treating the infection, the patient's physician has determined that the device system must be completely removed.

Description of Service for Code ●0269T

Please note that every surgeon has his or her preferred method to perform an open surgical operation. In addition, each patient's anatomy and pathology require individualization. Thus, the following is a generic description. Individual procedures will vary. Both sides of the neck are incised skin from ear lobe to clavicle. The soft tissue and scar are dissected until the common carotid artery is located avoiding the adherent neurovascular structures in the redo field. Circumferentially dissect artery. Dissect to expose carotid bifurcation, including lead attachment site. Repeat for contralateral neck/carotid artery. Incise the chest wall and open the subcutaneous pocket in the pectoral region for isolation of the implantable pulse generator. Free the lead from tunnel from neck incision to the pulse generator pocket. Repeat for contralateral neck/carotid artery. Remove implantable generator.

Irrigate incisions copiously with sterile saline. Use electrocautery or suture ligation to achieve final hemostasis. Close incisions in multiple layers with special attention. Close skin.

Clinical Example for Code ●0270T

A 58-year-old heart failure patient was previously implanted with an entire carotid sinus baroreflex activation system and has responded favorably to the therapy. The patient's lead positioning has begun to cause discomfort, possibly due to movement, scar formation or patient weight gain/loss, and needs to be corrected.

Description of Service for Code ●0270T

Please note that every surgeon has his or her preferred method to perform an open surgical operation. In addition, each patient's anatomy and pathology require individualization. Thus, the following is a generic description. Individual procedures will vary. The side of the neck with a malfunctioning lead is incised skin from ear lobe to clavicle. The soft tissue and scar are dissected until the common carotid artery is located avoiding the adherent neurovascular structures in the redo field. Dissect to expose carotid bifurcation, including distal common carotid, proximal external and internal carotid arteries. Incise the chest wall and open the subcutaneous pocket in the pectoral region for isolation of the implantable pulse generator. The malfunctioning lead is freed from the tunnel by neck incision to the pulse generator pocket.

Irrigate incisions copiously with sterile saline. Use electrocautery or suture ligation to achieve final hemostasis. Close incisions in multiple layers with special attention. Close skin.

Clinical Example for Code ●0271T

A 58-year-old adult patient was previously implanted with a total carotid sinus baroreflex activation system and has responded favorably to the therapy. The pulse generator has begun to cause the patient discomfort, possibly due to migration, scar formation or patient weight gain/loss, and needs to be corrected.

Description of Service for Code ●0271T

Please note that every surgeon has his or her preferred method to perform an open surgical operation. In addition, each patient's anatomy and pathology require individualization. Thus, the following is a generic description. Individual procedures will vary. Incise the chest wall and subcutaneous pocket in the pectoral region for isolation of the implantable pulse generator. The malfunctioning device is removed from pocket and disconnected from the leads.

CHAPTER 5

Irrigate incisions copiously with sterile saline. Use electrocautery or suture ligation to achieve final hemostasis. Close incisions in multiple layers with special attention. Close skin.

Clinical Example for Code ●0272T

A 53-year-old, hypertensive female was implanted with a total carotid sinus baroreflex activation system 5 months ago and is receiving baroreflex activation therapy. A programming device evaluation had been performed 2 months earlier. The patient returns to her physician for routine evaluation but not for therapy adjustment.

Description of Service for Code ●0272T

The programmer head is placed on the patient's skin over the implantable pulse generator to establish a telemetry communication. Information is retrieved from the pulse generator regarding the longevity of the pulse generator battery, the integrity of the implanted leads, and the full set of therapy programmed parameters. The documented information is interpreted by the physician and based on the results no programming is required.

Clinical Example for Code ●0273T

A 53-year-old, hypertensive female was implanted with a total carotid sinus baroreflex activation system 3 months ago and is receiving baroreflex activation therapy. The patient returns to her physician for routine evaluation and therapy optimization.

Description of Service for Code ●0273T

A patient has been implanted with a carotid sinus baroreflex activation therapy system. Either bedside for patients with a new implant or in the physician's office for existing patients, the programmer head is placed on the patient's skin over the implantable pulse generator to establish a telemetry communication. Software commands are issued through the programmer computer to the implantable pulse generator with a selected therapy. The patient's blood pressure and heart rate response are continuously monitored. The physician documents the results of the evaluation and interprets the results to determine the optimal setting parameters for the patient. Once determined, the device is programmed and the programmer head is removed from the pulse generator to discontinue communication.

CODING TIP For bilateral lead implantation or replacement, use code **0267T** with **modifier 50**.

CHAPTER 6

Modifiers

Modifiers are appended to a CPT code to more precisely describe the service indicated by that code. Modifiers are essential tools in the coding process.

To expand the information provided by the five-digit CPT codes, the American Medical Association (AMA), Centers for Medicare & Medicaid Services (CMS), and local Medicare carriers created a number of modifiers. These modifiers, in the form of two symbols (numbers, letters, or a combination of each) are intended to convey specific information regarding the procedure or service to which they are appended. Modifiers are attached to the end of a Healthcare Common Procedure Coding System (HCPCS) or CPT code to indicate that a service or procedure described in the code's definition has been modified by some circumstance but not changed in its definition or code.

As with the five-digit CPT codes, the use of modifiers (AMA, CMS, or locally defined modifiers) requires explicit understanding of the purpose of each modifier. It is also important to identify when the purpose of a modifier has been expanded or restricted by a third-party payer. It is essential to understand the specific meaning of the modifier to the payer for which a claim is being submitted. Within the context of reporting the provision of multiple services, without the addition of an appropriate modifier, there will be the appearance that the provider is engaging in the practice of unbundling. The appropriate use of modifiers indicates that the services were performed under circumstances that did not involve unbundling.

There are two levels of modifiers within the HCPCS coding system. Level I (CPT) and Level II (HCPCS national codes) modifiers are applicable nationally for many third-party payers and all Medicare Part B claims. Level I, or CPT modifiers, are developed by the AMA. The HCPCS Level II modifiers are developed by the CMS.

There will be times when the coding and modifier information issued by the CMS differs from the AMA's coding advice in its CPT manual regarding the use of modifiers. A clear understanding of the payer's rules is necessary to assign the modifier correctly.

Modifiers may be used to indicate the following:

- A service or procedure has both a professional and technical component.
- A service or procedure was performed by more than one physician.
- A service or procedure has been increased or reduced.
- Only part of a service was performed.
- An additional service was performed.
- A bilateral procedure was performed more than once.

General Guidelines for Ranking Modifiers[*]

When billing CPT codes with more than one modifier, the functional (pricing) modifier should be placed in the first modifier field. Statistical and informational modifiers should be placed in the second modifier field.

For example, when entering a pricing modifier and a statistical modifier that affects pricing, enter the pricing modifier in the first modifier field and the statistical modifier that affects pricing in the second modifier field: for the professional component (**modifier 26**) in a health professional shortage area (**modifier QB**), enter 26 in the first modifier field and QB in the second modifier field.

When entering a statistical modifier that affects pricing and a statistical or informational modifier, enter the statistical modifier in the first field and the statistical or informational modifier in the second field. For example, when billing for the professional component

[*] Confirm with your local carrier or payer. Payers are quite variable in their recognition of modifiers and payments. If you have questions or concerns about the application of modifiers, contact the professional/provider relations representative of the specific payer.

(**modifier 26**) and a repeated procedure by the same physician (**modifier 76**), enter 26 in the first modifier field and 76 in the second modifier field.

If more than one statistical or informational modifier with no modifiers that affect pricing is entered, it does not matter which modifier is entered first, except for the QT, QW, and SF modifiers. These three modifiers are valid in the first modifier field only.

When more than four modifiers apply, enter **modifier 99** in the first modifier field. In the narrative field

(item 19 on the claim form), list all modifiers in the correct ranking order, being sure to identify the detail line or procedure code to which the modifiers apply.

CPT Level I and HCPCS Modifiers

The following table lists Level I (AMA) modifiers.

TABLE 6-1. AMA Level I Modifiers

Modifier	Description
22	**Increased Procedural Services:** When the work required to provide a service is substantially greater than typically required, it may be identified by adding modifier 22 to the usual procedure code. Documentation must support the substantial additional work and the reason for the additional work (ie, increased intensity, time, technical difficulty of procedure, severity of patient's condition, physical and mental effort required). **Note:** This modifier should not be appended to an E/M service.
23	**Unusual Anesthesia:** Occasionally, a procedure, which usually requires either no anesthesia or local anesthesia, because of unusual circumstances must be done under general anesthesia. This circumstance may be reported by adding modifier 23 to the procedure code of the basic service.
24	**Unrelated Evaluation and Management Service by the Same Physician During a Postoperative Period:** The physician may need to indicate that an evaluation and management service was performed during a postoperative period for a reason(s) unrelated to the original procedure. This circumstance may be reported by adding modifier 24 to the appropriate level of E/M service.
25	**Significant, Separately Identifiable Evaluation and Management Service by the Same Physician on the Same Day of the Procedure or Other Service:** It may be necessary to indicate that on the day a procedure or service identified by a CPT code was performed, the patient's condition required a significant, separately identifiable E/M service above and beyond the other service provided or beyond the usual preoperative and postoperative care associated with the procedure that was performed. A significant, separately identifiable E/M service is defined or substantiated by documentation that satisfies the relevant criteria for the respective E/M service to be reported (see **Evaluation and Management Services Guidelines** for instructions on determining level of E/M service). The E/M service may be prompted by the symptom or condition for which the procedure and/or service was provided. As such, different diagnoses are not required for reporting of the E/M services on the same date. This circumstance may be reported by adding modifier 25 to the appropriate level of E/M service. **Note:** This modifier is not used to report an E/M service that resulted in a decision to perform surgery. See modifier 57. For significant, separately identifiable non-E/M services, see modifier 59.
26	**Professional Component:** Certain procedures are a combination of a physician component and a technical component. When the physician component is reported separately, the service may be identified by adding modifier 26 to the usual procedure number. **Note:** Modifier 26 should not be appended to procedure codes that represent a professional component (eg, **93010**).
32	**Mandated Services:** Services related to *mandated* consultation and/or related services (eg, third-party payer, governmental, legislative or regulatory requirement) may be identified by adding modifier 32 to the basic procedure.
33	**Preventive Services:** When the primary purpose of the service is the delivery of an evidence based service in accordance with a US Preventive Services Task Force A or B rating in effect and other preventive services identified in preventive services mandates (legislative or regulatory), the service may be identified by adding modifier 33 to the procedure. For separately reported services specifically identified as preventive, the modifier should not be used.

TABLE 6-1. AMA Level I Modifiers *(continued)*

Modifier	Description
47	**Anesthesia by Surgeon:** Regional or general anesthesia provided by the surgeon is designated using modifier 47. (This does not include local anesthesia.) **Note:** Modifier 47 would not be used as a modifier for the anesthesia procedures.
50	**Bilateral Procedure:** Unless otherwise identified in the listings, bilateral procedures that are performed at the same session, should be identified by adding modifier 50 to the appropriate 5-digit code.
51	**Multiple Procedures:** When multiple procedures, other than E/M services, Physical Medicine and Rehabilitation services, or provision of supplies (eg, vaccines), are performed at the same session by the same provider, the primary procedure or service may be reported as listed. The additional procedure(s) or service(s) may be identified by appending modifier 51 to the additional procedure or service code(s). **Note:** This modifier should not be appended to designated "add-on" codes.
52	**Reduced Services:** Under certain circumstances, a service or procedure is partially reduced or eliminated at the physician's discretion. Under these circumstances the service provided can be identified by its usual procedure number and the addition of modifier 52, signifying that the service is reduced. This provides a means of reporting reduced services without disturbing the identification of the basic service. **Note:** For hospital outpatient reporting of a previously scheduled procedure/service that is partially reduced or cancelled as a result of extenuating circumstances or those that threaten the well-being of the patient prior to or after administration of anesthesia, see modifiers 73 and 74 (see modifiers approved for ASC [ambulatory surgery center] hospital outpatient use).
53	**Discontinued Procedure:** Under certain circumstances, the physician may elect to terminate a surgical or diagnostic procedure. Due to extenuating circumstances or those that threaten the well being of the patient, it may be necessary to indicate that a surgical or diagnostic procedure was started but discontinued. This circumstance may be reported by adding modifier 53 to the code reported by the physician for the discontinued procedure. **Note:** This modifier is not used to report the elective cancellation of a procedure prior to the patient's anesthesia induction and/or surgical preparation in the operating suite. For outpatient hospital/ambulatory surgery center (ACS) reporting of a previously scheduled procedure/service that is partially reduced or cancelled as a result of extenuating circumstances or those that threaten the well being of the patient prior to or after administration of anesthesia, see modifiers 73 and 74 (see modifiers approved for ASC hospital outpatient use).
54	**Surgical Care Only:** When 1 physician performs a surgical procedure, and another provides preoperative and/or postoperative management, surgical services may be identified by adding modifier 54 to the usual procedure number.
55	**Postoperative Management Only:** When 1 physician performed the postoperative management and another physician performed the surgical procedure, the postoperative component may be identified by adding modifier 55 to the usual procedure number.
56	**Preoperative Management Only:** When 1 physician performed the preoperative care and evaluation and another physician performed the surgical procedure, the preoperative component may be identified by adding modifier 56 to the usual procedure number.
57	**Decision for Surgery:** An evaluation and management service that resulted in the initial decision to perform the surgery may be identified by adding modifier 57 to the appropriate level of E/M service.
58	**Staged or Related Procedure or Service by the Same Physician During the Postoperative Period:** It may be necessary to indicate that the performance of a procedure or service during the postoperative period was: (a) planned or anticipated (staged); (b) more extensive than the original procedure; or (c) for therapy following a surgical procedure. This circumstance may be reported by adding modifier 58 to the staged or related procedure. **Note:** For treatment of a problem that requires a return to the operating/procedure room (eg, unanticipated clinical condition), see modifier 78.

continued

TABLE 6-1. AMA Level I Modifiers *(continued)*

Modifier	Description
59	**Distinct Procedural Service:** Under certain circumstances, it may be necessary to indicate that a procedure or service was distinct or independent from other non-E/M services performed on the same day. Modifier 59 is used to identify procedures or services, other than E/M services, that are not normally reported together, but are appropriate under the circumstances. Documentation must support a different session, different procedure or surgery, different site or organ system, separate incision/excision, separate lesion, or separate injury (or area of injury in extensive injuries) not ordinarily encountered or performed on the same day by the same individual. However, when another already established modifier is appropriate, it should be used rather than modifier 59. Only if no more descriptive modifier is available, and the use of modifier 59 best explains the circumstances, should modifier 59 be used. **Note:** Modifier 59 should not be appended to an E/M service. To report a separate and distinct E/M service with a non-E/M service performed on the same date, see modifier 25.
62	**Two Surgeons:** When 2 surgeons work together as primary surgeons performing distinct part(s) of a procedure, each surgeon should report his/her distinct operative work by adding modifier 62 to the procedure code and any associated add-on code(s) for that procedure as long as both surgeons continue to work together as primary surgeons. Each surgeon should report the co-surgery once using the same procedure code. If additional procedure(s) (including add-on procedure(s)) are performed during the same surgical session, separate code(s) may also be reported with modifier 62 added. **Note:** If a co-surgeon acts as an assistant in the performance of additional procedure(s) during the same surgical session, those services may be reported using separate procedure code(s) with modifier 80 or modifier 82 added, as appropriate.
63	**Procedure Performed on Infants less than 4 kg:** Procedures performed on neonates and infants up to a present body weight of 4 kg may involve significantly increased complexity and physician work commonly associated with these patients. This circumstance may be reported by adding modifier 63 to the procedure number. **Note:** Unless otherwise designated, this modifier may only be appended to procedures/services listed in the **20005-69990** code series. Modifier 63 should not be appended to any CPT codes listed in the **Evaluation and Management Services, Anesthesia, Radiology, Pathology/Laboratory,** or **Medicine** sections.
66	**Surgical Team:** Under some circumstances, highly complex procedures (requiring the concomitant services of several physicians, often of different specialties, plus other highly skilled, specially trained personnel, and various types of complex equipment) are carried out under the "surgical team" concept. Such circumstances may be identified by each participating physician with the addition of modifier 66 to the basic procedure number used for reporting services.
76	**Repeat Procedure or Service by Same Physician or Other Qualified Health Care Professional:** It may be necessary to indicate that a procedure or service was repeated by the same physician or other qualified health care professional subsequent to the original procedure or service. This circumstance may be reported by adding modifier 76 to the repeated procedure or service. **Note:** This modifier should not be appended to an E/M service.
77	**Repeat Procedure or Service by Another Physician or Other Qualified Health Care Professional:** It may be necessary to indicate that a basic procedure or service was repeated by another physician or other qualified health care professional subsequent to the original procedure or service. This situation may be reported by adding modifier 77 to the repeated procedure or service. **Note:** This modifier should not be appended to an E/M service.
78	**Unplanned Return to the Operating/Procedure Room by the Same Physician or Other Qualified Health Care Professional Following Initial Procedure for a Related Procedure During the Postoperative Period:** It may be necessary to indicate that another procedure was performed during the postoperative period of the initial procedure (unplanned procedure following initial procedure). When this procedure is related to the first, and requires the use of an operating/procedure room, it may be reported by adding modifier 78 to the related procedure. (For repeat procedures, see modifier 76.)
79	**Unrelated Procedure or Service by the Same Physician During the Postoperative Period:** The physician may need to indicate that the performance of a procedure or service during the postoperative period was unrelated to the original procedure. This circumstance may be reported by using modifier 79. (For repeat procedures on the same day, see modifier 76.)
80	**Assistant Surgeon:** Surgical assistant services may be identified by adding modifier 80 to the usual procedure number(s).

TABLE 6-1. AMA Level I Modifiers *(continued)*

Modifier	Description
81	**Minimum Assistant Surgeon:** Minimum surgical assistant services are identified by adding modifier 81 to the usual procedure number.
82	**Assistant Surgeon (when a qualified resident surgeon not available):** The unavailability of a qualified resident surgeon is a prerequisite for use of modifier 82 appended to the usual procedure code number(s).
90	**Reference (Outside) Laboratory:** When laboratory procedures are performed by a party other than the treating or reporting physician, the procedure may be identified by adding modifier 90 to the usual procedure number.
91	**Repeat Clinical Diagnostic Laboratory Test:** In the course of treatment of the patient, it may be necessary to repeat the same laboratory test on the same day to obtain subsequent (multiple) test results. Under these circumstances, the laboratory test performed can be identified by its usual procedure number and the addition of modifier 91. **Note:** This modifier may not be used when tests are rerun to confirm initial results, due to testing problems with specimens or equipment; or for any other reason when a normal, one-time, reportable result is all that is required. This modifier may not be used when another code(s) describe a series of test results (eg, glucose tolerance tests, evocative/suppression testing). This modifier may only be used for laboratory test(s) performed more than once on the same day on the same patient.
92	**Alternative Laboratory Platform Testing:** When laboratory testing is being performed using a kit or transportable instrument that wholly or in part consists of a single use, disposable analytical chamber, the service may be identified by adding modifier 92 to the usual laboratory procedure code (HIV testing **86701-86703**, and **87389**). The test does not require permanent dedicated space, hence by its design it may be hand carried or transported to the vicinity of the patient for immediate testing at that site, although location of the testing is not in itself determinative of the use of this modifier.
99	**Multiple Modifiers:** Under certain circumstances, 2 or more modifiers may be necessary to completely delineate a service. In such situations modifier 99 should be added to the basic procedure, and other applicable modifiers may be listed as part of the description of the service.

CODING TIP Appendix A of the AMA CPT codebook lists all modifiers applicable to CPT codes. Payer recognition of modifiers and payment for modifiers are known to vary.

Modifiers Approved for Ambulatory Surgery Center (ASC) Hospital Outpatient Use

CPT LEVEL I MODIFIERS

TABLE 6-2. Level I Modifiers Approved for ASC Hospital Outpatient Use

Modifier	Description
25	**Significant, Separately Identifiable Evaluation and Management Service by the Same Physician on the Same Day of the Procedure or Other Service:** It may be necessary to indicate that on the day a procedure or service identified by a CPT code was performed, the patient's condition required a significant, separately identifiable E/M service above and beyond the other service provided or beyond the usual preoperative and postoperative care associated with the procedure that was performed. A significant, separately identifiable E/M service is defined or substantiated by documentation that satisfies the relevant criteria for the respective E/M service to be reported (see **Evaluation and Management Services Guidelines** for instructions on determining level of E/M service). The E/M service may be prompted by the symptom or condition for which the procedure and/or service was provided. As such, different diagnoses are not required for reporting of the E/M services on the same date. This circumstance may be reported by adding modifier 25 to the appropriate level of E/M service. **Note:** This modifier is not used to report an E/M service that resulted in a decision to perform surgery. See modifier 57. For significant, separately identifiable non-E/M services, see modifier 59.
27	**Multiple Outpatient Hospital E/M Encounters on the Same Date:** For hospital outpatient reporting purposes, utilization of hospital resources related to separate and distinct E/M encounters performed in multiple outpatient hospital settings on the same date may be reported by adding modifier 27 to each appropriate level outpatient and/or emergency department E/M code(s). This modifier provides a means of reporting circumstances involving evaluation and management services provided by physician(s) in more than one (multiple) outpatient hospital setting(s) (eg, hospital emergency department, clinic). **Note:** This modifier is not to be used for physician reporting of multiple E/M services performed by the same physician on the same date. For physician reporting of all outpatient evaluation and management services provided by the same physician on the same date and performed in multiple outpatient setting(s) (eg, hospital emergency department, clinic), see **Evaluation and Management, Emergency Department**, or **Preventive Medicine Services** codes.
50	**Bilateral Procedure:** Unless otherwise identified in the listings, bilateral procedures that are performed at the same operative session should be identified by adding modifier 50 to the appropriate 5 digit code.
52	**Reduced Services:** Under certain circumstances a service or procedure is partially reduced or eliminated at the physician's discretion. Under these circumstances the service provided can be identified by its usual procedure number and the addition of modifier 52, signifying that the service is reduced. This provides a means of reporting reduced services without disturbing the identification of the basic service. **Note:** For hospital outpatient reporting of a previously scheduled procedure/service that is partially reduced or cancelled as a result of extenuating circumstances or those that threaten the well-being of the patient prior to or after administration of anesthesia, see modifiers 73 and 74 (see modifiers approved for ASC hospital outpatient use).
58	**Staged or Related Procedure or Service by the Same Physician During the Postoperative Period:** It may be necessary to indicate that the performance of a procedure or service during the postoperative period was: (a) planned or anticipated (staged); (b) more extensive than the original procedure; or (c) for therapy following a surgical procedure. This circumstance may be reported by adding modifier 58 to the staged or related procedure. **Note:** For treatment of a problem that requires a return to the operating/procedure room (eg, unanticipated clinical condition), see modifier 78.

TABLE 6-2. Level I Modifiers Approved for ASC Hospital Outpatient Use *(continued)*

Modifier	Description
59	**Distinct Procedural Service:** Under certain circumstances, it may be necessary to indicate that a procedure or service was distinct or independent from other non-E/M services performed on the same day. Modifier 59 is used to identify procedures/ services, other than E/M services, that are not normally reported together, but are appropriate under the circumstances. Documentation must support a different session, different procedure or surgery, different site or organ system, separate incision/excision, separate lesion, or separate injury (or area of injury in extensive injuries) not ordinarily encountered or performed on the same day by the same individual. However, when another already established modifier is appropriate, it should be used rather than modifier 59. Only if no more descriptive modifier is available, and the use of modifier 59 best explains the circumstances, should modifier 59 be used. **Note:** Modifier 59 should not be appended to an E/M service. To report a separate and distinct E/M service with a non-E/M service performed on the same date, see modifier 25.
73	**Discontinued Out-Patient Hospital/Ambulatory Surgery Center (ASC) Procedure Prior to the Administration of Anesthesia:** Due to extenuating circumstances or those that threaten the well being of the patient, the physician may cancel a surgical or diagnostic procedure subsequent to the patient's surgical preparation (including sedation when provided, and being taken to the room where the procedure is to be performed), but prior to the administration of anesthesia (local, regional block(s), or general). Under these circumstances, the intended service that is prepared for but cancelled can be reported by its usual procedure number and the addition of modifier 73. **Note:** The elective cancellation of a service prior to the administration of anesthesia and/or surgical preparation of the patient should not be reported. For physician reporting of a discontinued procedure, see modifier 53.
74	**Discontinued Out-Patient Hospital/Ambulatory Surgery Center (ASC) Procedure After Administration of Anesthesia:** Due to extenuating circumstances or those that threaten the well being of the patient, the physician may terminate a surgical or diagnostic procedure after the administration of anesthesia (local, regional block(s), general) or after the procedure was started (incision made, intubation started, scope inserted, etc). Under these circumstances, the procedure started but terminated can be reported by its usual procedure number and the addition of modifier 74. **Note:** The elective cancellation of a service prior to the administration of anesthesia and/or surgical preparation of the patient should not be reported. For physician reporting of a discontinued procedure, see modifier 53.
76	**Repeat Procedure or Service by Same Physician or Other Qualified Health Care Professional:** It may be necessary to indicate that a procedure or service was repeated by the same physician or other qualified health care professional subsequent to the original procedure or service. This circumstance may be reported by adding modifier 76 to the repeated procedure or service. **Note:** This modifier should not be appended to an E/M service.
77	**Repeat Procedure by Another Physician or Other Qualified Health Care Professional:** It may be necessary to indicate that a basic procedure or service was repeated by another physician or other qualified health care professional subsequent to the original procedure or service. This circumstance may be reported by adding modifier 77 to the repeated procedure or service. **Note:** This modifier should not be appended to an E/M service.
78	**Unplanned Return to the Operating/Procedure Room by the Same Physician or Other Qualified Health Care Professional Following Initial Procedure for a Related Procedure During the Postoperative Period:** It may be necessary to indicate that another procedure was performed during the postoperative period of the initial procedure (unplanned procedure following initial procedure). When this procedure is related to the first, and requires the use of an operating/procedure room, it may be reported by adding modifier 78 to the related procedure. (For repeat procedures on the same day, see modifier 76.)
79	**Unrelated Procedure or Service by the Same Physician During the Postoperative Period:** The physician may need to indicate that the performance of a procedure or service during the postoperative period was unrelated to the original procedure. This circumstance may be reported by using modifier 79. (For repeat procedures on the same day, see modifier 76.)

continued

TABLE 6-2. Level I Modifiers Approved for ASC Hospital Outpatient Use *(continued)*

Modifier	Description
91	**Repeat Clinical Diagnostic Laboratory Test:** In the course of treatment of the patient, it may be necessary to repeat the same laboratory test on the same day to obtain subsequent (multiple) test results. Under these circumstances, the laboratory test performed can be identified by its usual procedure number and the addition of modifier 91. **Note:** This modifier may not be used when tests are rerun to confirm initial results; due to testing problems with specimens or equipment; or for any other reason when a normal, one-time, reportable result is all that is required. This modifier may not be used when other code(s) describe a series of test results (eg, glucose tolerance tests, evocative/suppression testing). This modifier may only be used for laboratory test(s) performed more than once on the same day on the same patient.

LEVEL II (NATIONAL) MODIFIERS

Codes and descriptors are approved and maintained jointly by the alphanumeric editorial panel (consisting of representatives from the CMS, the Health Insurance Association of America, and the Blue Cross and Blue Shield Association). These are 2-position alphanumeric codes.

TABLE 6-3. Level II (National) Modifiers

Modifier	Description
AI	Principal Physician of Record
LT	Left side (used to identify procedures performed on the left side of the body)
RT	Right side (used to identify procedures performed on the right side of the body)
LC	Left circumflex coronary artery
LD	Left anterior descending coronary artery
RC	Right coronary artery

Understanding Third-Party Reimbursement

What Is Third-Party Reimbursement?

Generally speaking, third-party payment is the process by which groups and individuals purchase health benefit products to insure themselves against future health care costs by paying premiums to an insurer. In the United States, most third-party payers are either public programs or private health insurance companies. Third-party payers include public, government-run programs such as Medicare, which is primarily for the elderly and disabled; Medicaid, for the poor and disabled; TriCare, for active military personnel and their families; and private health insurance companies such as AETNA, WellPoint, Blue Cross and Blue Shield, and UnitedHealthcare. In addition, some private health plans contract with government programs to process benefits and payments for their beneficiaries.

AN ENROLLMENT OVERVIEW

In the United States, health insurance covers an estimated 80 to 85% of the population. Approximately 15% of the United States population is Medicare-eligible, and approximately 25% of the population is covered by health maintenance organizations (HMOs). The vast majority of the insured population is covered through employer-purchased group insurance plans. Employers either purchase health benefit products (fully fund) or allocate monies to pay for their employees' health care costs directly (self-funded). Employers determine the level of benefits, the cost to the employee, and the types of plans offered. Increasingly, the level of benefits has become more restricted, larger cost-sharing models have emerged, and the types of plans offered have been restricted to HMOs or preferred provider organizations (PPOs). The 15 to 20% of the population that does not qualify for government insurance programs is typically unemployed or employed but does not earn enough money to purchase

health insurance. This portion of the population pays for all health services directly out of personal resources. Some states have begun to provide new programs to help the underinsured acquire more complete health coverage.

STATE REGULATION

Each state regulates the insurance companies and products that operate within its jurisdiction. The main function of state insurance regulatory agencies is to oversee the companies or payers that transact insurance business in their state. Agencies use various state laws, which differ from state to state, to oversee and monitor health plans. State laws such as insurance codes, prompt payment statutes, and laws governing unfair trade practices are all used to regulate health plans. Sometimes, states also enforce certain federal laws in cases where no state laws exist to address a certain dispute or when state laws are less comprehensive than federal laws. In other instances, states must defer to federal laws in cases where states do not have jurisdiction over a particular health plan (eg, Medicare, plans covering federal employees, or federally regulated plans). Many national for-profit insurance companies maintain separate business entities in each state to manage these varying requirements. Note that the same insurance company may sponsor or manage many insurance plans and products at the same time. For example, in Pennsylvania, Highmark Blue Cross and Blue Shield is a dominant commercial insurer in the state, the parent company of a separate large managed-care entity, and the provider of Medicare services.

PHYSICIAN PRACTICE OPERATIONS

A physician practice may have many separate contracts for different types of plans and products with the same parent company, each with a different fee schedule. As a result, each physician practice is likely to have at least

20 to 30 contracts with different health plans, and in some states, work directly with the Medicare carrier.

In addition, physician practices may have contractual arrangements with other providers in integrated delivery systems, networks or limited liability companies, or practice management companies to provide services to a select group. Currently, in some states, cardiovascular specialty practices are networking and expanding to be large enough to contract directly with large employers such as local governments to provide "carve-out" services to those populations.

The physician practice must become familiar with both the administrative and medical policy of each third-party payer. Ultimately, the physician who performs the service and submits the insurance claim is responsible for ensuring that information sent to third-party payers is accurate and appropriate. But practice staff must also be familiar with the process of claims preparation, coding, and reimbursement, because they are directly involved with the administrative and/or clinical steps that ensure the practice's success. Physicians and staff must therefore maintain current knowledge of both coding and documentation, along with a sound working knowledge of each payer's reimbursement and coverage policies.

The medical specialty societies, both national and local, can be helpful in addressing both medical policy issues as well as claims adjudication problems.

Submitting Claims

KEEPING TRACK OF PAYER REQUIREMENTS

The interests of all parties are best served if physicians and their staff have a good understanding of billing protocols used by third-party payers in their market area. There is often significant variation among health plans in terms of claims forms, preauthorizations, primary-care referrals, and other requirements. Familiarity with the procedures used by each plan will facilitate proper submission of claims and timely payments. Providing accurate and consistent descriptions of care provided and the justification for rendering such care are critical elements in third-party payer relations.

A tracking system—as simple as an index card for each payer and employer in the area or as sophisticated as a computerized system—can save time, money, and frustration. Information should include the payer's or employer's name, the name and telephone numbers of a

contact person (the person in charge of provider inquiries or services in the case of insurance companies and the employee benefits officer in the case of employers), and the address to which claims should be mailed. It may also help to include the telephone number patients should use for their own inquiries.

Files should include information concerning the types of written policies, deductibles, filing restrictions, any benefit verification requirements, and the managed-care plans' referral and authorization requirements, plus services that are not covered. The following specifics could be itemized and frequently updated:

- claim forms that are accepted and/or mandated (eg, CMS 1500);
- procedure for electronic claims submission (if any);
- procedure, service, and diagnosis codes that are accepted and/or mandated, including CPT, Healthcare Common Procedure Coding System (HCPCS), *International Classification of Diseases, Ninth Revision, Clinical Modification* (ICD-9-CM), modifiers, and narrative descriptions;
- standard provider inquiry forms that are accepted;
- restrictions regarding assigned claims;
- mechanism to verify patient eligibility;
- mechanism to check on patient benefits before claims are submitted;
- whether patient signatures are required on claim forms;
- whether checks are mailed directly to the physician;
- whether health plan offers electronic funds transfer option and related procedures;
- appeals protocols; and
- required patient copayment amounts.

COMPLYING WITH FRAUD AND ABUSE REGULATIONS

The federal government has taken an increasingly strict stance with regard to investigating and prosecuting alleged instances of Medicare fraud and abuse. As a result, physicians submitting claims to carriers for Medicare services need to be more aware of the requirements surrounding claims submission. Special attention should be paid to ensuring appropriate documentation of services, levels of supervision, and the evolving rules surrounding evaluation and management (E/M) codes. When submitting claims, an extra level of care can go a long way toward avoiding potential problems.

CLAIMS PROCESSING

There are many differences in the way third-party payers instruct personnel to process claims. Some payers may reimburse for the least expensive, similar procedure if conflicting information is reported, referred to as downcoding, or group similar procedures to provide a global payment, referred to as bundling. Both downcoding and bundling are problematic but can be mitigated by adhering to proper coding principles.

All third-party payers follow certain procedures when a claim is submitted. As soon as a payer receives a claim form, it is date-stamped. As a result of the Health Insurance Portability and Accountability Act (HIPAA), most claims-related transactions are electronic in nature. This paperless transmission eliminates many of the problems of mailed claims and allows for faster payment.

REASONABLE SERVICES

Regardless of the means of transmission, the claim is subjected to an automated review to determine whether beneficiary deductibles have been met, services are covered, and charges are reasonable. This stage of the process will also determine whether the services qualify as medically necessary.

Payers also have a built-in utilization screening step. Claims are screened for predetermined frequency parameters of specific services or procedures, and at which time, the claim may be identified for further review. The Centers for Medicare & Medicaid Services (CMS) has certain mandated screens that are observed by Medicare carriers; third-party payers may also employ local screens. Physicians may ask local third-party payers for a list of the screens they use; however, insurers, including Medicare carriers, may not release this information or provide only limited information.

Claims that are screened out for manual review are examined by a claims reviewer, employed by the insurance company and trained to review and process claims. In certain cases, clinical expertise may be required to fully review the claim. Payers employ nurses or physicians to handle this part of the process. For claims that are selected for review, established policies apply to each situation. Such policies have been developed by medical professionals—usually physicians and, in some instances, representatives of medical societies—in consultation with the payer.

Claims reviewers typically manually review all claim forms submitted with attached supporting documentation. But because a paper claim with attachments may be more likely to become separated or lost, necessitating resubmission of the claim and attachments, providers should send a paper claim without attachments or submit the claim electronically whenever possible. The payer's claims systems can then begin to adjudicate the claim: processing for reimbursement, denying unapproved or ineligible services, or holding the claim pending additional information. It will be particularly beneficial for physician office staff to perform additional follow-up for any denied services or claims requiring additional information, often times requiring escalation to the claim reconsideration process.

The best assurance for receiving reimbursement is accurate and appropriate coding communicated in a payer's required "language." The claim should describe the services performed—and why they were performed—to avoid denials of benefit payments for which physician practices are entitled.

Quality Coding

Accurate coding begins by translating the information from a patient's medical record into appropriate codes. Complete and legible documentation in charts is imperative. Physicians should help the billing staff by clearly and fully documenting each patient encounter and procedure.

The following list offers several helpful suggestions that may mean the difference between appropriately paid and denied claims:

- Identify the most appropriate code(s) to describe the services provided to the patient and clearly document the services—on both the patient's chart and on the claim form. Remember, submitting codes that do not accurately describe the service provided is considered fraud. An understanding of all coding systems recognized by payers in the area—CPT, HCPCS, ICD-9-CM, and others—is essential for anyone involved in the billing process.

- Approach every patient encounter as a unique coding situation. Habits of routine coding should be avoided.

- Confirm that appropriate billing identification numbers are included on all claim forms.

- Understand the correct use of modifiers and which modifiers are recognized by area payers. Modifiers alert claims processors to one or more unusual circumstances under which the service or procedure was performed.

- File claims quickly and regularly. Because many health insurance policies have caps, delays in filing could mean that a severely ill patient reaches his or her benefit limit before the claim is submitted. While indemnity plans allow up to one year to file claims, managed-care contracts may specify much shorter periods (eg, 60 days) for filing.

- Recognize that many carriers list denial codes on an explanation of benefits so that clerical errors can simply be retransmitted for correction, without necessitating an appeal.

- Take advantage of telephone reviews offered by many carriers to quickly correct clerical claims errors and simple medical necessity issues. This approach is not typically used for more complex medical necessity denials; these usually must be refiled on paper and/or accompanied by supporting documentation.

- Be sure all bills submitted for payment have signed documentation in the medical record to support the physician's request for payment. E/M visit notes should clearly indicate the level of service provided.

EDITOR'S NOTE Adequate documentation is the physician's only protection from downcoding, and/or repayment and fines, resulting from post-payment review. CMS had previously stated that each progress note "should stand alone without the need to page back through the medical record for reference or orientation purposes." To keep this requirement from making progress notes duplicative and therefore cumbersome, the latest E/M documentation guidelines allow reference to earlier notes. Notes should be legible and signed by the physician.

Claim Forms

Effective October 16, 2003, the Department of Health and Human Services (HHS) required that all claims be submitted electronically to Medicare unless a waiver is obtained. The Administrative Simplification Compliance Act (ASCA) defines who is exempt from submitting claims electronically. The electronic standard transaction for submitting claims is known as the 837. The CMS 1500 form for professional claims and the UB-04 form for institutional claims are still used to submit claims on paper. Additional information can be obtained at www.hhs.gov.

In addition, all health plans are required to use CPT-4 codes and modifiers for procedure coding, currently

ICD-9-CM, and futuristically ICD-10-CM for diagnosis coding. Plans can no longer generate local codes.

CHARGE CAPTURE PROCESS

The superbill (also called a charge ticket, fee slip, encounter form, or routing form) is a practice-specific form. Many medical practices actively and efficiently use superbills for capturing office and/or hospital service data. The superbill serves as a charge capture document because most practices use automated claims preparation that it is updated annually. Also, third-party payers are increasingly encouraging or mandating electronic submissions. For efficiency and timely cash flow, physicians should take advantage of electronic filing options whenever available. Manual claims processing is being phased out by the insurance industry and will virtually ensure a slowdown in payment.

Avoiding Claims Denials and Rejections

AVOIDABLE CAUSES OF DENIED CLAIMS

The following is a list of common problems that result in claims denial:

- incomplete, wrong, or truncated CPT code or ICD-9-CM diagnostic code;

- inadequate documentation to support medical necessity;

- use of outdated CPT, ICD-9-CM, or HCPCS codes;

- failure to obtain precertification or authorization;

- lack of correspondence between the place of service code and the procedure code;

- failure to include the referring or ordering physician's designated identification number (UPIN, Tax ID, NPI);

- incorrect linking of diagnostic codes to procedure codes;

- failure to document the consultative nature of a referral; and

- incomplete or inaccurate patient information.

Decisions on medical necessity or appropriateness vary from payer to payer, but, for the most part, all payer claim reviews are made on the basis of certain common criteria. The physician's sensitivity to these may avoid inquiries, denials, rejections, and even the need to appeal—and, in all of these instances, payment delays.

Payers check that all basic information, such as physician, patient, and insurance identification, has been included in the claim submission. Payers check as well for service or procedure and diagnostic codes and other supporting documentation. Moreover, they check to see that the codes match and are appropriate. If they find inconsistencies or discrepancies, the physician practice may receive a notice challenging the medical necessity requirements of the service or procedure. The level of service may be downcoded if the diagnosis does not justify the reported level of service.

Any physician who receives such a notice should first review the original claim and ensure that it includes all of the appropriate information and documentation. If the reason for the challenge is still unclear, the physician should contact the insurance company. The physician should ask what information the carrier requires to understand the medical necessity of the services provided. The physician should also document all transactions and correspondence, including any subsequent information received from the carrier.

Claims reviewers will make an initial determination concerning the medical necessity of the reported service based on the additional information the physician provides. The service will either be reimbursed or a denial notice will be issued that includes the reason for the decision.

The American Medical Association (AMA) describes the Medicare carrier review and appeals process in detail in its publication, *Medicare Carrier Review: What Every Physician Should Know About "Medically Unnecessary" Denials*. Other payers, lacking independent external reviewers in the appeals process, have faced litigation and penalties by state insurance regulatory agency. Monitoring documentation is essential to countering inappropriate denials.

The American College of Cardiology (ACC) has worked in conjunction with other national specialty societies and America's Health Insurance Plans (AHIP) to develop a form to assist in the appeals process. This form and other resources for working with third-party payers are available at www.cardiosource.org/Practice-Management/Working-With-Health-Plans.aspx.

PAYMENTS FOR MEDICALLY UNNECESSARY AND NONCOVERED SERVICES

Physicians and providers should not bill Medicare or any other payer for services that typically are not

eligible for benefit payments. If a patient insists that Medicare or another insurer be billed for services the physician believes will not be covered, the physician should obtain a signed waiver from the patient. This is essential to protect the physician from liability for the service under the waiver of liability provision. Physicians may bill patients for noncovered services, but it is prudent to have a signed advance notice from the patient for all of these circumstances.

If Medicare determines that a service was medically unnecessary, a refund must be made to the patient for any amount collected for the denied service. A refund is not required if either of the two following conditions is met:

- The physician did not know and could not have been expected to know that payment would be denied for the service or procedure because it was not reasonable.

- Before delivery of the service, the patient was informed via a signed advance notice that the payer would not reimburse because the service was considered unnecessary and the patient agreed to pay for the service.

A signed waiver form for these services will be needed to provide the appropriate documentation that the patient was properly advised of the expected reimbursement limitations as well as the patient's obligation to pay the physician directly for such services.

OFFICE OF INSPECTOR GENERAL: COMPLIANCE PROGRAM GUIDANCE FOR INDIVIDUAL AND SMALL GROUP PHYSICIAN PRACTICES

The Office of Inspector General (OIG) released its final "Compliance Program Guidance for Individual and Small Group Physician Practices" in September 2000. The OIG states that it recognizes that full implementation of the seven standard components of a full-scale compliance program may not be feasible for smaller physician practices and that some practices may never fully implement all components. The OIG instead suggests that practices follow a step-by-step approach to a compliance program, outlining the following:

1. Conduct internal monitoring and auditing through the performance of periodic audits.

2. Implement compliance and practice standards through the development of written standards and procedures.

3. Designate a compliance officer or contact(s) to monitor compliance efforts and enforce practice standards.

4. Conduct appropriate training and education on practice standards and procedures.

5. Respond appropriately to detected violations by investigating and disclosing incidents to appropriate government entities.

6. Develop open lines of communication.

7. Enforce disciplinary standards through well-publicized guidelines.

The final guidance discusses each of these steps in detail. The guidance also lists four specific compliance risk areas in which the OIG has focused its investigations and audits related to physician practices:

- Proper coding and billing;

- Ensuring that services are reasonable and necessary;

- Proper documentation; and

- Avoiding improper inducements, kickbacks, and self-referrals.

EDITOR'S NOTE For assistance in resolving recurring private-sector insurance claim issues for which you feel proper coding principles were applied, contact the College's Payer Advocacy department and the AMA's Private Sector Advocacy department at www.ama-assn.org/go/psa.

Chapter Involvement in Payer Relations

The College's chapters play a key role in payer relations at the local level. Many chapters have formed committees on private-sector relations, third-party payers, and government relations to address coding, billing, payment, and care-related issues of concern to cardiovascular specialists. In many cases, chapters have successfully resolved such issues through discussion and cooperation with private health plans and Medicare carriers. The personal relationships and understanding of local concerns which chapters bring to bear can greatly facilitate these endeavors.

A chapter committee that focuses on private-sector relations has significant potential for addressing the concerns of cardiovascular specialists by:

- establishing a dialogue with third-party payers on reimbursement and policy issues;

- educating payers on issues of quality care;

- working within College guidelines to establish algorithms on appropriateness of standards for quality care;

- advocating for patients on access to quality care;

- educating payers regarding the practice of cardiovascular medicine;

- serving as an advisor to the payer's or carrier's medical director in the interpretation of access, appropriateness, and standards of quality care;

- serving as an advocate for resolving conflicts, specifically between physicians and payers; and

- being the eyes, ears, and voice of the chapter membership in dealing with third-party payers, representing the membership-at-large by establishing key contacts with the appropriate representatives of HMOs, PPOs, Medicare, and commercial carriers.

The committee's knowledge of CPT coding, CMS guidelines, current reimbursement policies of all local carriers, and issues related to the Resource-Based Relative Value Scale (RBRVS) and Medicare fee schedule are important to effectively serve the interest of the chapter.

Many chapters have used the following framework for their third-party payer activities:

1. **Select a chairperson.** This physician chairs the committee and typically serves as the contact for negotiations with third-party payers.

2. **Develop mechanisms for collecting information on member concerns.** For example, a "hassle log" or complaint form is a useful tool to collect information. Determine how such tools will be distributed (eg, direct mail, newsletter, e-mail, through the ACC, etc).

3. **Hold the first organizational meeting without representation by third-party payers.** During this meeting, it is important to: (a) identify current issues; (b) prepare an agenda for the meeting with the payer; and (c) contact appropriate ACC committees, including Coding and Nomenclature, Government Relations, or Private Sector Relations, as well as ACC staff, for collateral data.

To ensure a productive meeting with third-party payers, appropriate representatives of the health plan should be identified. The committee should know the following individuals:

- the medical director;

- the individual(s) involved in deciding medical policy, including coverage and utilization;

- the individual(s) involved with administrative policy, including claims adjudication, appeals, and contracting; and

- the individual who serves as the cardiology representative on the Carrier Advisory Committee (CAC), which advises the medical director on medical policies.

Chapters that have established such programs have found them effective in expediting and clarifying many important issues.

APPENDIX B

Summary of CPT Codes Having Technical and Professional Components

Certain third-party payers require that submitted claims clearly define whether a complete technical or professional service was provided in order for physicians to receive appropriate reimbursement. Thus, an understanding of a complete service and its technical and professional components is critical to making an appropriate claim for reimbursement.

A *complete service*, as defined by the Centers for Medicare & Medicaid Services (CMS), is one in which the physician provides everything needed for the entire service, including equipment, supplies, technical personnel, and the physician's personal professional services. The complete service can then be divided into a technical component and a professional component. The following is a comprehensive list as determined by CMS.

93024	93287	93308	93451	93464	93602	93622
93025	93288	93312	93452	93505	93603	93623
93278	93289	93314	93453	93530	93609	93624
93279	93290	93315	93454	93531	93610	93631
93280	93291	93317	93455	93532	93612	93640
93281	93292	93318	93456	93533	93615	93641
93282	93293	93320	93457	93561	93616	93642
93283	93303	93321	93458	93562	93618	93660
93284	93304	93325	93459	93571	93619	93662
93285	93306	93350	93460	93572	93620	93724
93286	93307	93351	93461	93600	93621	93745

ICD-9-CM Coding

Mandate for ICD-10

Regulation naming the International Classification of Diseases, Tenth Revision, Clinical Modification and Procedure Coding System (ICD-10-CM and ICD-10-PCS) to replace the International Classification of Diseases, Ninth Revision, Clinical Modification (ICD-9-CM) was published on January 16, 2009. All hospital services provided and discharges on or after October 1, 2013, are required to be coded using the ICD-10 code sets. ICD-10-CM replaces ICD-9-CM Volumes 1 and 2 for reporting of diagnoses. ICD-10-PCS replaces ICD-9-CM Volume 3 for reporting of hospital procedures. ICD-10-PCS does *not* replace Current Procedural Terminology (CPT®) or Healthcare Common Procedure Coding System (HCPCS) for coding of procedures and services performed in outpatient and office settings.

ICD-10 code structures and coding guidelines vary greatly from ICD-9. Appropriate training on ICD-10 will be necessary for health care professionals to code properly.

Guidelines for Use of ICD-9-CM Codes

The following guidelines may be helpful when using ICD-9-CM codes:

- Identify each service, procedure, or supply with an ICD-9-CM code from 001.0 through V82.9 to describe the diagnosis, symptom, complaint, condition, or problem.

- Identify services or visits for circumstances other than disease or injury, such as follow-up care after chemotherapy, with V codes provided for this purpose.

- Code the primary diagnosis first, followed by the secondary, tertiary, and so on. The primary and first diagnostic code must describe the most important reason for the care provided. Code any coexisting conditions that affect the treatment of the patient for that visit or procedure as supplementary information. Do not code a diagnosis that is no longer applicable. Many patients will have a long list of chronic complaints. Code chronic complaints only when the patient has received treatment for the condition. If the patient has an acute condition, utilize codes that specify "acute" whenever available.

- Code to the highest degree of specificity. Carry the numerical code to the fourth or fifth digit when necessary. Occasionally, when patients are seen for ill-defined complaints such as backache, it will be necessary to use an unspecified code until test results confirm a diagnosis. Investigate the patient's record for documentation, which should provide definitive information and facts as to why the patient is being seen. If this information is not provided in the patient's record, seek information from the physician who provided care for the patient. However, remember to code only what is documented. Codes for symptoms can be found in categories 780 to 789. Remember to watch for the "excludes" notations to ensure correct use of all diagnostic codes. Claims coded to 0.9 specificity may result in slower payment.

- When only ancillary services are provided, list the appropriate V code first and the problem second. For example, if a patient is receiving only ancillary therapeutic services such as physical therapy, use the V code first followed by the code for the condition.

- For surgical procedures, code the diagnosis applicable to the procedure. If at the time the claim is filed the postoperative diagnosis is different than the preoperative diagnosis, use the postoperative diagnosis.

Primary Diagnosis

The first diagnostic code must describe the most important reason for the care provided (ie, chief complaint). Often, a single ICD-9-CM code adequately identifies the need for care. If additional facts are required to substantiate the care provided that day, list the ICD-9-CM codes in the order of importance. Report (code) only the current condition that prompted the patient's visit. If the patient has many chronic conditions, be sure to code these chronic complaints only when the patient has received treatment for the condition. If the diagnosis is an acute condition, use the code that specifies "acute" whenever it is available.

To revise and/or propose changes to the ICD-9-CM coding system, submit requests in writing to the co-chairman of the ICD-9-CM Coordination and Maintenance Committee, Department of Health and Human Services. These proposals should be submitted prior to a meeting of the Coordination Committee (usually by a published date). ICD-9-CM revisions are made once a year, effective October 1 of each year.

It is suggested you determine from your Medicare carrier and/or insurance companies which diagnosis codes are acceptable to report with the various procedure codes.

National Correct Coding Initiative

Coding Edits and Mutually Exclusive Code List for Cardiology-Related Codes

The Centers for Medicare & Medicaid Services (CMS) has implemented a correct coding program that includes the National Correct Coding Initiative (NCCI) for Medicare payment. The NCCI is intended to identify procedures and services that should not be billed at the same time when furnished by the same provider for the same patient on the same day. These correct coding limitations reflect services that are integral parts of larger services or that are considered mutually exclusive. The most recent quarterly updates are available on the CMS Web site at www.cms.gov/NationalCorrectCodInitEd/.

The NCCI is administered by CMS through an outside contractor. The American Medical Association (AMA) and the national medical specialty societies, including the American College of Cardiology (ACC), are given the opportunity to provide comment regarding proposed edits. CMS accepts many, but not all, of the recommendations of the ACC for inclusion in the NCCI. Cardiovascular specialists who encounter problems with reimbursement related to NCCI edits may contact the ACC for more information. ACC staff monitors complaints about inappropriate payment denials and provides regular updates to members in the publication *Cardiology* and on the ACC Web site (www.acc.org). The ACC staff also uses information obtained from members to propose revisions to the NCCI.

The NCCI contains a list of "column 1/column 2 codes" and "mutually exclusive codes" in a columnar format. Codes in the "column 1/column 2" pairs cannot be billed to Medicare on the same day. The "mutually exclusive codes" include procedures that

cannot be reasonably performed by a physician in the same patient encounter or at the same anatomic site.

Modifiers may be used to bypass the edit if the code pair has a correct coding modifier indicator of "1" and the clinical circumstances make it appropriate to use the modifier to bypass the edit. A listing of modifiers that may be appended to the code pair under appropriate clinical circumstances can be found in the NCCI guidelines located on the CMS Web site. The correct coding modifier indicator of "0" indicates code pairs for which no separate payment will be made. The "0" indicator signifies that no modifiers may be used with the NCCI code pair to bypass the edit and no separate payment will be made for both codes under any circumstance. Indicator "9" means that the code pair is no longer active; the code combination is billable separately, and no modifier is needed.

Physicians should be aware of the most common code pairs in the NCCI that may affect their practice. With this information, physicians should use care in documentation to support the necessity for diagnostic procedures and the reasons for separate services.

PAYMENT POLICY ALERT National Correct Coding Initiative (NCCI) edits are updated quarterly.

EDITOR'S NOTE ACC receives notification and reviews all proposed edits. ACC replies to all edits believed to be inappropriate. We encourage members to contact ACC with any concerns regarding NCCI edits.

APPENDIX E

Health Insurance Portability and Accountability Act (HIPAA)

The Health Insurance Portability and Accountability Act (HIPAA) was enacted in August 1996 in an effort to improve the efficiency and effectiveness of health care. Key provisions of the law require a federal floor for privacy protections for personal health information and adoption of national standards for electronic health care transactions by providers, health care clearinghouses, and payers. The purpose of the law is to protect individually identifiable health data and to streamline and provide uniform electronic filing and processing of health insurance claims and other administrative transactions.

The Department of Health and Human Services (HHS) has issued several major regulations to address the privacy and security of personal health information, as well as the administrative burden for providers and payers. The American Recovery and Reinvestment Act of 2009 (ARRA) made significant changes to HIPAA, requiring additional regulations. Some rules implementing these changes have been published.

Administrative Simplification Standards

ELECTRONIC TRANSACTION AND CODE SETS STANDARDS

In August 2000, HHS issued final electronic transaction standards to reduce paperwork and speed the processing and payment of health care claims. The new standards established standard data content, codes, and formats for submitting electronic claims and other administrative health care transactions. All health plans were required to accept these standard electronic transactions. The regulations went into effect as of October 16, 2003; however, several contingency plans have been enacted, so many of the new transactions are not yet required.

HHS issued two additional regulations in January 2009 to update the version of the electronic transaction standards and replace ICD-9 with ICD-10. Compliance with the new version (5010) of electronic transactions is January 1, 2012. ICD-10 must be used to code all services and discharges on or after October 1, 2013.

IDENTIFIERS

HIPAA also included provisions for developing standard identifiers for employers, providers, and health plans. Implementation of the employer identifier, the employer identification number (EIN) assigned by the Internal Revenue Service, was completed in 2005. The national provider identifier (NPI) regulation was issued in 2006, with a final compliance date of May 23, 2008. The Patient Protection and Affordability Care Act of 2010 (ACA) included a provision to implement the health plan identifier no later than October 1, 2012. Neither proposed nor final regulations have been issued to date.

Privacy Standards

In December 2000, HHS issued a final rule to protect the confidentiality of medical records and other personal health information. The rule limits the use and release of individually identifiable health information and provides patients increased access and control over their medical records. The deadline for compliance with the privacy rule took place on April 14, 2003.

The Health Information Technology for Economic and Clinical Health (HITECH) Act, enacted as part of ARRA, included additional privacy and security requirements. HHS has published a final rule addressing concerns pertaining to breaches of HIPAA-covered entities' (ie, payers, providers, and clearinghouses) records containing patients' protected health information (PHI), commonly known as the "breach notification" rule. HHS also published a proposed rule extending HIPAA requirements beyond covered entities to business associates, as well as modifying the current regulation for marketing, sale of PHI, use of a limited data set when complying with the release of the minimum amount of PHI, patient access to and accounting for disclosures of PHI, and enforcement. A final rule on this is forthcoming. See the HHS Web site for up-to-date information on these requirements (www.hhs.gov/ocr/privacy/hipaa/understanding/index.html).

Security Standards

In February 2003, HHS issued final standards for security, adopting national standards for safeguards to shield the confidentiality, integrity, and availability of electronic PHI. Previously, no model measures existed in the health care industry to address all aspects of the security of electronic PHI while it is in use, in storage, or during the exchange of such information between entities. HIPAA mandates security standards to protect an individual's health information while permitting the appropriate access and use of that information by health care providers, clearinghouses, and health plans. Compliance was required as of April 20, 2005.

Security standards were designed to be technology neutral in order to facilitate use of the latest and most promising technologies that meet the needs of different health care organizations. Any regulatory requirement for implementation of specific technologies would bind the health care community to specific systems and/or software that may be superseded by rapidly developing technologies and improvements.

As mentioned earlier, ARRA made several changes that affect the HIPAA security requirements.

Enforcement

In June 2005, the US Department of Justice outlined the requirements for criminal liability under HIPAA administrative simplification provisions. Those who "knowingly" obtain or disclose PHI can face fines up to $50,000 and prison time up to one year. Fines rise to $100,000 and prison terms increase to up to five years when the violations were made committed under "false pretenses." Crimes made with the intent to sell, transfer, or use PHI can result in fines up to $250,000 and imprisonment of up to 10 years. The same provisions of HITECH discussed under the Privacy section above also require clarification and updating of certain enforcement provisions.

Category II Codes and the Physician Quality Reporting System

CPT Category II Codes Defined

There are three categories of Current Procedural Terminology (CPT®) codes: Category I, Category II, and Category III. Category I codes are the ones used to report billable services provided by physicians and other professionals. Category III codes are similar to Category I codes but are used to report newer and developing techniques and technology.

Category II codes differ from Category I and Category III codes because they are not used to report a billable physician service. Instead they are used to report the provision of services that has been identified as optimal quality care for a given disease process, clinical condition, or patient population. An example might be providing aspirin to a patient who presents at the emergency room with an acute myocardial infarction. The measures assigned Category II codes are vetted through nationally recognized consensus organizations to ensure that they are based on current evidence. Category II codes may be used as part of pay-for-reporting and pay-for-performance programs, which are increasingly used to augment fee-for-service payments made to physicians.

One notable program that requires the use of CPT Category II codes is the Physician Quality Reporting System (PQRS) in the Medicare program. This program, which began in 2007, pays a bonus to physicians for submitting certain CPT Category II codes. The PQRS is **not** a pay-for-performance program in which physicians are paid on the basis of adherence to measures. Instead, it is a pay-for-reporting program in which physicians are paid for reporting data that indicates compliance with specific quality measures from

nationally recognized quality improvement organizations. PQRS uses measures to report the provision of certain evidence-based care not typically reflected in the payment and billing record.

Methods of Reporting

The following three reporting methods are used to document physician services:

- claims-based;
- electronic health record; and
- registry reporting.

CLAIMS-BASED REPORTING

Claims-based reporting enables physicians to use CPT Category II codes to report measure compliance by direct input on their claim form or electronic billing mechanism. Physicians may report on any three measures 50% of the time or report a group of measures for clinically similar patients. Most of the measures developed by the American College of Cardiology and the American Heart Association may not be reported through the claims-based method. Because of the limited numbers of measures available for reporting and greater chance of error compared to other methods of reporting, most cardiologists select other reporting methods.

ELECTRONIC HEALTH RECORD REPORTING

The Centers for Medicare & Medicaid Services (CMS) allow direct reporting of PQRS data from electronic health records from a limited number of electronic health record system. Measures relevant to cardiology are included in the program. (It is advised that physicians who use electronic health records check with their vendors to determine if Category II reporting is accepted using this method.)

REGISTRY REPORTING

CMS allows clinical registries to report PQRS data on behalf of physicians. There are many registries available, but two are sponsored by the ACC: (1) the PINNACLE registry; and (2) the ACC's PQRS Wizard. The PINNACLE registry is a comprehensive outpatient registry that interfaces with existing electronic medical records and calculates performance measures and translates them into PQRS data. The ACC's PQRS Wizard enables physicians to enter data into a Web-based tool. Because this tool enables physicians to report measures groups, data on only 30 patients is allowed for successful reporting.

EXAMPLE OF A PERFORMANCE MEASURE: ORAL ANTIPLATELET THERAPY PRESCRIBED FOR PATIENTS WITH CORONARY ARTERY DISEASE

Based on a review of the available evidence, the ACC and AHA, in collaboration with national stakeholder organizations, developed a performance measure on the prescription of oral antiplatelet therapy to patients with coronary artery disease (CAD). The measure identifies whether or not the patient was prescribed antiplatelet therapy. The denominator for this calculation is the number of eligible patients who received an outpatient evaluation and management (E/M) visit from the physician for which a diagnosis of CAD was reported. In the claims-based reporting method, physicians would report a CPT Category II code (**4011F**) to indicate the therapy was prescribed. If, however, the therapy was not prescribed, the physician would report the code along with one of four modifiers that indicate the reason(s) why the therapy was not prescribed.

There are three exclusions modifiers that are used to identify reasons for excluding the patient from consideration for the measure: **modifier 1P** indicates medical reasons for not prescribing the antiplatelet therapy; **modifier 2P** indicates patient reasons for not prescribing the therapy (eg, patient refusal); and modifier 3P reports system reasons for not prescribing the drug (eg, no prescription drug plan). **Modifier 8P** is an additional modifier for other reporting circumstances that do not qualify as exclusions from meeting the measure's recommendation (ie, other reasons for not prescribing antiplatelet therapy).

Some of the measures require more than one CPT Category II code be reported in claims-based reporting. An example of this is the use of denominator Category II codes to identify the specific patient population in question.

APPENDIX G

Moderate (Conscious) Sedation

Moderate (conscious) sedation, as described in the guidelines of the AMA's *CPT 2012* codebook, is defined as "a drug-induced depression of consciousness during which patients respond purposefully to verbal commands, either alone or accompanied by light tactile stimulation. No interventions are required to maintain a patient airway and spontaneous ventilation is adequate. Cardiovascular function is usually maintained. Moderate sedation does not include minimal sedation (anxiolysis), deep sedation, or monitored anesthesia care (**00100-01999**)" (*CPT Professional 2012*, page 531).

The *CPT 2012* codebook lists codes for which moderate sedation is an inherent part of the procedure. As such, it is expected that the moderate sedation service will be provided by the physician performing the procedure, and thus, it is not appropriate to submit the moderate (conscious) sedation codes for these procedures. However, inclusion of a code on this list does not preclude the separate reporting of an anesthesia procedure or service (codes **00100-01999**) when provided by a physician other than the operating physician.

The following cardiology codes are included on the list of procedures for which moderate (conscious) sedation is considered part of the procedure. Please refer to Appendix G of the *CPT 2012* codebook for the complete guidelines and list of codes that include moderate (conscious) sedation.

The inclusion of a procedure on this list does not prevent separate reporting of an associated anesthesia procedure/service (CPT codes **00100-02999**) when performed by a physician other than the health care professional performing the diagnostic or therapeutic procedure. In such cases the person providing anesthesia services shall be present for the purpose of continuously monitoring the patient and shall not act as a surgical assistant. When clinical conditions of the patient require such anesthesia services, or in the circumstances when the patient does not require sedation, the operating physician is not required to report the procedure as a reduced service using **modifier 52**.

TABLE G-1 Cardiology Codes with Inherent Moderate (Conscious) Sedation

33010	33011	33206	33207	33208	33210	33211	33212	33213	33214	33216
33217	33218	33220	33221	33222	33223	33227	33228	33229	33230	33231
33233	33234	33235	33240	33241	33244	33249	33262	33263	33264	35471
35472	35475	35476	36147	36148	36200	36245	36246	36247	36248	36251
36252	36253	36254	36481	36555	36557	36558	36560	36561	36563	36565
36566	36568	36570	36571	36576	36578	36581	36582	36583	36585	36590
36870	37183	37184	37185	37186	37187	37188	37191	37192	37193	37203
37210	37215	37216	92953	92960	92961	92973	92974	92975	92978	92979
92980	92981	92982	92984	92986	92987	92995	92996	93312	93313	93314
93315	93316	93317	93318	93451	93452	93453	93454	93455	93456	93457
93458	93459	93460	93461	93462	93463	93464	93505	93530	93561	93562
93563	93564	93565	93566	93567	93568	93571	93572	93609	93613	93615
93616	93618	93619	93620	93621	93622	93624	93640	93641	93642	93650
93651	93652	-	-	-	-	-	-	-	-	-

Medicare Part B Carriers

The Medicare Prescription Drug Improvement and Modernization Act of 2003 (MMA) enabled the Centers for Medicare & Medicaid Services (CMS) to make significant changes to the administrative structure of the Medicare fee-for-service program. The MMA mandated that CMS restructure and combine its Parts A and B contractors to create new entities called Medicare Administrative Contractors (MACs).

The MACs serve as the providers' primary point-of-contract for enrollment; training on Medicare coverage and billing requirements; and receipt, processing, and payment of Medicare fee-for-service claims within their respective jurisdictions. These contractors perform all core claims processing operations for both Part A and Part B.

The MACs are listed below. This listing of contractors was complete as of the publication of this book. The most up-to-date MAC listing is available on the CMS Web site at www.cms.gov/InfoExchange/Downloads/cmddirectory.pdf.

CMS Carrier Medical Director (CMD) Directory

Awodele, Olatokunbo, MD, MPH
Wisconsin Physician Services Corp
3333 Farnam Street
Omaha, NE 68131
Tel: (402) 351-2585
Fax: (402) 351-8047
Email: olatokunbo.awodele@wpsic.com
Jurisdiction: Legacy A
Specialty: Family Practice w/ OB

Boren, Stephen D, MD, MBA
Wisconsin Physician Services Corp
111 East Wacker Drive, Suite 950
Chicago, IL 60601
Tel: (312) 228-6254
Fax: (312) 228-6280

Email: Stephen.boren@wpisc.com
Jurisdiction: Part B IL, MI, MN
Specialty: Emergency Medicine

Burken, Mitchell, MD
Riverbend GBA
1 Cameron Hill Circle
Chattanooga, TN 37402
Tel: (423) 535-5332
Fax: (423) 535-3435
Email: mitchell_burken@bcbst.com
Jurisdiction: J-15 Part A
Specialty: Clinical Pathology

Bussan, Kenneth L, MD
Wisconsin Physician Services Corp
1717 W. Broadway, PO Box 1787
Madison, WI 53701
Tel: (608) 301-2604
Fax: (608) 301-2625
Email: Kenneth.bussan@domino.wpsic.com
Jurisdiction: J-5 MAC
Specialty: Internal Medicine

Clark, Laurence, MD, FACP
Highmark Medicare Services
1800 Center Street
Camp Hill, PA 17011
Tel: (717) 302-4199
Fax: (717) 302-4165
Email: Laurence.clarkmd@highmarkmedicareservices
.com
Jurisdiction: J-12 MAC
Specialty: Not available

Cope, James W, MD
AdvanceMed Corp
1530 East Parham Road
Henrico, VA 23228
Tel: (804) 864-9935
Fax: (804) 264-8191
Email: copej@admedcorp.com
Jurisdiction: CERT
Specialty: Emergency Medicine

Corcoran Jr, James J, MD, MPH
First Coast Service Options, Inc.
532 Riverside Avenue 20T
Jacksonville, FL 32202
Tel: (904) 791-8211
Fax: (904) 361-0327
Email: James.Corcoran@fcso.com
Jurisdiction: J9 MAC
Specialty: Internal Medicine, Public Health

Cunningham, Carolyn, MD
National Government Services
8115 Knue Road, INA102-AF10
Indianapolis, IN 46250
Tel: (317) 841-4607
Fax: (317) 841-4600
Email: Carolyn.cunningham@anthem.com
Jurisdiction: Part A & B IN, KY; Part A IL, OH
Specialty: Internal Medicine

Deutsch, Paul, MD
National Government Services
PO Box 4767
Syracuse, NY 13221-4767
Tel: (914) 801-3567
Fax: (914) 801-3600
Email: Paul.deutsch@empireblue.com
Jurisdiction: J13 MAC
Specialty: Cardiology

Feliciano, Harry, MD, MPH
Palmetto GBA
PO Box 1437
Augusta, GA 30903-1437
Tel: (803) 763-5007
Fax: (803) 462-3917
Email: Harry.Feliciano@PalmettoGBA.com
Jurisdiction: J1 MAC
Specialty: Internal Medicine, Public Health

Haley, Charles, MD, MS, FACP
Trailblazer Health Enterprises, LLC
8330LBJ Freeway, Executive Center III
Dallas, TX 75243-1213
Tel: (469) 372-0992
Fax: (469) 372-2649
Email: Charles.Haley@trailblazerhealth.com
Jurisdiction: J4 MAC, TX, CO, NM, OK
    and Part B VA
Specialty: Internal Medicine, Epidemiology

Jeter, Elaine, MD
Palmetto GBA
PO Box 100190, AG-300
Columbia, SC 29202-3190
Tel: (803) 763-5059

Fax: (803) 935-0199
Email: Elaine.jeter@palmettogba.com
Jurisdiction: J-11
Specialty: Pathology

Kamps, Robert R, MD
Palmetto GBA
4249 Easton Way, Suite 400
Columbus, OH 43219
Tel: (614) 473-6424
Fax: (614) 473-6204
Email: Robert.kamps@palmettogba.com
Jurisdiction: OH
Specialty: Oncology/Hematology

Ludwig, Robert, MD
Palmetto GBA
4249 Easter Way
Columbus, OH 43219
Tel: Not available
Fax: Not available
Email: Not available
Jurisdiction: WV
Specialty: Gastroenterology

Lurvey, Arthur N, MD
Palmetto GBA
PO Box 1476 Medical Review Part B
Augusta, GA 30903-1476
Tel: (310) 476-5760
Fax: (803) 462-3918
Email: Arthur.Lurvey@PalmettoGBA.com
Jurisdiction: J1 MAC
Specialty: Endocrinology Internal Medicine

Hoover Jr, Robert (Bob) D, MD, MPH, FACP
CIGNA Government Services
Two Vantage Way RTG 795
Nashville TN 37228
Tel: (615) 385-2476
Fax: (860) 731-3065
Email: robert.hoover@cigna.com
Jurisdiction: DME MAC - C
Specialty: Internal Medicine

Hughes, Paul, MD
National Heritage Insurance Co
75 Sgt William B Terry Drive
Hingham, MA 02043
Tel: (803) 315-5311
Fax: (803) 264-2753
Email: paul.hughesmd@eds.com
Jurisdiction: DME MAC - A
Specialty: Family Practice

Szczys, Robert F, MD, FACS
Noridian Administrative Services, LLC
901 40th Street South
Fargo, ND 58108-6757
Tel: (701) 433-3100
Fax: (701) 433-3100
Email: robert.szczys@noridian.com
Jurisdiction: PDAC
Specialty: General Surgery

QUALITY IMPROVEMENT ORGANIZATION (QIO) AND QUALIFIED INDEPENDENT CONTRACTOR (QIC) CMDS

Church, Laura K, MD
MAXIMUS Federal Services
50 Square Drive Suite 210
Victor, NY 14564
Tel: (585) 425-5219
Fax: (585) 425-5292
Email: LauraChurch@MAXIMUS.com
Jurisdiction: QIC Part C
Specialty: Emergency Medicine

Cook, Cathy, MD
Q2 Administrators, LLC
5151 E Dublin-Granville Road, Suite 200
Westerville, OH 43081
Tel: (614) 775-5311
Fax: (614) 775-5798
Email: MaryCCook@Maximus.com
Jurisdiction: QIC Part B South
Specialty: Family Medicine

Delli Carpini, Frank A, MD
C2C Solutions, Inc
11 Lake Avenue Extension
Danbury, CT 06810
Tel: (203) 739-0130
Fax: (203) 739-0405
Email: Frank.dellicarpini@fcso.com
Jurisdiction: QIC B North
Specialty: Internal Medicine

Dunn, Cindy, MD
MAXIMUS Federal Services
800 Cross Keys Office Park
Fairport, NY 14450
Tel: (585) 425-5201
Fax: (585) 425-5292
Email: CindyDunn@MAXIMUS.com
Jurisdiction: QIC Part D
Specialty: Not available

Eckhert, Sandra, MD
MAXIMUS Federal Services
860 Cross Keys Office Park
Fairport, NY 14450
Tel: (585) 598-9236
Fax: (585) 425-0635
Email: Not available
Jurisdiction: QIC Part A East
Specialty: Internal Medicine

Evans, Ellen R, MD
HealthDataInsights
7501 Trinity Peaks Avenue, Suite 120
Las Vegas, NV 89128
Tel: (866) 376-2319
Fax: (702) 240-5510
Email: HDI_CMD@emailhdi.com
Jurisdiction: Region D RAC
Specialty: Geriatrics and Family Practice

Norris, Robert E, MD
Q2Administrators, LLC
PO Box 183092
Columbus, OH 43218
Tel: (614) 775-5797
Fax: Not available
Email: Not available
Jurisdiction: QIC Part B South
Specialty: Internal Medicine

O'Neal, Barbara Meyer, MD
Rivertrust Solutions
801 Pine Street
Chattanooga, TN 37401
Tel: (423) 535-6659
Fax: Not available
Email: Barbara.ONeal@rtrust.org
Jurisdiction: DME QIC
Specialty: Emergency Medicine

Sheridan, David P, MD, MS
Q2 Administrators, LLC
300 Arbor Lake Drive, Suite 1350
Columbia, SC 29223-4582
Tel: (803) 234-5802
Fax: (571) 266-3141
Email: David.Sheridan@q2a.com
Jurisdiction: AdQIC
Specialty: Preventive Medicine

Stein, Bernice, MD
MAXIMUS Federal Services
1040 First Avenue, Suite 400
King of Prussia, PA 19406
Tel: Not available
Fax: Not available
Email: BerniceStein@Maximus.com
Jurisdiction: QIC Part A West
Specialty: Not available

OTHER AGENCIES

Cope, James W, MD
AdvanceMed Corp
1530 East Parham Road
Henrico, VA 23228
Tel: (804) 864-9935
Fax: (804) 264-8191
Email: copej@admedcorp.com
Jurisdiction: CERT
Specialty: Emergency Medicine

Grisell, Ted W, MD
IntegrGuard, LLC
10551 N 800 W
Fairland, IN 46126
Tel: (317) 313-9320
Fax: Not available
Email: tgrisell@integriguard.org
Jurisdiction: ZPIC Zone 7, DME BISC
Specialty: General Surgery (Abdominal)

Oleck, Adrian, MD
Correct Coding Solutions, LLC
Carmel, IN 46082-0907
Tel: Not available
Fax: (317) 571-1745
Email: adrian.oleck@correctcodingsolutions.com
Jurisdiction: NCCI/MUE
Specialty: Internal Medicine

Perez, E David, MD
AdvanceMed Corp
1530 East Parham Road
Henrico, VA 23228
Tel: (804) 864-9885
Fax: (804) 264-8191
Email: perezd@admedcorp.com
Jurisdiction: CERT
Specialty: Not available

Rosen, Niles R, MD
Correct Coding Solutions, LLC
PO Box 907
Carmel, IN 46082-0907
Tel: Not available
Fax: (317) 571-1745
Email: Niles.rosen@correctcodingsolutions.com
Jurisdiction: NCCI/MUE
Specialty: Pathology

Code Index

93600–93652 196
93602 197, 198, 201, 235
93603 197, 201, 235
93609 196, 199, 201, 204, 206, 235, 245
93610 197, 198, 201, 235
93610–93612 197, 198, 199
93612 197, 198, 199, 201, 235
93613 196, 199, 201, 204, 206, 245
93615 199, 200, 235, 245
93615–93618 199
93616 199, 200, 235, 245
93618 200, 201, 203, 235, 245
93618–93624 126, 207
93619 196, 198, 200, 201, 202, 203, 235, 245
93619–93622 199, 200, 201
93620 198, 199, 200, 201, 202, 203, 208, 235, 245
93620–93622 201
93620–93624 196, 205
93621 199, 200, 201, 202, 203, 208, 235, 245
93621–93622 201, 202
93621–93623 203
93622 199, 200, 201, 202, 208, 235, 245
93623 202, 203, 235
93624 203, 235, 245
93631 126, 203, 204, 207, 235
93640 46, 57, 203, 204, 205, 245
93640–93641 57
93640–93642 126, 196, 198, 204, 207
93641 46, 57, 58, 59, 60, 204, 205, 235, 245
93642 204, 205, 207, 235, 245
93650 205, 206, 207, 245
93650–93652 126, 198, 203, 205, 206, 207
93651 175, 197, 199, 206, 207, 208, 245
93651–93652 197
93652 175, 197, 199, 205, 206, 207, 208, 245
93660 207, 235
93662 126, 194, 207, 208, 235
93668 208
93701 209
93720 127

93721 127
93722 127
93724 209, 210, 235
93741 203
93742 203
93744 203
93745 153, 209, 235
93750 80, 84, 209, 210
93799 2, 8, 127, 139, 145
93875 211
93922 127, 210, 211, 212, 213, 214
93922–93924 210, 211
93923 211, 212, 213, 214
93924 211, 213, 214
93965 211
93967 188
94002–94004 36
94660 36
94662 36
94760 36
94761 36
94762 36
95921–959233 207
96365–96366 142
96365–96379 126
96464 176
97016 127
98966 39
98966–98969 38
98967 39
98968 39
98969 39
99090 36
99143–99150 166
99201 27, 31, 38
99201–99205 23, 30, 37
99201–99499 7
99202 27, 31, 38
99203 6, 26, 27, 31, 33, 38
99204 27, 31
99205 27, 31
99211 27, 31
99211–99215 23, 30
99212 27, 31
99212–99215 37
99213 26, 27, 31
99214 27, 31
99215 27, 31
99217 23, 34, 35
99217–99220 33
99217–99239 38
99218 28
99218–99220 23, 33, 34, 35, 37
99219 28

99220 28
99221 27, 31
99221–99223 23, 30, 34, 35, 37
99222 27, 31
99223 27, 31
99224 28
99224–99226 23, 33, 34, 35
99225 28
99226 28
99231 28
99231–99233 23, 30
99232 28
99233 28, 32
99234 29
99234–99236 23, 34, 35
99235 29
99236 29
99238 29, 34
99238–99239 23, 35
99239 29, 34
99241 29, 32
99241–99245 23, 30, 33, 37, 39
99242 29, 32
99243 29
99244 29, 32, 33
99245 29, 32
99251 30, 33
99251–99255 23, 30, 37
99252 30, 33
99253 30, 33, 33
99254 30, 33
99255 30, 33
99281–99288 23
99288 125
99291 35, 36, 124, 125
99291–99292 23, 35, 36, 38, 124
99292 35, 36, 39, 124, 125
93000 138
99304–99306 23
99304–99310 37
99304–99318 38
99305 138
99307–99310 23
99308 25, 38, 39
99310 138
99315–99316 23
99324–99328 23
99334–99337 23, 37
99339–99340 23, 40
99341–99345 24
99341–99350 37
99347–99350 24
99354 36, 37

99354–99355 36
99354–99357 24, 36, 37
99354–99359 36
99354–99360 142
99355 36, 37
99356 36, 37
99356–99357 36
99357 36, 37
99358–99359 24, 37
99359 37
99360 24
99363 38, 138
99363–99364 24, 38, 40
99364 38, 138
99366–99368 24
99374–99380 24, 38, 40
99379 38
99380 38
99381–99387 24
99391–99397 24
99401–99404 24
99406–99409 24
99411–99412 24
99420–99429 24
99441 39
99441–99443 24, 39, 40
99441–99444 38, 39
99442 39
99443 39
99444 24, 39, 40
99450–99456 24
99460–99463 24
99464–99465 24
99466 36, 124, 125
99466–99467 124, 125
99466–99480 24
99467 36, 124, 125
99468–99476 124, 125
99471 26, 39, 108
99471–99480 38
99499 24

CATEGORY III
NEW/EMERGING
TECHNOLOGY CODES

0048T 78, 79
0050T 78, 79
0075T 98, 100
0076T 98, 100
0078T 97
0079T 97
0159T 115
0188T–0189T 36
0234T 82
0234T–0238T 91, 95

Index

Comprehensive examination, 13, 14, 17, 25

Comprehensive history, 11, 24

Computed tomographic angiography (CTA)
  abdominal aorta and extremity runoff, 106, 108
  abdominal, pelvis, and lower extremities, 108
  CT imaging compared to, 107
  definition of, 106
  distinction between CT and, 107
  with and without contrast material, 106

Computed tomography (CT), heart
  with contrast material, 106, 107
  without contrast material, 106, 107

Computed tomography (CT), three-dimensional rendering with interpretation and reporting of, 114–115

Congenital anomalies, 72, 160

Congenital heart disease, 162–164
  cardiac catheterization for patients with, 180–183
  cyanotic, 192

Conscious sedation. *See* Moderate sedation

Consultative services, Medicare discontinuance of payment for, 30

Coordination of care component for E/M service level, 26
  documentation of encounter dominated by, 21
  extent of, 26
  time in, 25

Coronary angiography, 86–88. *See also* Angiography; Computed tomographic angiography (CTA)

Coronary artery bypass
  arterial grafting for, 69–72
  combined arterial-venous grafting for, 67–69
  determining number of bypass grafts for, 68
  venous grafting only for, 64–67

Coronary artery disease (CAD), therapy for, 244

Coronary artery stenting, 130–131

Coronary brachytherapy, 130

Coronary thrombectomy, 127–128

Coronary thrombolysis, 128–129

Co-surgeons, 49

Counseling component for E/M service level, 25–26
  areas of discussion for, 25–26

documentation of encounter dominated by, 21
time in, 11, 21

CPT codebook
  appendixes in, 30, 223
  Cardiovascular System section of, 43
  Surgery section of, 43
  symbols used in, 8

Critical care, definition of, 35

Critical care services, 35–36

Current Procedural Terminology (CPT) code set
  applying for codes in, 2, 3, 4
  basics of, 7–8
  definition of, 1
  guidelines for, 7
  history of, 1
  modifiers for, 219, 220–223, 224–226
  organization of, 7–8
  perspective for, 1–8
  purpose of, for reporting services, 7
  symbols used for, 8
  updates to, 2, 3, 8
  use by major carriers of, 6

D

Defibrillation
  as component of other procedure, 126
  definition of, 125

Department of Health and Human Services (HHS), 7

Detailed examination, 13, 14, 17, 25

Detailed history, 11, 24

Diagnostic radiologic services, 103–122

Distal embolic protection, 128, 135

Documentation Guidelines (·DG) for E/M services, 10, 11, 17

Documentation, medical record
  of complexity of medical decision making, 19–21
  definition of, 11
  of E/M services, 9–21
  of encounter, inclusions in, 10
  of examination, 13–17
  of extent of counseling and/or coordination of care, 26
  general principles of, 10
  guidelines for, ·DG representation of, 10
  of history, 11–13
  importance of, 9–10

of medical necessity, 230
Medicare requirements for, 35, 230
of online medical evaluation, 40
payer requirements for, 10
of prolonged services, 37
as protection from downcoding, 230, 231
of referral, 230
of renal angiography at cardiac catheterization procedure, 186
signed, 230
SOAP method of, 10
supporting, 231

Domiciliary, 10, 13, 23

Downcoding, protection from, 230, 231

Drug infusion, testing for, 202–203

E

Echocardiography
  Doppler, 159, 160, 163–154
  ICD-9-CM codes to justify, 161
  intracardiac (ICE), 194–195, 208
  noncongenital, 160
  procedures bundled with, 159
  stress, 159–160
  transesophageal (TEE), 83, 162–163, 194–195
  transthoracic (TTE), 158–162, 194

Electrocardiogram (ECG, EKG)
  complete service for, 139, 160
  data interrogation of, 158
  definition of, 123
  example of, 124
  monitor connection for, 148
  professional component in monitoring, 139, 144
  rhythm, 142, 144–145
  signal-averaged, 145–146
  stress, 161–162
  telephonic transmission of, 139, 144
  tracing (technical component only) for, 138, 139
  waves recorded by, 123

Electrocardiographic rhythm, 142
  elements derived from, 142, 143, 146

Electrograms
  esophageal, 199, 200
  to detect arrhythmias, 154
  intracardiac, 198

Electronic health record reporting, 243–244

Electronic transactions standard (5010), 241

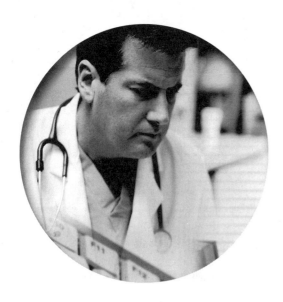

ADVANCE YOUR CAREER AS A CARDIOVASCULAR ADMINISTRATOR MEMBER OF THE AMERICAN COLLEGE OF CARDIOLOGY

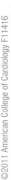

THE ACC NOW WELCOMES PRACTICE AND CARDIOVASCULAR SERVICE LINE ADMINISTRATORS TO MEMBERSHIP!

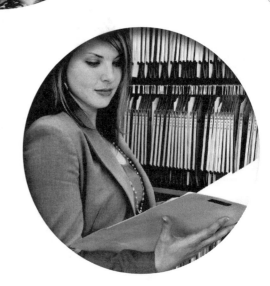

Managing a cardiology practice in a changing healthcare and economic environment can be challenging. The ACC can help support you as you navigate these challenges with tools and resources for everyday practice support, networking opportunities with all members of the care team and information to help you stay up to date.

To find out more and to join as a Cardiovascular Administrator member today, visit *www.CardioSource.org/JoinCA.*

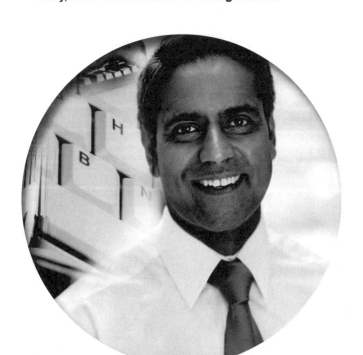

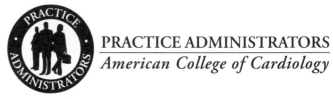

PRACTICE ADMINISTRATORS
American College of Cardiology